Prescription for Drug Alternatives

All-Natural Options for Better Health without the Side Effects

JAMES F. BALCH, M.D.

MARK STENGLER, N.D.

ROBIN YOUNG BALCH, N.D.

WILEY

John Wiley & Sons, Inc.

Published by John Wiley & Sons, Inc., Hoboken, New Jersey
Published simultaneously in Canada

Limit of Liability/Disclaimer of Warranty: While the publisher and the author have used their best efforts in preparing this book, they make no representations or warranties with respect to the accuracy or completeness of the contents of this book and specifically disclaim any implied warranties of merchantability or fitness for a particular purpose. No warranty may be created or extended by sales representatives or written sales materials. The advice and strategies contained herein may not be suitable for your situation. You should consult with a professional where appropriate. Neither the publisher nor the author shall be liable for any loss of profit or any other commercial damages, including but not limited to special, incidental, consequential, or other damages.

The information contained in this book is not intended to serve as a replacement for professional medical advice. Any use of the information in this book is at the reader's discretion. The author and the publisher specifically disclaim any and all liability arising directly or indirectly from the use or application of any information contained in this book. A health care professional should be consulted regarding your specific situation.

For general information about our other products and services, please contact our Customer Care Department within the United States at (800) 762-2974, outside the United States at (317) 572-3993 or fax (317) 572-4002.

Wiley also publishes its books in a variety of electronic formats. Some content that appears in print may not be available in electronic books. For more information about Wiley products, visit our web site at www.wiley.com.

Library of Congress Cataloging-in-Publication Data:

Balch, James F., date.
  Prescription for drug alternatives : all-natural options for better health without the side effects / James F. Balch, Mark Stengler, Robin Young-Balch.
        p. ; cm.
  Includes bibliographical references and index.
  ISBN 978-0-470-18399-1 (paper)
  1. Naturopathy. 2. Alternative medicine. 3. Drugs—Side effects—Prevention. I. Stengler, Mark. II. Young-Balch, Robin. III. Title. [DNLM: 1. Naturopathy—methods—Popular Works. 2. Diet Therapy—Popular Works. 3. Pharmaceutical Preparations—adverse effects—Popular Works. 4. Pharmacognosy—methods—Popular Works. 5. Phytotherapy—methods—Popular Works. WB 935 B174p 2008]
  RZ440.B284 2008
  615.5'35—dc22
                                                                2008031707

Printed in the United States of America

10 9 8 7 6 5 4 3 2

CONTENTS

PREFACE

With the success of our best-selling book *Prescription for Natural Cures*, we found that many people have been helped by having access to concise, effective information on natural medicine for a variety of health conditions. From our discussions with patients, the public, and doctors, we saw a great need for a book comparing commonly used pharmaceutical medications and effective natural alternatives. With the explosion in scientific validation of natural therapies, combined with public concern over potential side effects of pharmaceutical drugs, the current medical climate has created an unprecedented demand for natural alternatives to pharmaceutical medications. This book provides a resource for patients and doctors alike to bridge the gap between these two fields of medicine.

Chances are that you or someone you know takes one or more medications. Many of these come with a long list of potential side effects, some of which can be life-threatening. The question we are often asked is, "Are there any natural alternatives I can use instead?" Depending on the situation, the answer can be yes. There are also cases in which the answer is no. There are, however, many circumstances where a combination of both pharmaceutical and natural medicines can be used together to best help a patient. *Prescription for Drug Alternatives* provides readers with the most up-to-date and time-tested natural alternatives for today's most commonly used drugs.

Knowledge is the key to empowerment for those wanting to take charge of their health. To help readers understand and assess various pharmaceuticals, we have provided an extensive amount of information on these drugs. This will help readers assess whether a certain pharmaceutical may be causing undesirable side effects. Readers can also review potential interactions with other drugs, supplements, and foods. How a drug works and its potential benefits are also addressed. We have done our best to provide unbiased information for each of the covered pharmaceuticals. It is up to patients and their doctors to assess a drug's benefits compared to its risks. Taking this a step further, the benefits and risks of a particular drug can be compared to those of commonly available natural medicines.

With all of the pertinent information about a class of drugs and corresponding natural alternatives, we now have the ability to make fully informed decisions. Gone are the days when we had to rely upon traditional use or folklore as the sole means of choosing natural options. We believe that *Prescription for Drug Alternatives* will provide the information needed to help people use pharmaceuticals more effectively. In addition, many readers will discover safer, natural alternatives that can accomplish their health goals just as effectively as their pharmaceutical counterparts. For people who require pharmaceutical treatment, we have provided information on nutrients that may be depleted by these medications, so further health problems caused by nutritional deficiencies can be prevented.

Through common grace, our Creator has provided us with healing remedies found in nature as well as the ability of human beings to create pharmaceutical medications.

ACKNOWLEDGMENTS

From all three authors: Thanks to our book agent, Jeff Herman, and our editor, Tom Miller, and the staff at John Wiley & Sons for their support in publishing *Prescription for Drug Alternatives.*

I thank my Lord Jesus Christ for expanding my knowledge about
health and healing over thirty-three years ago.
James F. Balch, M.D.

To my Lord and Savior Jesus Christ, the One who
sustains me and all things.
(Colossians 1:17)
Mark Stengler, N.D.

My thanks to Jehovah Rapha, the Lord who heals us all.
Robin Young Balch, N.D.

Introduction: How to Use This Book

This book has been organized to help you access the information you need in a timely and precise manner. Part one, "What You Need to Know about Pharmaceutical Drugs," is a review of the benefits of pharmaceuticals as well as their risks. We also give a behind-the-scenes view of how some dangerous pharmaceuticals get into the hands of consumers. There is also a summary of popular drugs from recent years that were either pulled from the market or given new warnings on the serious risks they carry. Finally, we provide some important tips on how to stay safe when using pharmaceuticals. The end of part one summarizes our thoughts on the benefits of natural medicine and the role it should play in health care.

The largest component of the book is part two, "Pharmaceuticals and Their Natural Alternatives," which includes information condition by condition.

At the end of the book we provide additional resources for our readers, including:

- A listing of holistic doctor associations
- A glossary of the terms used in this book
- Resources and recommended reading that include further information to complement what is provided in this book

Pharmaceuticals

For each condition there is a variety of classes of drugs that can be used to treat it. We list the pharmaceutical names and common brands for each class of drugs. For example, in the common cold chapter, we cover all the drug classes that are used for colds, including analgesics, topical nasal decongestants, oral decongestants, antihistamines, mucus thinners, and cough suppressants. For each of these classes of drugs we provide information on:

- How do these drugs work?
- What are the benefits?
- What symptoms can be reduced or health benefits gained from this class of pharmaceuticals?
- Potential side effects. This section covers the common or nonlethal side effects that are known to occur with this class of drugs.
- Major cautions. This section covers serious risks such as organ damage or potentially lethal side effects.
- Drug interactions. This section covers the drugs that are known to have potentially harmful interaction with this class of drugs.
- Food or supplement interactions. This section covers foods and supplements known to have potentially harmful interaction with this class of drugs.
- Nutrient depletion/imbalance. This section covers nutrients that are known to be depleted or imbalanced from this class of drugs, along with recommendations for supplementation.

There may be differences for some of the individual drugs within a category. Our summary covers the information common to the drugs in each class. However, there can be individual differences that are not covered within the summary.

Natural Alternatives

This section describes natural supplements and therapies that are recommended as alternatives, including dosages and cautions. Key studies on these natural alternatives are summarized in an easy-to-read format.

PART ONE

What You Need to Know about Pharmaceutical Drugs

Drugs: The Good and the Bad

Pharmaceuticals certainly have their place in health care. For example, drug therapy saves lives in cases of infections, certain cancers, and insulin-dependent diabetes, and it relieves suffering for those in acute and chronic pain. The fact is, we need pharmaceuticals for the proper treatment of a wide variety of illnesses. It is obvious, however, that we in the United States have put too much faith in drug therapy. The "pop a pill and everything will be fine" mentality has led many to an early death or suppressed the health and vitality of others. The fact is that few magic bullets exist in the drug industry. Our health care system has gotten out of balance. We need a shift toward preventing and treating the root cause of illness with diet, lifestyle changes, stress reduction, and natural remedies. Pharmaceutical medications should complement this approach and be used judiciously.

Astoundingly, Americans spend close to $200 billion each year on prescription drugs. This number does not include over-the-counter medications. The United States is the world leader when it comes to popping pharmaceuticals. Did you know that in 1986 there were fewer than 900 prescription medications in existence, but that currently there are over 8,000? There is a drug for everything. Critics argue that new disease labels are being created under the influence of pharmaceutical companies so that pharmaceutical markets can expand.

The *Journal of the American Medical Association* published an eye-opening report stating that 106,000 patients die each year from adverse reactions caused by drugs administered by medical professionals. In addition, 5 percent of hospital admissions are due to adverse drug reactions. Many researchers believe the incidence is likely much higher.

Over-the-counter or nonprescription drugs are not without risk, either. Many people assume that an over-the-counter item is safe because it does not require a prescription. While there is truth to that perception, nonprescription medications still carry a risk of serious side effects. For example, approximately 16,000 people in the United States die each year from adverse reactions to over-the-counter nonsteroidal anti-inflammatory drugs (NSAIDs), such as aspirin and ibuprofen, which can cause gastrointestinal bleeding and kidney and cardiovascular problems. Again, many researchers feel this number is conservative and could easily be two to three times higher.

How do the numbers of fatal adverse reactions compare for nutritional supplements? There simply is no comparison. The American Association of Poison Control Centers reports that dietary supplements lead to about 10 deaths yearly, most of which are iron overdoses. As you can see, the risk of serious harm from nutritional supplements out of the millions of doses taken daily is a drop in a lake compared to the risk from pharmaceuticals. Therefore, nutritional supplements should be used instead of pharmaceutical medications whenever possible.

Our children are also at risk from adverse reactions from pharmaceuticals. It makes logical sense that a child's developing body can be more easily harmed by drugs. While you won't see it in media headlines, the risk is very clear. A study published in the prestigious journal *Pediatrics* in 2002 concluded, "Adverse reactions to drug therapy are a significant cause of death and injury in infants and children under two years of age." It is outrageous, but the truth is that most drugs given to children have never undergone pediatric-related studies! In 2007, Food and Drug Administration (FDA) experts published a 365-page report showing that decongestants and antihistamines have been linked with 123 pediatric deaths since 1969. Pharmaceutical companies announced a voluntary withdrawal of oral cough and cold medicines marketed for use in infants. The FDA also announced that almost 200 unapproved prescription medicines containing hydrocodone, a narcotic that is used to ease pain and cough, must be taken off the market for children under age 6. Frighteningly, pharmaceutical companies had extrapolated data from adult studies to estimate dosages for children. These doses may or may not be accurate.

At the other end of the spectrum, there is concern about the vulnerability of seniors to the toxicity of pharmaceuticals. As people age, the kidneys and liver process pharmaceuticals less efficiently. This means the drugs' effects are more potent, last longer, and are more likely to cause adverse or fatal reactions.

Many consider the FDA lax in its protection of the public against dangerous drugs. Ongoing congressional hearings on financial interests between FDA employees and drug companies continue to expose a flawed agency. Many drug company executives are former FDA employees, and the FDA gets much of its funding from drug company research fees. The November 2004 edition of the *Journal of the American Medical Association* disclosed that "an investigation of 18 FDA expert advisory panels revealed that more than half of the members of these panels had direct financial interests in the drug or topic they were evaluating and for which they were making recommendations." The same report also noted that in 2003 "the pharmaceutical industry earmarked $4.9 million to lobby the FDA."

The FDA drug approval system is far from where it needs to be. This is evident from the numerous recalls of popular drugs. You may wonder how the drugs we list below could have been on the market if the testing procedures are so stringent. Two (sometimes one) Phase 3 clinical human trials are required for drug approval by the FDA. This involves a few hundred to a few thousand patients. The trials allow researchers to identify the most common but not always the most serious side effects a drug may have. The problem is that less than 50 percent of all serious adverse reactions to a new drug are identified before it enters the marketplace. This means at least half of the serious adverse reactions are discovered by you—the public.

Following is a brief summary of drugs that were either withdrawn from the market or given new warnings in recent years. Although not an exhaustive list, it demonstrates the point that FDA-approved drugs can be dangerous.

- Erectile dysfunction drugs, including:

    Sildenafil (Viagra)

    Vardenafil (Levitra)

    Tadalafil (Cialis)

    Use: Treatment of erectile dysfunction (ED).

    In 2007, the FDA informed doctors of reports of sudden decreases or loss of hearing following the use of these drugs.

- Thiazolidinedione class of antidiabetic drugs, including:

    Rosiglitazone maleate (Avandia)

    Pioglitazone hydrochloride (Actos)

    Rosiglitazone maleate and glimepiride (Avandaryl)

    Rosiglitazone maleate and metformin hydrochloride (Avandamet)

    Pioglitazone hydrochloride and glimepride (Duetact)

    Use: Type 2 diabetes.

    In 2007, the FDA requested an updated label with a boxed warning on the risks of heart failure.

- Tegaserod maleate (Zelnorm)

    Use: Irritable bowel syndrome and constipation.

    In 2007, this drug was removed from the market due to serious cardio-vascular problems, including myocardial infarction (heart attack), unstable angina (chest pain), and stroke.

- Antidepressant medications

    Use: Treatment of depression.

In 2007, the FDA notified the makers of all antidepressant medications to update the existing black box warning on the prescribing information for their products to include warnings about the increased risks of suicidal thinking and behavior in young adults ages 18 to 24 years during the first one to two months of treatment.

- Amphetamine with dextroamphetamine (Adderall), methylphenidate (Ritalin, Concerta)

    Use: Pediatric and adult attention deficit/hyperactivity disorder treatment.

    In 2006, a black box warning was given for cardiovascular risk.

- Pimecrolimus (Elidel) and tacrolimus (Protopic)

    Use: Topical eczema treatments.

    In 2006, these were given a black box warning after researchers found a link between these drugs and increased risk of lymphoma and skin cancer.

- Celecoxib (Celebrex)

    Use: Anti-inflammatory.

    In 2005, a boxed warning was required regarding potentially serious adverse cardiovascular events and possibly life-threatening gastrointestinal events.

- Valdecoxib (Bextra)

    Use: Anti-inflammatory.

    In 2005, this was withdrawn due to lack of data on the cardiovascular safety of long-term use of Bextra, along with increased risk of adverse cardiovascular events, possibly associated with chronic Bextra use. There also were reports of rare, but serious, potentially life-threatening skin reactions.

- Rofecoxib (Vioxx)

    Use: Nonsteroidal anti-inflammatory.

    In 2004, this drug was withdrawn due to increased risk of serious cardiovascular events, including heart attacks and strokes.

- Cerivastatin (Baycol)

    Use: Cholesterol-lowering.

    In 2001, it was withdrawn due to reports of sometimes fatal rhabdomyolysis, a severe muscle adverse reaction.

- Phenylpropanolamine (PPA) and phenylpropanolamine hydrochloride (the active ingredient in PPA)

    Use: Ingredients in cold and cough medicines, nasal decongestants, and over-the-counter appetite suppressants and weight-loss products.

    In 2000, they were withdrawn due to risk of hemorrhagic stroke.

- Troglitazone (Rezulin)

    Use: Treatment of type 2 diabetes.

    In 2000, it was withdrawn due to severe liver toxicity.

- Cisapride (Propulsid)

    Use: Treatment of acid reflux.

    Serious cardiac arrhythmias (irregular heart rhythms) and cardiac arrest. In 2000, it was withdrawn from the market.

Staying Safe with Pharmaceuticals

Get educated. Read as much information as you can on any drug before taking it. Learn the possible dangers and weigh them against the potential benefits. Ask your doctor and pharmacist about their experiences with patients who have used this medication. Find out whether to take the drug with meals or on an empty stomach, side effects to watch for, and what to do in case of an adverse reaction.

Create a "medication card." Make a list that summarizes all prescription and over-the-counter (OTC) drugs and all supplements you take. Include the name of the product, its strength, the dose and frequency at which you use it, your reason for taking it, the date when you first started it, and the names and phone numbers of your doctors and pharmacist. Keep this card in your wallet as a ready reference. You can also receive a free medication card by mail from the University of Connecticut Health Center. Call 800-535-6232 or download it from http://health.uchc.edu/medicard/index.htm.

Learn about drug interactions. Tell your doctor and pharmacist about all your drugs and supplements. Inquire about possible interactions. Read the drug package inserts. This book also discusses possible drug interactions.

Replenish nutrients known to be depleted by the medications you are taking. This book is a good resource for that purpose.

Be extra-cautious with new drugs. As you read earlier in this chapter, adverse reactions are often discovered after new drugs have been on the market for a few years or longer. Stick with tried-and-true drugs. If you must use a new one, request the lowest starting dose possible.

Choose natural therapies. Whenever you can safely do so, try natural remedies instead of drug therapies. Work with a doctor who will support this decision, and make a holistic doctor a part of your health care team.

References

Fontanarosa, PB, D Rennie, and CD DeAngelis. 2004. Postmarketing surveillance—lack of vigilance, lack of trust. *Journal of the American Medical Association.* 292(21): 2647–50.

2

Natural Medicine: A Necessity for Good Health

We are in the midst of a revolution in our nation's health care. We live in an era when there are more office visits to complementary and alternative medicine practitioners than to primary care medical doctors. The public has demanded safer, less expensive, and more nonsuppressive therapies to prevent disease and restore their health. We have come to the conclusion that as individuals, we want to have control over our own health care decisions. Doctors are to be partners in the decision-making and healing process. As a consequence, we are seeing more and more complementary medicine health care providers in all spheres of medicine. Although there are not enough to meet the demand, we are moving in the right direction.

The fundamental question is, Why is natural medicine a necessity for good health? A 2007 report gave some insight into this question. It disclosed that Americans have a shorter life expectancy than people in 41 other countries. This is eye opening, considering that we in the United States on average spend more on health care than people anywhere else. What's behind this discouraging statistic? There are various possibilities, including the fact that almost 70 percent of U.S. adults are now overweight, with 32 percent of these considered obese. Lack of medical insurance is another likely reason. A third reason, which you won't read about in the press, is the suppression of nutritional and holistic therapies in mainstream U.S. health care. Approximately 80 percent of the world's population rely on plants and other holistic medicines as a primary form of medicine. For people in many cultures, medicine begins in the backyard, where family gardens yield plentiful fruits, vegetables, and healing herbs; and natural, nontoxic therapies such as massage and nutritional therapy are widely used. We encourage you to incorporate holistic healing into your health care—and to urge your insurance carrier to cover these therapies.

Can you have confidence in the dietary and supplement approaches recommended in this book? You certainly can. We have cited key studies and scientific references validating their effectiveness. In addition, among this book's three authors, we have well over a combined 75 years of clinical experience. It is one thing to read a study on the effectiveness of a particular natural medicine, it is another to monitor a patient and see a health transformation take place.

There is a lot more science behind natural and nutritional therapies than most people, including medical doctors, are aware of. Thousands of scientific studies from around the world are published monthly validating the effectiveness and safety of natural medicine.

Natural medicine is a diverse system of medicine that offers a variety of healing therapies. While there are different philosophies and styles of natural therapies, they have common principles. The following six principles are embraced by modern-day naturopathic and holistic doctors.

1. **First, do no harm.** Whenever possible, use therapies that have the lowest risk of causing adverse effects. In general, nutritional and other natural approaches are quite safe.

2. **Use the healing power of nature.** Our bodies have an inherent healing mechanism. We can aid that healing mechanism through the use of nutritional and various natural (as well as conventional) therapies. From a divinely complex design, we see how the medicinal properties of foods, herbs, and other natural substances nourish and stimulate the healing ability of the body.

3. **Find the cause.** The best way to help individuals with their health needs is to treat their root causes. Holistic doctors are generally very effective at identifying and treating the root cause of an illness. When possible, we should strive to remove the underlying cause of an illness rather than just eliminate or suppress its symptoms.

4. **Treat the whole person.** Wellness or illness comes from a complex interaction of physical, emotional, dietary, genetic, environmental, lifestyle, and other factors. One is best helped by taking all these factors into account. This includes the physical, mental, emotional, and spiritual aspects of a person.

5. **Practice preventive medicine.** Illness is often caused by diet, habits, poor stress-coping mechanisms, environmental pollutants, and lifestyle. Good holistic doctors assess risk factors and susceptibility to disease and make appropriate recommendations to prevent illness, or to keep a minor illness from developing into a more serious or chronic disease. The emphasis is on building health rather than on treating symptoms.

6. **Practice the principle of doctor as teacher.** The original meaning of the word "doctor" is teacher. A good doctor will educate patients on what they should do to achieve health as opposed to just relying on medical intervention.

Now we move on to discuss a variety of health conditions.

References

Ohlemacher, Stephen. 2007. U.S. life expectancy lags behind 41 nations. *USA Today*, August 11, Health and Behavior section.

PART TWO

Pharmaceuticals and Their Natural Alternatives, Condition by Condition

3

Acne Drugs and Their Natural Alternatives

What Is Acne?

Acne is a common skin condition caused by oils that get trapped in the pores, forming whiteheads or blackheads (comedones), which can subsequently become infected and inflamed, resulting in pimples or cysts. Because they contain the highest concentration of oil glands, the face, neck, chest, shoulders, and back are usually the most affected areas of the body. Acne ranges in development from very mild to extremely severe. Although generally not dangerous, it can cause scarring and emotional trauma.

Common acne usually affects people in their teen years, with three out of four developing symptoms. Although both sexes develop acne, boys tend to have more severe, longer-lasting acne. While teens are the most affected group, acne is also common in people in their twenties, and can even occur in children, or in adults in their thirties, forties, or fifties.

What Causes Acne?

Statistics suggest that heredity (family history) is a strong predisposing factor for the development of acne. The major physiological factors contributing to the formation of acne are overactive oil glands, blocked skin pores, activity of normal skin bacteria, overgrowth of fungal organisms, diet, hormonal stimulation of the oil glands, and inflammation.

Overactive Oil Glands

Oil glands (or sebaceous glands) produce sebum, which flows to the surface of the skin through canals containing hair follicles, to lubricate the hair follicles and the surrounding skin. Oil glands are stimulated to produce sebum by androgens, which are hormones produced by both males and females. Puberty, stress, and hormonal shifts can cause the body to produce more androgens, and subsequently more oil.

Blocked Skin Pores

If oil cannot flow through the follicular canal and out of the pore due to blockage, it becomes trapped and builds up within the pore. Such blockage is caused by skin cells that have been shed, but which bunch together at the pore for unknown reasons. People with acne tend to produce more dead skin cells, but do not shed them properly. A simple blocked pore will manifest as a whitehead or a blackhead.

Activity of Normal Skin Bacteria

The bacterium *Propionibacterium acnes* is a healthy, normal part of the skin surface; it prevents harmful bacteria from entering the skin. Although it is not the cause of acne, it can play a role in making it worse. When oil becomes trapped, *P. acnes* grows in the blocked pore, ultimately resulting in inflammation and pimple formation.

Inflammation

In the case of acne, the body's immune system works to rid itself of bacteria or irritating substances in the pores. The resulting inflammation is characterized by redness, swelling, warmth, and discomfort. Once infection and inflammation have taken hold, the problem can become deeper than a pimple, and pustules, nodules, and/or cysts can develop in the pores.

Things that can additionally stimulate the above processes include oily cosmetics, comedogenic (blackhead-producing) skin care or hair care products, nutritional deficiencies, candida overgrowth, certain drugs such as steroids or estrogen medications, and friction or pressure caused by clothing, helmets, phones, and so on. In some people, food sensitivities may also play a role. Most over-the-counter and prescription medications for acne such as benzoyl peroxide, salicylic acid, antibiotics, and retinoids address one or more of the root causes discussed above in a noncurative fashion.

Acne Drugs

Benzoyl Peroxide Topical

Benoxyl

Benzac AC

Benzagel

Brevoxyl

Persa-Gel

HOW DO THESE DRUGS WORK?

Benzoyl peroxide works by removing cells from the top layer of the skin surface. This action unclogs the pores so that oil (sebum) can escape. In addition, it has antibacterial action, thereby helping to clear the pores of infection by *Propionibacterium acnes*. Many acne preparations incorporate benzoyl peroxide because research indicates that it increases the effectiveness of some medicines. For instance, when used in combination with antibiotics, benzoyl peroxide reduces the likelihood of a patient developing resistance to the antibiotic.

WHAT ARE THE BENEFITS?

These topical medications can reduce mild to moderate acne without the risk of systemic side effects.

POTENTIAL SIDE EFFECTS

Stinging, dryness, and peeling tend to occur initially. Irritation, redness, scaly eruptions, darkening or lightening of the skin, or rash can be more serious side effects.

MAJOR CAUTIONS

Benzoyl peroxide can make the skin more sensitive to sunlight, so avoid prolonged sun exposure and tanning lights. It should not be used on sunburned, windburned, dry, chapped, or irritated skin. Research conducted on lab mice, and in some instances hamsters, indicates that benzoyl peroxide has led to the rapid development of carcinoma (skin cancer). Avoid contact with wounds, the eyes, the mouth, and mucous membranes.

MEDICAL PRECAUTIONS

If you are pregnant or lactating, you should discuss the risks of using benzoyl peroxide with your doctor.

KNOWN DRUG INTERACTIONS

Benzoyl peroxide should not be used with other topical treatments unless indicated by your doctor. If used with tretinoin (Avita, Renova, Retin-A), it may cause severe skin irritation.

FOOD OR SUPPLEMENT INTERACTIONS

There are no known food or supplement interactions or nutrient depletions and/or imbalances associated with the use of topical benzoyl peroxide treatments.

Salicylic Acid Topical

Oxy Clean Maximum Strength

Oxy Clean Medicated

Salex

Sebasorb

Stri-Dex

HOW DO THESE DRUGS WORK?

Salicylic acid is a peeling agent found in many over-the-counter and some prescription acne treatments. It causes the cells of the epidermis to become "unglued," allowing the dead skin cells to slough off. As these skin cells are shed and removed, pores unclog.

WHAT ARE THE BENEFITS?

These topical medications can reduce mild to moderate acne without the risk of systemic side effects.

POTENTIAL SIDE EFFECTS

Common side effects include burning, stinging, itching, dryness, redness, peeling, or irritation. More serious, but less common, side effects may include severe skin irritation or allergic reaction.

MAJOR CAUTIONS

Avoid all mucous membranes when applying salicylic acid. Also, do not use on sunburned, windburned, dry, chapped, irritated, or broken skin, or on open wounds.

MEDICAL PRECAUTIONS

People with the following conditions or disorders should discuss their risks with their physician:

- Liver disease
- Kidney disease

- Diabetes
- Poor circulation
- Pregnancy
- Breast-feeding

KNOWN DRUG INTERACTIONS

Using other topical preparations may interfere with the effectiveness of salicylic acid or increase skin irritation; do not use other topical preparations on the treated area unless directed by your doctor. Talk with your doctor if you are taking aspirin, diuretics, and methyl salicylate (found in some muscle rubs); he/she may need to change the doses of your medications or monitor you carefully for side effects.

FOOD OR SUPPLEMENT INTERACTIONS

None known.

Antibiotics: Topical and Oral

Topical

Erythromycin (Akne-Mycin, Staticin, Erygel, EryDerm)

Clindamycin (C/T/S, Cleocin T, Clinda-Derm, Clindets Pledget)

Erythromycin and benzoyl peroxide (Benzamycin)

Clindamycin and benzoyl peroxide (Benzaclin)

Oral

Erythromycin (E-Mycin, Eryc, Ery-Tab, PCE, Pediazole, Ilosone)

Tetracycline (Achromycin, Sumycin)

HOW DO THESE DRUGS WORK?

Antibiotics stop the growth of bacteria. In the case of acne, they help rid the pores of *P. acnes* and reduce inflammation. Topical antibiotics, which have fewer side effects, are generally tried first; and if the patient does not respond, oral antibiotics are often the next step. Oral antibiotics have been the mainstay of treatment for years in patients with persistent moderate to severe acne. Treatment usually begins with a higher dosage that is reduced as acne resolves. Treatment can be continued for up to six months. Unfortunately, as with all antibiotics, the bacteria can develop resistance, making it necessary to switch to a different antibiotic or treatment.

WHAT ARE THE BENEFITS?

Topical antibiotics are helpful in reducing mild to moderate acne, and oral antibiotics are generally effective for moderate to severe acne.

POTENTIAL SIDE EFFECTS

With topical antibiotics, common side effects may include burning, itching, dryness, redness, oiliness, or peeling where applied.

With oral antibiotics, the most frequently observed, and usually dose-related, side effects are dizziness, nausea, vomiting, loss of appetite, diarrhea, and abdominal pain. A less common side effect with oral antibiotics is blurred vision, primarily associated with tetracycline. Photosensitivity can also occur with tetracycline, so it is advisable to reduce sun exposure.

More serious side effects associated with oral antibiotics that may require medical attention include severe allergic reactions; other infections; vaginal irritation or discharge; bloody stools; red, swollen, or blistered skin; severe diarrhea; severe stomach pain or cramps; and yellowing of the skin or eyes.

MAJOR CAUTIONS

Antibiotics can cause a severe intestinal condition (pseudomembranous colitis) that may occur during treatment or even several weeks after treatment has stopped. Symptoms of this condition may include persistent diarrhea, abdominal or stomach pain or cramping, or blood or mucus in the stool. Clindamycin is particularly associated with this condition, but it can be caused by any antibiotic.

In rare cases, erythromycin has been associated with the production of cardiac ventricular arrhythmias. There have also been reports of reversible hearing loss primarily in people with renal insufficiency or in those taking high doses of erythromycin. Abnormal liver tests and hepatic dysfunction can also occur.

Tetracycline and its derivatives (doxycycline, minocycline) should not be taken by children younger than 8 years of age because they can affect growth and stain teeth, and there have been reports of severe gastrointestinal problems occurring in infants following erythromycin therapy. Rare instances of esophagitis and esophageal ulceration have been reported in patients receiving the capsule and tablet forms of tetracycline.

Antibiotics may cause *Candida albicans* or other *Candida* species to overgrow in the digestive, respiratory, urinary, and vaginal areas of the body. They destroy friendly flora that keeps these yeast organisms in check. (Friendly flora also is involved in the synthesis of various nutrients, aids in detoxification, and supports normal immunity.)

Microbial resistance to antibiotics is a major concern and problem associated with antibiotic use.

MEDICAL PRECAUTIONS

People with the following conditions or disorders should discuss their risks with their physician:

- Allergy to any component of the antibiotic
- History of allergies

- Impaired liver function
- Impaired renal function
- History of heart problems
- Porphyria (blood disorder)
- Myasthenia gravis
- History of intestinal disease (e.g., ulcerative colitis, enteritis, etc.)
- Diabetes
- Pregnancy
- Breast-feeding
- History of *Candida albicans* infection

KNOWN DRUG INTERACTIONS

Topical Antibiotics

Using other topical therapies may cause irritation. Research suggests that clindamycin has neuromuscular-blocking properties. Therefore, it should be used with caution in patients receiving such agents because it may enhance their action.

Oral Antibiotics

Erythromycin administered together with theophylline (an asthma treatment) can lead to elevated blood levels of theophylline and subsequent toxicity. Erythromycin can also raise blood levels and cause toxic reactions with digoxin, warfarin (Coumadin), and antiseizure medications such as phenytoin (Dilantin) and carbamazepine (Tegretol). Serious arrhythmias and even cardiac arrest have been observed when erythromycin and terfenadine (Seldane) are used together. Erythromycin can also interact with lovastatin (Mevacor), causing muscle inflammation. Erythromycin may interact with many other common medications prescribed for a variety of conditions, due to its effects on certain liver enzymes. Talk to your doctor about your medication. If your medication is metabolized by a CYP3A enzyme system, you should discuss possible interactions.

Bismuth subsalicylate (Pepto-Bismol) and antacids containing aluminum, calcium, or magnesium bind tetracycline in the intestines, reducing its effectiveness. Like erythromycin, tetracycline may enhance the activity of warfarin (Coumadin), causing excessive blood thinning. Phenytoin (Dilantin), carbamazepine (Tegretol), and barbiturates (such as phenobarbital) can enhance the metabolism of tetracycline. Avoid acitretin (psoriasis medication) or isotretinoin (Accutane) because side effects, such as increased pressure in the fluid surrounding the brain, may occur. Concurrent use of tetracycline may reduce the effectiveness of oral contraceptives and penicillin.

FOOD OR SUPPLEMENT INTERACTIONS

Tetracycline should not be taken with dairy products or with minerals such as calcium, magnesium, zinc, or iron; these cause binding of tetracycline in the intestinal tract and may reduce its effectiveness. There is some evidence that berberine-containing herbs such as goldenseal, barberry, and oregon grape may also reduce the effectiveness of tetracycline. Avoid alcohol, as it may increase dizziness associated with tetracycline use.

Digitalis lanata and *Digitalis purpurea*, herbs commonly known as foxglove, contain digitalis glycosides. (These herbs are not commonly available but may be prescribed by some natural health care providers.) These chemicals have similar actions and toxicities to the prescription drug digoxin and should not be used with erythromycin. These herbs, though, are not available over the counter. Erythromycin should be taken without food to avoid breakdown before it reaches the intestines.

Research has demonstrated that consuming yogurt or supplements containing probiotics such as bifidobacterium, *Lactobacillus acidophilus*, and *Saccharomyces boulardii* can help prevent symptoms of antibiotic-induced diarrhea and reduce the likelihood of antibiotic-induced infection by clostridium or candida. In other research, the enzyme bromelain showed beneficial effects on the activity of erythromycin.

NUTRIENT DEPLETION/IMBALANCE

Erythromycin may interfere with the absorption and/or activity of calcium, folic acid, B12, B6, and magnesium. And tetracycline can interfere with the activity of folic acid, potassium, vitamin B2, vitamin B6, vitamin B12, and vitamin C. In addition, excessive bleeding has been reported in people using antibiotics; this effect is believed to be a result of reduced vitamin K activity and/or production associated with the antibiotic-related loss of "friendly" bacteria in the colon. We recommend the following supplements:

- Multivitamin and mineral.
- Vitamin C—take 500 mg.
- Probiotic that contains friendly bacteria with 5 billion or more active organisms. Take daily, two hours or more away from taking antibiotics.

Retinoids

Topical
Tretinoin (Retin-A, Avita, Renova)
Adapalene (Differin)
Isotretinion (Isotrex gel)

Oral
Isotretinion (Accutane)

HOW DO THESE DRUGS WORK?

Retinoids are a derivative of vitamin A. In topical form, they work by increasing skin cell turnover and promoting the release of the plugged material in the follicle. They also prevent the formation of new whiteheads and blackheads (comedones) because the rapid turnover of cells prevents new pimples from forming. Some retinoids (oral isotretinoin specifically) also reduce the amount of sebum produced by the sebaceous glands and stop *P. acnes* growth.

WHAT ARE THE BENEFITS?

Although the list of side effects and precautions is daunting, the long-term effectiveness of Accutane (isotretinoin) is extremely positive. Seventy percent of patients receiving Accutane will be acne-free for more than 10 years. However, about 25 percent of patients who have used Accutane will see acne symptoms return after two years, and 10 percent will see acne return after just one year. A normal treatment period is about four to six months.

POTENTIAL SIDE EFFECTS

With topical retinoids, local inflammation commonly occurs with application and resolves when treatment is stopped. Mild stinging and a sensation of warmth also occur with application. Dryness, scaling, and redness are considered common side effects. However, severe redness, vesicles, or crusting are signs that a lower-concentration treatment should be considered.

Isotretinoin can cause dry nose, nosebleeds, cracks in the corners of the mouth, dry mouth, inflammation of the whites of the eyes, thinning hair, bone loss, and joint aches. More rare side effects can include skin infections, excessive peeling, sun sensitivity, hearing impairment, and hepatitis.

MAJOR CAUTIONS

It cannot be guaranteed that any topical retinoid would not have an adverse effect on a developing human fetus. Isotretinoin must not be used by females who are pregnant. Major human fetal abnormalities related to isotretinoin administration in females have been documented. There is also an increased risk of spontaneous abortion (miscarriage) and premature births.

Patients using isotretinoin may develop elevated blood sugar, triglycerides, and cholesterol. In addition, psychiatric problems (e.g., depression, hallucinations, suicidal behavior) have been reported. Severe allergic reaction may also occur. In rare cases, isotretinoin can cause brain swelling, producing nausea, vomiting, headache, and changes in vision.

MEDICAL PRECAUTIONS

People with the following conditions or disorders should discuss their risks with their physician:

- Pregnant or planning to become pregnant

- Lactating
- Eczema
- Mental problems
- Asthma
- Liver disease
- Diabetes
- Heart disease
- Bone loss or weak bones
- Anorexia nervosa
- Food or medicine allergies

KNOWN DRUG INTERACTIONS

Topical retinoids should not be used with any other topical skin treatments unless otherwise instructed. Tetracycline should not be given at the same time as isotretinoin due to the risk of brain swelling. Dilantin or corticosteroids taken with isotretinoin may weaken bones. Coadministration of isotretinoin and carbamazepine has resulted in a reduced carbamazepine plasma level.

FOOD OR SUPPLEMENT INTERACTIONS

Isotretinoin is closely related to vitamin A. Therefore, the use of vitamin A and isotretinoin at the same time may lead to vitamin A toxicity effects. The combined administration of isotretinoin and vitamin E may significantly reduce the initial toxicity of high-dose isotretinoin without affecting its efficacy.

NUTRIENT DEPLETION/IMBALANCE

None known.

Natural Alternatives to Acne Drugs

Diet and Lifestyle Changes

For some people with acne, a healthy diet can do wonders to clear up their complexion. Conventional medicine has traditionally held to the notion that acne is not related to diet. Nutrition-oriented doctors such as ourselves have found that diet plays a major role in acne for some but not all individuals. An emerging body of scientific evidence is demonstrating that diet does indeed have an impact on acne. For example, researcher Loren Cordain, professor of health and exercise science at Colorado State University, teamed up with five scientists from around the country to look at the more than 1,300 Kitivan Islanders of Papua New Guinea and Ache hunter-gatherers of Paraguay. They could not find a single case of active acne in either Kitivan Islanders or Ache hunter-gatherers. According to Cordain, the perfect skin of the two unrelated groups in the study was not due to genetics, but likely was the result of different environmental factors, especially diet. Unlike the high simple sugar content of U.S. foods, the diet of the Kitivans in Papua, New Guinea, consists mainly of fruit, fish, and tubers. The diet of the Ache hunter-gatherers of Paraguay includes wild and foraged foods, locally cultivated food, and a small percentage of Western foods obtained from external sources.

A Western diet boosts the hormone insulin, which promotes inflammation of the skin as well as the overproduction of oil and skin cells in pores that lead to bacteria overgrowth on the skin and acne formation. In addition, the Western diet increases growth factors and other hormones such as testosterone that contribute to acne.

A recent study in the *American Journal of Clinical Nutrition* confirmed the benefits of a low-glycemic diet for improving acne vulgaris. Foods in a low-glycemic diet are less likely to increase glucose and insulin levels. The twelve-week study involved 43 male acne patients 15 to 25 years of age. The participants were put on a low-glycemic-load diet composed of 25 percent energy from protein and 45 percent from low-glycemic-index carbohydrates, while the control group was on a typical U.S. carbohydrate-rich diet. Acne lesion counts and severity were assessed during monthly visits, and insulin sensitivity was measured at baseline and at 12 weeks. Researchers found that total lesion counts decreased by 22 in the study group, whereas the control group had a decrease of approximately 12. Also, the low-glycemic diet group had a greater improvement in insulin sensitivity. Thus we recommend eliminating junk and processed foods such as white flour products as much as possible from the diet. Focus on whole foods, cold-water fish, and lean poultry. We have also found that cow's milk aggravates acne in some patients and should be avoided. Choose hormone-free meats, poultry, and eggs, since acne is influenced greatly by hormonal factors. Drink 8 ounces of quality water every two to three waking hours to maintain good detoxification and skin health.

Stress can bring on or worsen acne. High levels of the stress hormone cortisol can lead to hormonal changes that worsen acne. Therefore stress-reduction techniques such as exercise, prayer, and biofeedback can be helpful in treating acne.

Zinc

Several small double-blind clinical trials have shown that zinc supplements are effective for acne. Zinc is involved in skin healing and improved immunity. Zinc also reduces the skin levels of the testosterone metabolite dihydrotestosterone, which can aggravate acne. Studies show that people with acne tend to have lower serum and skin levels of zinc. We have observed zinc supplementation to be effective for numerous patients. A study published in *Dermatology* compared the effectiveness and safety of zinc versus antibiotic therapy (minocycline) in the treatment of acne vulgaris. In this multicenter randomized, double-blind trial, 332 patients received either 30 mg of elemental zinc or 100 mg of minocycline over 3 months. The clinical success rate was 31.2 percent for zinc and 63.4 percent for minocycline. The zinc group had 5 dropouts; the minocycline group, 4 dropouts. Most of the adverse effects were related to gastrointestinal upset. The conclusion of this study was that both zinc and minocycline were effective in the treatment of acne, with minocycline having a better effect. However, it should be noted the zinc dosage was quite low compared to what nutrition-oriented doctors typically use to treat acne.

DOSAGE

Take 50 mg of zinc twice daily with meals for three months, and then reduce to 50 mg daily as a maintenance dosage if your acne is improved.

SAFETY

Zinc may have immune-suppressing effects when taken at dosages larger than 150 mg. Taking more than 100 mg daily for 10 or more years may increase the risk of prostate cancer. Zinc may deplete copper levels so take 2 to 3 mg of copper daily with long-term zinc supplementation. This amount is available in some multivitamins. Zinc may cause digestive upset in some users.

The History of Tea Tree Oil

Tea tree oil (*Melaleuca alternifolia*), also known as cajeput oil, has a long history of use in Australia. The leaves of the Australian *Melaleuca alternifolia* tree contain this medicinal oil. Scientific investigations of tea tree oil began in the city of Sydney back in 1922. A government researcher had noticed that the oils were antiseptic yet nontoxic. Tea tree oil was used by the Australian army during World War II. Today, researchers have found over 100 chemicals in tea tree oil. It is used topically for skin conditions other than acne such as fungal infections, warts, cuts, burns, and gingivitis. It is available as an oil, a cream, a gel, a soap, and other topical applications.

Tea Tree Oil

The topical application of tea tree oil is effective for the treatment of acne. Tea tree oil reduces bacteria and other microbes associated with acne vulgaris. It is available in a variety of topical creams or facial rinses. One Australian single-blind, randomized clinical trial on 124 patients found results from a 5 percent tea tree oil gel extract comparable to the effects of benzoyl peroxide in the treatment of mild to moderate acne. Although the onset of action was slower with tea tree oil, it had fewer side effects such as dryness, burning, redness, and itching.

Guggul

This herb native to India is commonly used in the United States to reduce cholesterol. It has been shown to be effective for difficult-to-treat cystic acne. A study in the *Journal of Dermatology* involved 20 patients with cystic acne. They received either tetracycline 500 mg or tablets of guggul (equivalent to 25 mg guggulsterone), taken twice daily for three months. The reduction of inflammatory lesions in the tetracycline group was 65.2

percent as compared to 68 percent with the gugulipid group. In addition, researchers observed that the patients with oily faces responded remarkably better to gugulipid.

DOSAGE

Take a standardized guggul product that gives a daily dosage of 25 mg of the active constituent guggulsterone daily.

SAFETY

Guggul is quite safe. It should not be combined with cholesterol-lowering medications. Rare side effects include rash and digestive upset such as diarrhea.

Vitamin A

Large doses of vitamin A have been found to be effective for the treatment of acne vulgaris. We have found it to be effective in patients who are nonresponsive to other natural treatments.

DOSAGE

Under a doctor's supervision take 100,000 to 150,000 IU daily along with 800 IU of vitamin E for three to five months.

SAFETY

High doses of vitamin A should not be used by women of childbearing age who are not on birth control, as it can cause birth defects. Dosages higher than 5,000 IU per day should not be used by pregnant or nursing women. One controversial study concluded that vitamin A can increase the risk of osteoporosis and hip fracture in postmenopausal women. Other side effects can include joint pain, dry and cracked skin, elevated liver enzymes, fatigue, headache, and

---

Like her mother, aunts, and sister, Lisa, 42, had been afflicted with adult-onset acne. Her face was constantly broken out with acne, including the cystic form. For years she had cycled on and off antibiotics with temporary benefits. We put her on a diet that limited simple sugars as well as gluten-containing foods. This gave her mild improvement. She was also prescribed a high daily dose of vitamin A. Since her husband had had a vasectomy, the vitamin A therapy was deemed to be safe as far as the potential for birth defects. Taking 100,000 IU of vitamin A along with 800 IU of vitamin E was quite helpful, with improvements noticed within four weeks. In addition, the hard-to-treat cystic acne greatly improved. The treatment worked so well, it was also prescribed to her 17–year-old son, who also had significant benefit.

LISA'S STORY

other symptoms. While we have not commonly observed these symptoms while monitoring patients on high-dose vitamin A, they are reported in the literature. Therefore anyone using high-dose vitamin A therapy must be under the supervision of a doctor.

References

Bassett, IB, DL Pannowitz, RS Barnetson. 1990. A comparative study of tea-tree oil versus benzoyl peroxide in the treatment of acne. *Medical Journal of Australia.* 153:455–8.

Dreno, B, et al. 2001. Multicenter randomized comparative double-blind controlled clinical trial of the safety and efficacy of zinc gluconate versus minocycline hydrochloride in the treatment of inflammatory acne vulgaris. *Dermatology.* 203(2):135–40.

Smith, RN, et al. 2007. A low-glycemic-load diet improves symptoms in acne vulgaris patients: A randomized controlled trial. *American Journal of Clinical Nutrition.* July;86(1):107–15.

Thappa, DM, J Dogra. 1994. Nodulocystic acne: Oral gugulipid versus tetracycline. *Journal of Dermatology.* October;21(10):729–31.

4

Allergy Drugs and Their Natural Alternatives

What Are Allergies?

Allergies are a very common health problem in the United States; approximately one out of five people is affected by hay fever. With this condition sufferers react to substances in the environment such as grass or tree pollens. This is usually seasonal. Some people react year-round to things such as dust mites, pet dander, or mold. Common symptoms include sneezing, runny nose, congested sinus, watery and/or itchy eyes, and sinus pressure and pain. Allergies can also cause sinus headaches, fatigue, inability to focus, itchy mouth and throat, sore throat, sleep problems, asthma, eczema, and a variety of other health problems.

Causes and timing of seasonal hay fever:
- Tree pollen, common in the spring
- Grass pollen, common in the late spring and summer
- Weed pollen, common in the fall
- Fungi and mold spores, often worse during warm weather months

Causes of year-round environmental allergies:
- Dust mites
- Animal dander
- Cockroaches
- Fungi and mold spores (indoor and outdoor)

While drug therapies can be quite effective for relieving allergy symptoms, many of the medications can have a number of undesirable side effects. Several nutritional supplements in this chapter can safely and effectively reduce allergy symptoms for most people.

Allergy Drugs

Antihistamines

Brompheniramine (BroveX, BroveX CT, Lodrane 12 Hour ER Tablet)

Chlorpheniramine (Aller-Chlor, Allergy, Chlo-Amine, Chlor-Trimeton, Chlor-Trimeton Allergy, Efidac 24)

Promethazine Oral (Phenergan)

Azelastine Nasal Spray (Astelin)

Fexofenadine (Allegra)

Loratadine (Alavert, Claritin)

Dexchlorpheniramine oral syrup

Desloratadine (Clarinex)

Brompheniramine Oral Suspension (BroveX Oral Suspension)

Cetirizine (Zyrtec)

Clemastine (Dayhist-1, Tavist, Tavist Allergy)

Diphenhydramine Oral (AllerMax, Banophen, Benadryl, Diphenhist, Genahist)

Dexchlorpheniramine ER

Carbinoxamine (Histex CT)

HOW DO THESE DRUGS WORK?

Antihistamines work by preventing histamine from binding to histamine receptors. This prevents the release of chemicals in cells that cause allergy symptoms.

WHAT ARE THE BENEFITS?

This class of allergy medications is effective in reducing the symptoms of sneezing, itchiness, and a runny nose.

POTENTIAL SIDE EFFECTS

- Drowsiness
- Dizziness

- Headache
- Loss of appetite
- Stomach upset
- Vision changes
- Irritability
- Dry mouth
- Dry eyes
- Dry nose
- Unusual restlessness or nervousness in children

MAJOR CAUTIONS
- Breathing difficulties
- Pounding or irregular heartbeat
- Ringing in the ears
- Difficulty urinating
- Seizures

KNOWN DRUG INTERACTIONS
- Barbiturate medicines
- Doxercalciferol (Hectorol)
- Anxiety medications
- Antidepressants and other psychiatric medications
- Parkinson's disease medications

Additional drug interactions for fexofenadine (Allegra):
- Antacids
- Erythromycin
- Grapefruit, apple, or orange juice
- Ketoconazole (Nizoral)
- Rifampin (Rifadin, Rimactane)

FOOD OR SUPPLEMENT INTERACTIONS
- Alcohol: can magnify drowsiness or dizziness of allergy medications
- St. John's wort specifically for fexofenadine (Allegra)

NUTRIENT DEPLETION/IMBALANCE
None known.

Decongestants

Pseudoephedrine

Actifed Daytime Allergy

Cenafed, Decofed

Dimetapp Decongestant Pediatric

Dimetapp Maximum Strength 12-Hour Non-Drowsy Extentabs

Dimetapp Maximum Strength Non-Drowsy Liqui-Gels

Dorcol Children's Decongestant

Efidac 24-Hour Relief

Genaphed

Kid Kare

PediaCare Infants Decongestant

Silfedrine Children's

Simply Stuffy

Sinustop

Sudafed Children's Non-Drowsy

Triaminic Allergy Congestion

HOW DO THESE DRUGS WORK?

Decongestants work by constricting blood vessels of the nose, which reduces swelling and stuffiness.

WHAT ARE THE BENEFITS?

Reduction of nasal and sinus stuffiness and sinus pain.

POTENTIAL SIDE EFFECTS

- Insomnia
- Headache
- Loss of appetite
- Nausea, stomach upset
- Restlessness or nervousness

MAJOR CAUTIONS

- Anxiety
- Fast or irregular heartbeat, palpitations
- Increased blood pressure

- Increased sweating
- Pain or difficulty passing urine
- Sleeplessness (insomnia)
- Tremor
- Vomiting
- Chest pain
- Bloody diarrhea and abdominal pain
- Confusion
- Dizziness or fainting spells
- Hallucinations
- Numbness or tingling in the hands or feet
- Rapid or troubled breathing
- Seizures (convulsions)
- Severe, persistent, or worsening headache

KNOWN DRUG INTERACTIONS

- Ammonium chloride
- Amphetamine or other stimulant drugs
- Bicarbonate, citrate, or acetate products (such as sodium bicarbonate, sodium acetate, sodium citrate, sodium lactate, and potassium citrate)
- Bromocriptine (Parlodel)
- Cocaine
- Furazolidone (Furoxone)
- Linezolid (Zyvox)
- Some cough and cold medicines
- Diabetic medications
- Antidepressants including MAO inhibitors such as phenelzine (Nardil), tranylcypromine (Parnate), isocarboxazid (Marplan), and selegiline (Carbex, Eldepryl)
- Migraine medications such as amitriptyline (Elavil)
- Procarbazine (Matulane)
- Cardiovascular medications for high blood pressure, chest pain, heart arrhythmias
- Theophylline (Theo-Dur, Respbid, Slo-Bid, Theo-24, Theolair, Uniphyl, Slo-Phyllin)
- Thyroid hormones

FOOD OR SUPPLEMENT INTERACTIONS

- Caffeine (coffee, tea, chocolate, guarana)
- St. John's wort
- High-tannin-containing herbs may interfere with absorption. Examples include green tea, black tea, uva ursi *(Arctostaphylos uva-ursi),* black walnut *(Juglans nigra),* red raspberry *(Rubus idaeus),* oak *(Quercus* spp.), and witch hazel *(Hamamelis virginiana).*

NUTRIENT DEPLETION/IMBALANCE

Folic acid—take 400 micrograms as part of a multivitamin or B complex.

Leukotriene Modifiers

Montelukast granules (Singulair granules)

Montelukast (Singulair)

HOW DO THESE DRUGS WORK?

These medications block the action or production of inflammatory compounds known as leukotrienes. These compounds are normally released during infection or an allergic response.

WHAT ARE THE BENEFITS?

They reduce allergy symptoms and are safer than steroids for long-term use by those with asthma caused by allergies.

POTENTIAL SIDE EFFECTS

- Cough
- Insomnia
- Dizziness
- Drowsiness
- Headache
- Heartburn
- Hoarseness or sore throat
- Indigestion or stomach upset
- Muscle aches or cramps
- Nausea
- Runny nose
- Unusual dreams

MAJOR CAUTIONS

- A feeling of pins and needles or numbness of the arms and legs
- Dark brown or yellow urine
- Diarrhea
- Easy bruising or bleeding
- Edema or swelling of the legs or ankles
- Fatigue
- Fever
- Flu-like illness
- Muscle aches or cramps
- Seizure
- Skin rash and itching
- Severe stomach pain
- Swelling of the face, lips, tongue, and/or throat, which may cause difficulty breathing or swallowing
- Vomiting
- Wheezing or continued coughing
- Yellowing of the eyes or skin

KNOWN DRUG INTERACTIONS

- Carbamazepine (Tegretol)
- Paclitaxel (Taxol)
- Phenobarbital
- Phenytoin (Dilantin)
- Repaglinide (Prandin)
- Rifabutin (Mycobutin)
- Rifampin (Rifadin, Rimactane)
- Rosiglitazone (Avandia)

FOOD OR SUPPLEMENT INTERACTIONS

None known.

NUTRIENT DEPLETION/IMBALANCE

None known.

Nasal Anticholinergics

Ipratropium nasal (Atrovent nasal)

HOW DOES THIS DRUG WORK?

This drug blocks the effect of the cholinergic nerves. This causes the muscles to relax and the lung bronchi to dilate for improved breathing. It also relieves a runny nose.

WHAT ARE THE BENEFITS?

Treats a runny nose and improves breathing that is affected by allergies.

POTENTIAL SIDE EFFECTS

- Cough
- Dry mouth, metallic taste in the mouth
- Dry nose, irritation, burning or itching in the nose
- Stuffy nose
- Dizziness
- Headache
- Infection in the respiratory tract
- Nausea
- Nosebleeds

MAJOR CAUTIONS

- Blurred vision
- Skin rash or hives
- Swelling of the lips, tongue, or face
- Vomiting

DRUG INTERACTIONS

- Atropine, hyoscyamine, or related medications; cromolyn sodium

FOOD OR SUPPLEMENT INTERACTIONS

None known.

NUTRIENT DEPLETION/IMBALANCE

None known.

Nasal Corticosteroids

Triamcinolone nasal inhalation (Nasacort HFA)

Mometasone nasal spray (Nasonex)

Fluticasone nasal inhalation (Flonase)

Beclomethasone nasal inhalation (Beconase AQ)

Triamcinolone nasal spray (Nasacort AQ)

Budesonide nasal inhaler (Rhinocort Aqua)

Flunisolide nasal inhalation (Nasarel)

HOW DO THESE DRUGS WORK?

This class of allergy medications reduces substances that promote allergy reactions such as a runny nose and swelling.

WHAT ARE THE BENEFITS?

Decreased runny nose and nasal congestion.

POTENTIAL SIDE EFFECTS

- Burning, dryness, or irritation inside the nose
- Headache
- Nosebleed
- Unpleasant taste
- Throat irritation

MAJOR CAUTIONS

- Blurred vision or other vision change
- Dizziness or light-headedness
- Nausea, vomiting
- Frequent nosebleeds
- Stomach pain
- Unusual tiredness or weakness
- White patches or sores in the mouth or nose (fungal infection)

KNOWN DRUG INTERACTIONS

None known.

FOOD OR SUPPLEMENT INTERACTIONS

None known.

NUTRIENT DEPLETION/IMBALANCE

Probiotic-friendly flora in the nasal cavity may become depleted. Take a probiotic orally that contains 5 billion or more active organisms daily.

The Sinus Fungal Connection

The Mayo Clinic has conducted studies demonstrating an association between sinus fungal infection and chronic sinusitis. Nasal steroidal sprays destroy the good flora of the nasal cavity, which predisposes one to a fungal infection of the sinus. One such study looked at the ability to test for sinus fungal infections in 54 patients who had a history of chronic sinusitis. Researchers found that with one of the testing methods, 100 percent of participants tested positive for fungus, while with another testing method, 76 percent showed signs of fungus.

Nasal Decongestants

Oxymetazoline (Afrin)

Phenylephrine nasal (4-Way Fast Acting, Afrin Children's Pump Mist, Ah-chew D, Little Colds, Little Noses Gentle Formula, Infants & Children, Neo-Synephrine 4-Hour, Rhinall, Vicks Sinex Ultra Fine Mist)

HOW DO THESE DRUGS WORK?

Nasal decongestants are sprayed directly into the nose to constrict blood vessels. Therefore, when you use a nasal decongestant, the blood vessels in your nose tighten, causing the linings of your nose to be less swollen. This makes your nose feel less stuffy.

WHAT ARE THE BENEFITS?

Decreased nasal congestion within a short period of time (a few minutes).

POTENTIAL SIDE EFFECTS

Burning, stinging, dryness, or irritation of the nose.

MAJOR CAUTIONS

- Dizziness
- Fainting spells
- Difficulty breathing
- Irregular heartbeat
- Palpitations
- Chest pain
- Swelling of the inside of the nose

Phenylephrine and Pseudoephedrine

Phenylephrine and pseudoephedrine are both decongestants. Historically, pseudoephedrine has been the more commonly used decongestant in many nonprescription cold and allergy medications. However, pseudoephedrine is also a key ingredient in making methamphetamine, a highly addictive illegal stimulant. Federal law now requires all nonprescription medications containing pseudoephedrine to be unavailable over the counter and kept behind the counter in the pharmacy. To purchase pseudoephedrine, one must show some form of government-issued identification and sign a logbook. Most products have been or are being reformulated with phenylephrine.

KNOWN DRUG INTERACTIONS

- Atropine
- Bromocriptine (Parlodel)
- Linezolid (Zyvox)
- Maprotiline (Ludiomil)
- Antidepressants
- Migraine medications
- High blood pressure medications
- Oxytocin
- Vasopressin
- Diuretic medications

FOOD OR SUPPLEMENT INTERACTIONS

None known.

NUTRIENT DEPLETION/IMBALANCE

None known.

Nasal Mast Cell Stabilizers

Cromolyn nasal spray (Nasalcrom)

HOW DO THESE DRUGS WORK?

These medications stabilize mast cell membranes, which prevents the release of inflammatory and allergy-producing substances known as histamines and leukotrienes.

WHAT ARE THE BENEFITS?

These drugs prevent allergy symptoms, although they can take up to four weeks to be fully effective.

POTENTIAL SIDE EFFECTS

- Bad taste in the mouth
- Cough, dry throat
- Headache
- Nosebleeds or runny nose
- Sneezing
- Stinging, burning, or irritation inside the nose

MAJOR CAUTIONS

- Difficulty breathing

KNOWN DRUG INTERACTIONS

None known.

FOOD OR SUPPLEMENT INTERACTIONS

None known.

NUTRIENT DEPLETION/IMBALANCE

None known.

Natural Alternatives to Allergy Drugs

Diet and Lifestyle Changes

Drink plenty of water to remain hydrated. Herbal teas such as ginger and peppermint are great to keep the sinuses clear. Avoid or reduce foods that commonly increase nasal congestion, such as cow's milk and gluten. Warm sinus irrigation rinses are helpful in reducing allergen exposure and reaction.

Butterbur

This plant extract is commonly used in Europe for the treatment of hay fever. A prospective, randomized, double-blind study compared butterbur to fexofenadine (Allegra) and placebo in 330 participants with allergies (allergic rhinitis). The butterbur group took one tablet (8 mg of the active ingredient petasine) three times daily. Both fexofenadine (Allegra) and butterbur were superior to placebo in relieving symptoms. Another study found butterbur extract to be effective in relieving nasal symptoms associated with allergies. It was also shown after five days of use to significantly reduce the allergenic substance histamine. In addition, a randomized, double-blind, parallel group comparison found butterbur to be as effective as cetirizine (Zyrtec) in treating seasonal allergic rhinitis (hay fever).

DOSAGE

For allergic rhinitis, use a standardized extract containing 8 to 16 mg of petasine taken three to four times daily. Also, a whole butterbur root extract at a dose of 50 mg twice daily has been studied and can be used as well.

SAFETY

Butterbur is well tolerated. It can cause digestive upset, headache, fatigue, and itchy eyes.

Tinospora Cordifolia

An extract of this plant has been shown to significantly decrease sneezing and nasal itching, discharge, and obstruction. A randomized, double-blind placebo-controlled trial published in the *Journal of Ethnopharmacology* involved 75 people with allergic rhinitis. They were given *Tinospora cordifolia* (TC) or a placebo for eight weeks. Those given TC had a significant decrease in all symptoms of allergic rhinitis. This included a 100 percent decrease in sneezing in 83 percent of participants, a 69 percent decrease in nasal discharge, a 61 percent decrease in nasal obstruction, and a 71 percent decrease in nasal pruritus (itching). Those given placebo had little improvement in the same symptoms that were monitored.

DOSAGE

Take 300 mg three times daily of a TC extract.

SAFETY

TC is well tolerated. Side effects reported in a clinical trial include headache and nasal pain. TC may reduce glucose levels; therefore caution is advised for people on diabetic drugs.

Thymus Extract

The thymus gland produces thymic hormones, which help to regulate immunity. Thymus extracts are used as nutritional support for those with allergies. Thymus extract has been shown in one study to be effective in the treatment of allergic rhinitis.

DOSAGE

Take 750 mg of crude thymus polypeptide fraction or 120 mg of pure thymus polypeptides (thymomodulin) daily, or as directed on the label.

SAFETY

No adverse effects have been reported.

Stinging Nettle

This plant has been used by naturopathic doctors in the United States over several decades for the treatment of allergies. A randomized, double-blind study at the National College of Naturopathic Medicine tested the benefit of freeze-dried nettles for the treatment of hay fever. In the study, 58 percent of participants given stinging nettle had a reduction in sneezing and itching.

The Sting in Stinging Nettle

Stinging nettle (*Urtica dioica*) has long been used by holistic doctors and traditional herbalists. It grows in North America, particularly in Oregon and other Northwestern states. It is also found throughout Europe. Its Latin name "*Urtica*," meaning "to sting," comes from its small spines that sting the skin. (These are removed for the supplement form.) The leaves are rich in minerals, especially potassium, along with anti-allergy compounds. The root contains unique substances that benefit the prostate.

DOSAGE

Take 300 mg three times daily.

SAFETY

No adverse effects are known for the aboveground parts of stinging nettle, the part of the plant used in the mentioned study.

Quercetin

This naturally occurring flavonoid, found in foods and available as a nutritional supplement, has anti-allergy and anti-inflammatory properties. Preliminary research shows that it reduces histamine release from mast cells While we are unaware of any studies, we find it to be helpful clinically for our patients.

DOSAGE

Take 500 to 1,000 mg three times daily.

SAFETY

Rare instances of headaches and tingling of the extremities have been reported.

JENNY'S STORY

Jenny, a 40-year-old teacher, suffered from allergies and sinus headaches on and off throughout the year. Dietary changes were of little benefit to her. After taking 500 mg three times daily of quercetin for two weeks, her allergies and headaches were greatly improved. She no longer requires pharmaceutical treatment for acute allergy-related headaches.

References

Badar, VA, et al. 2005. Efficacy of Tinospora cordifolia in allergic rhinitis. *Journal of Ethnopharmacol.* January 15;96(3):445–9.

Marzari, R, et al. 1987. Perennial allergic rhinitis. Prophylaxis of acute episodes using thymomodulin. *Minerva Medica.* 78:1675–81.

Schapowal, A. 2002. Petasites Study Group. Randomised controlled trial of butterbur and cetirizine for treating seasonal allergic rhinitis. *British Medical Journal.* 324:144–6.

———. 2005. Study Group. Treating intermittent allergic rhinitis: A prospective, randomized, placebo and antihistamine-controlled study of Butterbur extract Ze 339. *Phytotherapy Research.*19:530–37.

Taylor, MJ, et al. 2002. Detection of fungal organisms in eosinophilic mucin using a fluorescein-labeled chitin-specific binding protein. *Archives of Otolaryngology-Head and Neck Surgery.* November;127(5):377–83.

Thomet, OA, et al. 2002. Anti-inflammatory activity of an extract of Petasites hybridus in allergic rhinitis. *International Immunopharmacology.* 2:997–1006.

5

Antacid and Reflux Drugs and Their Natural Alternatives

Gastroesophageal reflux disease, commonly referred to as GERD or acid reflux, is a common condition that affects more than 60 million Americans at least once a month. It occurs when the liquid content of the stomach backs up into the esophagus. This backflow occurs when the valve between the lower esophageal sphincter and the stomach fails to close properly, permitting stomach acid and other liquid contents to back up. The stomach acid irritates and can damage the lining of the esophageal tissues and causes pain.

Common GERD symptoms include:

- Persistent heartburn (burning pain or pressure in chest and throat)
- Chest pain
- Dry cough
- Bad breath
- Hoarseness in the morning

Untreated, GERD can scar the lining of the esophagus, making it hard to swallow. It can also increase the risk of esophageal cancer.

Each year in the United States, 100 million prescriptions are given for proton pump inhibitors, which suppress the stomach's production of acid. There are other classes of antacid medications that will be discussed in this chapter. These medications do not come without some serious risks. For example, a 2006 study published in the *Journal of the American Medical Association* reviewed an analysis of 16 years of medical records of people over the age of 50, 13,556 with hip fractures and 135,836 patients without fractures. Researchers found that those patients who had taken proton pump inhibitors at average doses for more than a year had a 44 percent increased risk of breaking a hip. Those who took higher than average doses more than doubled their risk of hip fracture.

The prevailing thought is that these commonly used medications decrease calcium absorption. Our concern is that they also inhibit the absorption of many other minerals that require stomach acid for absorption. In addition, the decreased breakdown of protein foods into smaller amino acids is an issue. Protein that is not broken down effectively contributes to malabsorption and a host of other problems, including digestive symptoms (cramps, bloating, gas) and allergy symptoms as the immune system reacts to these larger-than-normal protein molecules. Natural therapies as outlined in this chapter should definitely be a preferred method of treatment whenever possible.

Antacid and Reflux Drugs

Antacids

Aluminum and magnesium hydroxide (Maalox, Mylanta)

Aluminum carbonate gel (Basajel)

Aluminum hydroxide (Amphojel, AlternaGEL)

Calcium carbonate (Tums, Titralac, Calcium-Rich Rolaids)

Magnesium hydroxide (Phillips' Milk of Magnesia)

Sodium bicarbonate

HOW DO THESE DRUGS WORK?

Antacids may be aluminum-, magnesium-, or calcium-based salts that temporarily neutralize stomach acid. They are usually taken within one hour after meals.

WHAT ARE THE BENEFITS?

Users can achieve short-term relief of heartburn with relatively safe medications.

POTENTIAL SIDE EFFECTS

Antacids containing aluminum and calcium carbonate may cause constipation. Antacids containing magnesium have a tendency to cause diarrhea.

MAJOR CAUTIONS

Regular consumption of aluminum is not healthy since accumulation is toxic to the brain and nervous system.

KNOWN DRUG INTERACTIONS

The following medications may have their absorption reduced by calcium-containing antacids: antibiotics (e.g., tetracyclines, quinolones), demeclocycline, methacycline, verapamil (a calcium channel blocker), quinidine, sodium polystyrene sulfonate, iron-containing products, and thyroid medications.

FOOD OR SUPPLEMENT INTERACTIONS

None known.

H2 Blockers

Cimetidine (Tagamet, Tagamet HB)

Famotidine (Pepcid, Pepcid AC)

Nizatidine (Axid)

Ranitidine (Zantac)

HOW DO THESE DRUGS WORK?

This group of acid-blocking medications works by blocking the receptors for histamine receptors in the stomach wall. Histamine is a chemical that stimulates the acid-producing cells of the stomach. These drugs are also known as histamine antagonists because they block the histamine type 2 receptor. They are best taken 30 minutes before meals and at nighttime before bed to prevent heartburn. These medications are available in lower doses over the counter or at higher doses by prescription only.

WHAT ARE THE BENEFITS?

H2 blockers are effective for relieving the symptoms of GERD, especially heartburn. They are easily accessible over the counter. They are not effective in the prevention or treatment of inflammation and erosion of the esophagus (esophagitis) that can occur with GERD.

POTENTIAL SIDE EFFECTS

Side effects may include constipation, diarrhea, fatigue, headache, insomnia, muscle pain, nausea, and vomiting. Other side effects include irregular heartbeat, impotence, rash, visual changes, allergic reactions, and hepatitis.

Side effects due to cimetidine are rare and generally are reversible once the medication is stopped. Minor side effects include constipation, diarrhea, fatigue, headache, insomnia, muscle pain, nausea, and vomiting. Major side effects include confusion and hallucinations (usually in elderly or critically ill patients); enlargement of the breasts; impotence (usually seen in patients on high doses for prolonged periods); decreased white blood cell counts. Other side effects include irregular heartbeat, rash, visual changes, allergic reactions, and hepatitis.

MAJOR CAUTIONS

A study in the *Journal of the American Geriatrics Society* found that long-term use of H2 blockers may increase the risk of mental decline in later life. Researchers looked at the use of H2 blockers among 1,558 over-65 African Americans enrolled in a study of aging. The study showed that after taking into account other factors, elderly people who reported "continuous use" of H2 blockers had a 2.4-fold higher chance of some form of cognitive impairment. This risk included mild to potentially severe dementia similar to Alzheimer's disease. Researchers speculate the impairment of B12 absorption may be the reason for the increased chance of mental impairment.

Other major cautions may include confusion and hallucinations (usually in elderly or critically ill patients), enlargement of the breasts, impotence, or decreased white blood cell counts.

KNOWN DRUG INTERACTIONS

These drugs may increase the blood levels of several drugs by reducing liver metabolism and excretion. These include warfarin (Coumadin), phenytoin, theophylline, lidocaine, amiodarone, metronidazole, loratadine, calcium channel blockers (e.g., diltiazem, felodipine, nifedipine), bupropion, carbamazepine, and fluvastatin. Drugs that require an acidic condition may have impaired absorption if taken with H2 blockers. One example is ketoconazole. These types of medications should be taken at least two hours before an H2 blocker. There have not been adequate studies in pregnant women, and the drug is excreted in breast milk.

FOOD OR SUPPLEMENT INTERACTIONS

Avoid ingesting caffeine-containing foods when using these medications. Avoid taking magnesium at the same time as these medications, as it may interfere with absorption.

NUTRIENT DEPLETION/IMBALANCE

While various nutrients may be depleted, the following are of most concern:

- Calcium—take 500 to 1,200 mg daily.
- Vitamin B12—take 100 to 200 micrograms daily.
- Vitamin D—take 1,000 IU daily.
- Iron—check with your doctor to see if you are anemic before supplementing.

Proton Pump Inhibitors

Lansoprazole (Prevacid)

Omeprazole (Prilosec)

Pantoprazole (Protonix)

Rabeprazole (Aciphex)

Esomeprazole (Nexium)

HOW DO THESE DRUGS WORK?

Proton pump inhibitors (PPIs) block the secretion of acid into the stomach by the acid-secreting cells with a different mechanism than H2 blockers. More specifically, PPIs inhibit the proton pump of the parietal cells (the stomach's acid-producing cells). The proton pump secretes hydrogen ions into the stomach lining for the production of hydrochloric acid, making it an ideal target for inhibiting acid secretion.

WHAT ARE THE BENEFITS?

PPIs suppress stomach acid production more completely and for a longer period of time than H2 blockers. PPIs alleviate heartburn and can protect the esophagus from the damaging effects of stomach acid. They are commonly used when H2 blockers are not effective enough or for those individuals with evidence of esophageal damage (ulcers, erosions, strictures, or Barrett's esophagus). They also are used in combination with antibiotics for treating *Helicobacter pylori*, a bacterium that together with acid causes ulcers of the stomach and duodenum.

POTENTIAL SIDE EFFECTS

The most common side effects of PPIs are headache, diarrhea, constipation, abdominal pain, nausea, and rash.

MAJOR CAUTIONS

Increased fracture risk with long-term use (see the chapter introductory section).

In addition, acid-suppressing medications such as PPIs and H2 blockers increase the risk of pneumonia. Reviews of medical records of more than 360,000 people compiled between 1995 and 2002 found that those using acid blockers were 4.5 times more likely to develop pneumonia than people of the same age and gender who had never used these drugs. The researchers also matched each of 475 individuals using acid blockers with 10 people of the same age, gender, and general health who had stopped taking the drugs at an earlier date. This analysis found that those taking an acid blocker had twice the risk of getting pneumonia compared to someone who had stopped taking the drug. Stomach acid not only is important for digestion, but is part of the immune system. Stomach acid kills microbes and may prevent harmful bacteria from entering the esophagus and lungs.

KNOWN DRUG INTERACTIONS

PPIs reduce the absorption and concentration in the blood of ketoconazole (Nizoral) and increase the absorption and concentration of digoxin (Lanoxin). Omeprazole is more likely than the other PPIs to reduce the breakdown of drugs by the liver. Omeprazole (Prilosec) can increase the blood levels of diazepam (Valium), warfarin (Coumadin), and phenytoin (Dilantin).

FOOD OR SUPPLEMENT INTERACTIONS

St. John's wort may decrease the absorption or utilization of PPI medications.

NUTRIENT DEPLETION/IMBALANCE

PPIs can inhibit the absorption of various nutrients, particularly the following:

- Calcium—take 500 to 1,200 mg daily.
- Vitamin B12—take 100 to 200 micrograms daily.
- Folic acid—take 400 micrograms daily.
- Vitamin C—take 500 mg daily.

Pro-motility Drugs

Metoclopramide (Reglan)

HOW DOES THIS DRUG WORK?

Metoclopramide (Reglan) is one in the class of pro-motility drugs approved for GERD. It works by mildly increasing the pressure in the lower esophageal sphincter, which strengthens contractions of the esophagus and speeds up emptying of the stomach. All these actions are thought to reduce reflux. It is most effective when taken 30 minutes before meals.

WHAT ARE THE BENEFITS?

This drug reduces symptoms of GERD. It is not very effective for treating the symptoms of GERD, however, and is usually prescribed as an addition to other GERD medications or for those who do not respond to common GERD medications.

POTENTIAL SIDE EFFECTS

- Nausea
- Diarrhea
- Headache
- Dizziness
- Drowsiness

- Dry mouth
- Restlessness
- Involuntary movements of the eyes/face/limbs
- Muscle spasms
- Trembling of the hands
- Personality changes such as depression or thoughts of suicide
- High fever
- Sweating
- Muscle stiffness
- Confusion
- Unusually fast heartbeat

MAJOR CAUTIONS

Let your doctor know if you have a medical history of adrenal tumors, seizure disorders, Parkinson's disease, high blood pressure, heart disease, liver disease, kidney disease, mental problems or depression, intestinal/stomach blockage or bleeding, diabetes, asthma, enzyme deficiency (e.g., NADH-cytochrome b5 reductase, G6PD). Also, use caution when engaging in activities requiring alertness such as driving or using machinery. Caution for use in the elderly who may be more sensitive to the side effect of drowsiness. If you are scheduled for surgery with general anesthesia, let your doctor know you are taking this medication. Before taking metoclopramide, tell your doctor or pharmacist if you are allergic to it, or if you have any other allergies.

KNOWN DRUG INTERACTIONS

The following medicines may interact adversely with this medication: cimetidine, insulin, cabergoline, cyclosporine, digoxin, levodopa, and MAO inhibitors (e.g., furazolidone, linezolid, moclobemide, phenelzine, procarbazine, selegiline). Drugs that may add to the drowsiness effect of metoclopramide are narcotic pain medications, tranquilizers, sleep medicines, antidepressants, and drowsiness-causing antihistamines such as diphenhydramine.

FOOD OR SUPPLEMENT INTERACTIONS

Avoid alcohol while taking this medication, as it can worsen the drowsiness caused by this drug. People with lactose intolerance may experience more severe symptoms while on this medication. Also, avoid the supplement n-acetylcysteine and the herb vitex (chasteberry) while on this medication.

NUTRIENT DEPLETION/IMBALANCE

None known.

Foam Barriers

Aluminum hydroxide gel, magnesium trisilicate, and alginate (Gaviscon)

HOW DO THESE DRUGS WORK?

Foam barriers are tablets composed of an antacid and a foaming agent.

Foam barriers provide a unique form of treatment for GERD. As the tablet disintegrates and reaches the stomach, it turns into foam that floats on top of the liquid contents of the stomach. The foam forms a physical barrier to the reflux of liquid. At the same time, the antacid bound to the foam neutralizes acid that comes in contact with the foam. The tablets are best taken after meals (when the stomach is distended) and when you are lying down, both times when reflux is more likely to occur.

WHAT ARE THE BENEFITS?

Foam barriers are not often used as the first or only treatment for GERD. Rather, they are added to other drugs for GERD when the other drugs are not adequately effective in relieving symptoms.

POTENTIAL SIDE EFFECTS

- Loss of appetite
- Constipation or diarrhea
- Weakness
- Headache

MAJOR CAUTIONS

Since this medication contains aluminum and magnesium, consult with your doctor first before using it if you have kidney disease. Also, those on a sodium-restricted diet should not take Gaviscon without consulting with their doctor first.

KNOWN DRUG INTERACTIONS

- Cellulose sodium phosphate (Calcibind)
- Isoniazid (Rifamate)
- Ketoconazole (Nizoral)
- Mecamylamine (Inversine)
- Methenamine (Mandelamine)
- Sodium polystyrene sulfonate resin (Kayexalate)
- Tetracycline antibiotics (Achromycin, Minocin)

FOOD OR SUPPLEMENT INTERACTIONS

The following nutrients should be taken four hours apart from Gaviscon, as they can interfere with absorption of the drug:

- Cherokee rosehip
- Rosehip
- Strontium

NUTRIENT DEPLETION/IMBALANCE

None known.

Natural Alternatives to Antacid and Reflux Drugs

Diet and Lifestyle Changes

For some people, changing their diet makes all the difference in their GERD symptoms. It is worth trying dietary changes to see how much your symptoms improve. Foods that commonly initiate or aggravate GERD include carbonated beverages, alcohol, coffee, nonherbal tea, cow's milk, citrus, chocolate, peppermint, and spicy foods. Make sure to chew your food thoroughly and eat in a calm, relaxed atmosphere. Do not overeat, as this can worsen symptoms. Eating raw foods or those lightly cooked is recommended. Drinking juices containing cabbage and carrot is helpful for many.

Losing weight, coping with stress effectively, and stopping smoking are helpful in eliminating or improving GERD.

Avoid eating within two hours of bedtime. Also, raise the head of your bed six inches by placing wooden blocks beneath the bed frame's head two legs.

Deglycyrrhizinated Licorice Root (DGL)

This herbal extract is very soothing to the lining of the esophagus and stomach. It also has natural anti-inflammatory effects. Studies have shown DGL to be effective for healing ulcers, and many practitioners find it helpful for GERD. There have been no direct studies of DGL for GERD.

Licorice Root

Licorice root is the most common herb used in traditional Chinese medicine. Approximately 50 percent of Chinese combination herbal formulas contain licorice root (although the Chinese species is a different species from the Western version, they have similar tastes and medicinal effects). It has an anti-inflammatory effect on the lining of the digestive tract and supports the turnover of healthy intestinal cells. It has also been shown to heal sores of the mouth caused by chemotherapy.

DOSAGE

Chew one to two 400-mg tablets three times daily, 20 minutes before meals. DGL is also available in powder form.

SAFETY

While higher doses of regular licorice root may elevate blood pressure and cause water retention, this is not a concern with DGL. Glycyrrhizin, the constituent that may elevate blood pressure and cause water retention, has been removed.

Aloe Vera

This plant has soothing and healing effects on the lining of the digestive tract. Herbalists throughout history traditionally have recommended aloe vera for the treatment of stomach acidity.

DOSAGE

Take 600 mg of the capsule form, or 2 tablespoons of the liquid form, or 2 tea-spoons of the powder form in water 20 minutes before each meal three times daily. Make sure you are using aloe with the bitter latex portion removed; aloe products containing this substance are used as a laxative. Unless identified as a product for constipation, most internally consumed aloe products have the bitter latex portion removed or substantially removed.

SAFETY

Consult with your doctor first before using aloe if you are on the following medications:

- Cardiac glycosides such as digoxin (Lanoxin)
- Diabetic medications

Aloe, an Ancient Plant

Aloe is a popular medicinal plant that is used medicinally around the world. Ancient Egyptian texts describe its use for skin conditions. It has a historical use in China, India, Europe, and North America. It has anti-inflammatory effects when applied topically and taken internally. It also contains 20 amino acids that help with tissue repair.

Nux Vomica

This is the most common homeopathic medicine used for GERD. For many it relieves symptoms quickly and without any side effects. Though no formal studies have been done, we believe it normalizes the function of the lower esophageal sphincter.

DOSAGE

Take two tablets of a 30C potency twice daily until symptoms are gone. Thereafter, use as needed for occasional symptoms. If there is no improvement within one week, stop using it.

SAFETY

Since it is in homeopathic form and highly diluted, there are no safety concerns with this medicine. The only factor to be aware of is that if the medicine is not helping within a week, stop using it. Continuous use without benefit could aggravate your symptoms.

Slippery Elm

This plant has a long tradition of use for acid reflux and a variety of other digestive conditions. It is soothing to the lining of the esophagus and stomach. The mucilage it contains acts as a barrier against the damaging effects of acid on the esophagus. It is generally more effective for occasional or mild GERD.

DOSAGE

Suck on a lozenge after each meal or as needed. It is also available in capsule form. Take 500 to 1,000 mg after each meal.

SAFETY

This herb is extremely safe. However, avoid taking medications at the exact same time; they should be taken at least one hour apart.

Slippery Elm

Slippery elm has traditionally been used among Native Americans for several medicinal purposes—including conditions such as sore throat and diarrhea. This herb contains mucilaginous compounds that reduce inflammation of the mucous membranes, including the throat and the rest of the digestive tract. Slippery elm lozenges are commonly found in pharmacies and health food stores.

PHILIP'S STORY

Philip, a 65-year-old judge, had been dealing with GERD for six months. At the urging of a friend who was a patient of Dr. Stengler's, he came in to evaluate his natural options.

Although skeptical of natural therapies, he was open to trying a simple natural solution. My recommendation was homeopathic Nux Vomica. This is a good medicine for those who have developed GERD from chronic stress. Within four weeks, Philip's GERD was resolved. He only required the Nux Vomica occasionally and was grateful for the results it achieved.

References

Boustani, M. 2007. The association between cognition and histamine-2 receptor antagonists in African Americans. *Journal of the American Geriatrics Society.* 55(8): 1248–1253.

Seppa, N. 2004. Affairs of the heartburn. *Science News*, Oct. 30, p. 277.

Yang, YX, et al. 2006. Long-term proton pump inhibitor therapy and risk of hip fracture. *Journal of the American Medical Association.* 296(24):2947–53.

6

Anxiety Drugs and Their Natural Alternatives

What Is Anxiety?

It is normal to feel anxiety or worry at times. However, feeling anxious without reason or having it disrupt functioning in daily life can be signs of a generalized anxiety disorder. Symptoms may include:

- Restlessness
- Being keyed up or feeling on edge
- Sensation of a lump in your throat
- Difficulty concentrating
- Fatigue
- Irritability
- Impatience
- Being easily distracted
- Muscle tension
- Trouble falling or staying asleep
- Excessive sweating
- Shortness of breath
- Stomachache
- Diarrhea
- Headache

Conventional treatment usually consists of anti-anxiety medications and psychotherapy. Natural medicines offer a much safer long-term approach. Addressing underlying psychological and spiritual imbalances is the key to prevention.

Anxiety Drugs

Benzodiazepines

Alprazolam Extended-Release (Xanax XR)

Alprazolam oral solution (Alprazolam Intensol)

Alprazolam tablets (Niravam, Xanax)

Chlordiazepoxide (Libritabs, Librium)

Clonazepam (Klonopin)

Clorazepate (Tranxene, Tranxene T, Tranxene-SD)

Diazepam (Valium)

Lorazepam (Ativan)

Oxazepam (Serax)

HOW DO THESE DRUGS WORK?

Benzodiazepines enhance the effect of the neurotransmitter known as gamma-aminobutyric acid (GABA). They bind to GABA receptors, which slows down the activity of nerve cells. This causes an inhibitory and relaxant effect.

WHAT ARE THE BENEFITS?

These drugs provide rapid relief for those with anxiety.

POTENTIAL SIDE EFFECTS

- Agitation
- Increased anxiety
- Confusion
- Memory impairment
- Lack of coordination
- Speech difficulties
- Light-headedness
- Constipation

MAJOR CAUTIONS

Benzodiazepines can be addictive, particularly in those with a history of drug or alcohol dependency. Also, people can experience withdrawal symptoms when stopping their use suddenly, such as blurred vision, decreased concentration, decreased mental clarity, diarrhea, increased awareness of noise or bright light, loss of appetite and weight, and seizures. Work with a doctor to gradually wean yourself off these medications to avoid their withdrawal effects.

Combining these drugs with alcohol is potentially lethal.

KNOWN DRUG INTERACTIONS

- Ketoconazole (Nizoral)
- Itraconazole (Sporanox)
- Some HIV or AIDS medications

FOOD OR SUPPLEMENT INTERACTIONS

Do not combine with alcohol, as the interaction can be deadly. Alcohol can increase drowsiness, confusion, and dizziness. Do not take grapefruit juice while on this class of medications. Do not combine with kava supplements.

NUTRIENT DEPLETION/IMBALANCE

This class of drugs can deplete the following:
- Calcium—take 500 to 1,200 mg daily.
- Folic acid—take 400 mcg daily
- Vitamin D—take 1,000 IU daily.
- Vitamin K—take 500 mcg daily.
- Melatonin—use under the guidance of a doctor if you are on an anxiety medication.

Beta-Blockers

Atenolol (Tenormin)

Nadolol (Corgard)

Pindolol (Visken)

Propranolol (Inderal)

Timolol oral (Blocadren)

HOW DO THESE DRUGS WORK?

Beta-blockers are a class of drugs commonly used for cardiovascular conditions such as hypertension, congestive heart failure, and heart arrhythmias. They reduce the force and rate of the heartbeat and decrease muscular tone in blood vessels. They inhibit beta-adrenergic receptors located throughout the body so that stressors such as adrenaline and noradrenaline cannot activate these receptors. This prevents symptoms such as heart palpitations, sweating, tremors, and other anxiety symptoms.

They often are prescribed for individuals with social phobias and to reduce performance anxiety in musicians and professional speakers.

WHAT ARE THE BENEFITS?

Reduction in anxiety symptoms.

POTENTIAL SIDE EFFECTS

- Digestive upset (abdominal cramps, diarrhea, constipation, nausea)
- Fatigue
- Insomnia
- Depression
- Memory loss
- Fever
- Erectile dysfunction
- Light-headedness
- Slow heart rate
- Low blood pressure
- Numbness
- Tingling
- Cold extremities
- Sore throat
- Shortness of breath or wheezing

MAJOR CAUTIONS

These medications may worsen the symptoms of congestive heart failure. For those with heart disease, stopping these medications suddenly may worsen angina or cause a heart attack.

KNOWN DRUG INTERACTIONS

- Calcium channel blockers such as digoxin (Lanoxin) and haloperidol (Haldol)
- Use with caution for those on diabetic medications
- Alcohol and aluminum-containing antacids may reduce absorption
- Phenytoin (Dilantin)
- Phenobarbital

- Rifampin
- Cimetidine (Tagamet)
- Chlorpromazine
- Theophylline
- Lidocaine
- Potassium

FOOD OR SUPPLEMENT INTERACTIONS

Do not take potassium supplements or consume large amounts of high-potassium foods while on these medications. Also, do not use black pepper within 2 hours of taking one of these medications, as it can increase their absorption.

NUTRIENT DEPLETION/IMBALANCE

Beta-blockers have been shown to deplete the body of coenzyme Q10. We recommend supplementing coenzyme Q10 while on these medications. A good dosage is 100 to 200 mg.

Selective Serotonin Reuptake Inhibitors (SSRIs)

Citalopram (Celexa)

Escitalopram (Lexapro)

Fluoxetine tablets or capsules (Prozac)

Fluvoxamine (Luvox)

Paroxetine (Paxil, Paxil CR, Pexeva)

Sertraline (Zoloft)

HOW DO THESE DRUGS WORK?

These drugs block the reuptake of serotonin so that it remains active in the brain longer before being broken down and reabsorbed. The neurotransmitter serotonin gives the sensation of well-being.

WHAT ARE THE BENEFITS?

Improvement in depression, generally with fewer side effects than other categories of antidepressants. SSRIs have fewer side effects than the tricyclic antidepressants and monoamine oxidase (MAO) inhibitors, which we discuss below. Unlike MAO inhibitors, SSRIs do not interact with the amino acid tyramine found in certain foods. Also, SSRIs do not cause orthostatic hypotension and heart rhythm disturbances, as tricyclic antidepressants can. SSRIs are often the first-line pharmaceutical choice for depression.

POTENTIAL SIDE EFFECTS

- Nausea
- Diarrhea
- Agitation
- Insomnia
- Decreased sexual desire
- Delayed orgasm or inability to have an orgasm

MAJOR CAUTIONS

Tremors can be a side effect of SSRIs. Serotonergic syndrome, in which serotonin levels are too high, is a serious but rare condition associated with the use of SSRIs. Symptoms can include high fevers, seizures, and heart rhythm disturbances.

There is an association between bone loss and the use of SSRIs in older men and women. Suicidal thoughts or increased risk of suicide may occur with these medications.

KNOWN DRUG INTERACTIONS

- Astemizole (Hismanal)
- Cisapride (Propulsid)
- Pimozide (Orap)
- Terfenadine (Seldane)
- Thioridazine (Mellaril)
- MAO inhibitors—phenelzine (Nardil), tranylcypromine (Parnate), isocarboxazid (Marplan), selegiline (Eldepryl)

FOOD OR SUPPLEMENT INTERACTIONS

Alcohol should be avoided while on these medications.

The following supplements also increase neurotransmitter levels, and the cumulative effect with SSRIs may be too strong. They should be avoided.

- 5-HTP
- L-tryptophan
- St. John's wort

NUTRIENT DEPLETION/IMBALANCE

In one study, women taking 500 mcg of folic acid daily in addition to fluoxetine (Prozac) experienced significant improvement in their symptoms and fewer side effects compared to women taking the drug only.

Fluoxetine (Prozac) has been shown to significantly lower melatonin levels. It has not been determined whether simultaneous supplementation is appropriate.

Ginkgo biloba extract has been shown to reduce sexual side effects in elderly men and women taking SSRIs. Participants in the study used 200 to 240 mg of ginkgo biloba extract.

Selective Serotonin and Norepinephrine Reuptake Inhibitors (SNRIs)

Duloxetine (Cymbalta)

Venlafaxine (Effexor)

HOW DO THESE DRUGS WORK?

SNRIs work mainly by increasing the amounts of two neurotransmitters in the brain, serotonin and norepinephrine. This improves alertness, energy, mood, and motivation.

WHAT ARE THE BENEFITS?

These drugs can be effective for severe and chronic cases of depression.

POTENTIAL SIDE EFFECTS

- Abdominal (stomach) pain or tenderness
- Itching
- Rash
- Dry mouth
- Constipation
- Dizziness
- Drowsiness
- Headache
- Increased sweating or flushing
- Loss of appetite, loss of weight
- Loss of sexual desire, erectile, or orgasm dysfunction
- Nausea
- Weakness or tiredness
- Weight gain or weight loss

MAJOR CAUTIONS

- Dark or brown urine
- Difficulty breathing
- Fainting spells
- Mania (overactive behavior)
- Restlessness, inability to sleep, or severe loss of sleep

- Suicidal thoughts
- Unexplained flu-like symptoms
- Vomiting
- Yellowing of the skin or whites of the eyes
- Increased blood pressure
- Seizures

KNOWN DRUG INTERACTIONS

Do not take while on MAO inhibitors or Haldol, and for at least two weeks after their discontinuation. Caution should be used when taking these medications with the heart drug Lanoxin and the blood thinner Coumadin.

FOOD OR SUPPLEMENT INTERACTIONS

Do not combine these medications, as there can be overproduction of certain neurotransmitters such as serotonin:

- 5-hydroxytryptophan (5-HTP)
- L-tryptophan
- Sour date nut (*Ziziphus jujube*)
- St. John's wort

NUTRIENT DEPLETION/IMBALANCE

None known.

Monoamine Oxidase Inhibitors (MAOIs)

Isocarboxazid (Marplan)

Phenelzine (Nardil)

Tranylcypromine (Parnate)

HOW DO THESE DRUGS WORK?

This group of antidepressants has been used since the 1950s. They increase the brain's level of neurotransmitters such as norepinephrine. They do this by inhibiting the enzyme monoamine oxidase that breaks down norepinephrine. Thus the amount of norepinephrine in the brain is increased.

WHAT ARE THE BENEFITS?

This class of drug can relieve depression as well as panic disorder and social phobias.

POTENTIAL SIDE EFFECTS

- Blurred vision or change in vision
- Constipation or diarrhea

- Difficulty sleeping
- Drowsiness or dizziness
- Dry mouth
- Increased appetite; weight increase
- Increased sensitivity to sunlight
- Muscle aches or pains, trembling
- Nausea or vomiting
- Sexual dysfunction
- Swelling of the feet or legs
- Tiredness or weakness

MAJOR CAUTIONS

MAOIs can impair the ability to break down tyramine, an amino acid found in aged cheese, wines, most nuts, chocolate, and some other foods. Like norepinephrine, tyramine can elevate blood pressure. MAOIs are not as commonly prescribed as other antidepressants. Other possible side effects are:

- Agitation, excitability, restlessness, or nervousness
- Chest pain
- Confusion or changes in mental state
- Convulsions or seizures (uncommon)
- Difficulty breathing
- Difficulty passing urine
- Enlarged pupils, sensitivity of the eyes to light
- Fever, clammy skin, increased sweating
- Headache or increased blood pressure
- Light-headedness or fainting spells
- Muscle or neck stiffness or spasm
- Slow, fast, or irregular heartbeat (palpitations)
- Sore throat and fever
- Yellowing of the skin or eyes

KNOWN DRUG INTERACTIONS

MAOIs can interact with over-the-counter cold and cough medications to cause dangerously high blood pressure.

FOOD OR SUPPLEMENT INTERACTIONS

- Aspartame
- Ephedra
- Scotch broom

- St. John's wort
- Tyramine-containing foods

NUTRIENT DEPLETION/IMBALANCE

Vitamin B6 may be depleted by these medications.

Atypical Antidepressants

Drugs in this class of antidepressants work in a variety of ways. They act like SSRIs and TCAs but have different mechanisms of action, and they have similar side effects as those from SSRIs and TCSs. Common examples include:

Bupropion (Wellbutrin)

Nefazodone (Serzone)

Trazodone (Desyrel)

Venlafaxine (Effexor)

HOW DO THESE DRUGS WORK?

Bupropion (Wellbutrin) works by inhibiting the reuptake of dopamine, serotonin, and norepinephrine, and therefore increases the brain's levels of these neurotransmitters. This medication is unique in that its major effect is on dopamine.

Nefazodone (Serzone) works by inhibiting the reuptake of serotonin and norepinephrine and therefore increases the brain's levels of these neurotransmitters.

Trazodone's (Desyrel) mechanism is not known exactly, but it likely inhibits the reuptake of serotonin and therefore increases the brain's levels of these neurotransmitters.

Venlafaxine (Effexor) increases the brain's levels of serotonin and norepinephrine.

WHAT ARE THE BENEFITS?

These medications can relieve depression and offer treatment for people who do not respond to other pharmaceutical antidepressants.

POTENTIAL SIDE EFFECTS

Bupropion (Wellbutrin)

- Agitation
- Dry mouth
- Insomnia
- Headache
- Nausea
- Constipation

- Tremor
- Weight loss

Nefazodone (Serzone)

- Nausea
- Dizziness
- Insomnia
- Agitation
- Tiredness
- Dry mouth
- Constipation
- Light-headedness
- Blurred vision
- Confusion

Trazodone (Desyrel)

- Nausea
- Dizziness
- Insomnia
- Agitation
- Tiredness
- Dry mouth
- Constipation
- Light-headedness
- Headache
- Low blood pressure
- Blurred vision
- Confusion
- Impaired ejaculation, orgasm, and libido

Venlafaxine (Effexor)

- Nausea
- Headaches
- Anxiety
- Insomnia
- Drowsiness
- Loss of appetite
- Increased blood pressure

MAJOR CAUTIONS

Bupropion (Wellbutrin)

- Seizures
- Suicidal thinking and behavior
- Manic episodes or hallucinations

Nefazodone (Serzone)

- Rarely associated with priapism (prolonged penile erection) and blood clot formation within the penis
- Suicidal thinking and behavior

Trazodone (Desyrel)

- Priapism, a painful condition in which the penis remains in an erect position for a prolonged period
- Suicidal thinking and behavior

Venlafaxine (Effexor)

- Suicidal thinking and behavior
- Confusion
- Seizures
- Mydriasis (prolonged dilation of the pupils of the eyes)

KNOWN DRUG INTERACTIONS

Bupropion (Wellbutrin)

- Prochlorperazine (Compazine)
- Chlorpromazine (Thorazine) and other antipsychotic medications in the phenothiazine class
- During withdrawal from benzodiazepines such as diazepam (Valium), alprazolam (Xanax)
- Carbamazepine (Tegretol)
- Monoamine oxidase inhibitors
- Warfarin (Coumadin)

Nefazodone (Serzone)

- MAO inhibitor antidepressants such as isocarboxazid (Marplan), phenelzine (Nardil), tranylcypromine (Parnate), and procarbazine (Matulane)
- Selegiline (Eldepryl)
- Fenfluramine (Pondimin), dexfenfluramine (Redux)

- Terfenadine (Seldane)
- Triazolam (Halcion)
- Alprazolam (Xanax)
- Digoxin (Lanoxin)

Trazodone (Desyrel)
- MAO inhibitor antidepressants such as isocarboxazid (Marplan), phenelzine (Nardil), tranylcypromine (Parnate), and procarbazine (Matulane)
- Selegiline (Eldepryl)
- Digoxin
- Phenytoin (Dilantin)
- Carbamazepine (Tegretol)
- Ketoconazole (Nizoral)
- Ritonavir (Norvir)
- Indinavir (Crixivan)

Venlafaxine (Effexor)
- MAO inhibitor antidepressants such as isocarboxazid (Marplan), phenelzine (Nardil), tranylcypromine (Parnate), and procarbazine (Matulane)

FOOD OR SUPPLEMENT INTERACTIONS
Avoid the following, as they increase neurotransmitter levels and the combination may be too much:
- 5-hydroxytryptophan (5-HTP)
- L-tryptophan
- Sour date nut (*Ziziphus jujube*)
- St. John's wort

NUTRIENT DEPLETION/IMBALANCE
None known.

Tricyclic Antidepressants (TCAs)

This older group of antidepressants is used to treat depression and other mental conditions such as obsessive-compulsive disorder, panic attacks, posttraumatic stress disorder, attention deficit hyperactivity disorder, bed-wetting, and nerve pain.

Amitriptyline (Elavil, Endep, Vanatrip)

Amitriptyline injection (Elavil injection, Vanatrip injection)

Amoxapine (Asendin)

Clomipramine (Anafranil)

Desipramine (Norpramin)

Doxepin (Adapin, Sinequan)

Imipramine (Tofranil)

Imipramine Pamoate (Tofranil PM)

Nortriptyline (Aventyl, Pamelor)

Nortriptyline oral solution (Aventyl oral solution)

Protriptyline (Vivactil)

HOW DO THESE DRUGS WORK?

TCAs work mainly by increasing the level of norepinephrine in the brain. They may also increase serotonin levels.

WHAT ARE THE BENEFITS?

They are used to treat moderate to severe depression.

POTENTIAL SIDE EFFECTS

- Blurred vision
- Constipation
- Dizziness
- Drowsiness
- Dry mouth
- Impaired sexual function
- Weight gain

MAJOR CAUTIONS

- Low blood pressure
- Glaucoma

KNOWN DRUG INTERACTIONS

These medications should not be combined with monoamine oxidase (MAO) inhibiting drugs as described in this chapter. Also do not combine with epinephrine, and use caution when also taking cimetidine (Tagamet).

FOOD OR SUPPLEMENT INTERACTIONS

Do not combine with alcohol.

NUTRIENT DEPLETION/IMBALANCE

The following nutrients may be depleted and should be supplemented while on these medications:

- Coenzyme Q10—take 100 mg daily
- Niacinamide
- Vitamin B1
- Vitamin B12
- Vitamin B2
- Vitamin B3
- Vitamin B5
- Vitamin B6

Take a B complex supplement to increase the levels of the many B vitamins that can become depleted.

Buspirone

Buspirone is marketed under the brand name Buspar.

HOW DOES THIS DRUG WORK?

This medication works by stimulating serotonin type 1A receptors on nerves, leading to a relaxation effect.

WHAT ARE THE BENEFITS?

Buspirone reduces the symptoms of anxiety. Unlike benzodiazepines, it does not cause sedation and is not considered addictive.

POTENTIAL SIDE EFFECTS

- Dizziness
- Nausea
- Headache
- Nervousness
- Light-headedness
- Excitement
- Insomnia
- Nasal congestion
- Nightmares

MAJOR CAUTIONS

- Blurred vision or other vision changes
- Difficulty breathing

- Chest pain
- Confusion
- Feelings of hostility or anger
- Muscle aches and pains
- Numbness or tingling in hands or feet
- Ringing in the ears
- Skin rash and itching (hives)
- Sore throat
- Vomiting
- Weakness

KNOWN DRUG INTERACTIONS

- Monoamine oxidase (MAO) inhibitors such as isocarboxazid (Marplan), phenelzine (Nardil), tranylcypromine (Parnate), and procarbazine (Matulane)
- Trazodone (Desyrel)
- Warfarin (Coumadin)
- Phenytoin (Dilantin)

FOOD OR SUPPLEMENT INTERACTIONS

Do not combine with grapefruit juice. Do not combine with kava supplements.

NUTRIENT DEPLETION/IMBALANCE

Melatonin—take 0.5 to 3 mg a half hour before bedtime.

Natural Alternatives to Anxiety Drugs

Diet and Lifestyle Changes

Make sure to eat regular meals throughout the day, as low blood sugar levels can worsen anxiety. Consume a diet with high-quality proteins such as fish, turkey, eggs, legumes, and chicken along with nonstarchy vegetables such as salads, broccoli, cauliflower, and green beans. An adequate amount of fat in the diet is important to reduce anxiety.

Caffeine sources should be reduced or eliminated, as they may worsen the symptoms of anxiety. This includes coffee, chocolate, and many teas. The same can be true of simple sugar products, so it is best to reduce your intake of candy, soda pop, fruit juices, and white flour products. Avoid deep-fried foods, as they can interfere with your body's ability to utilize essential fatty acids.

Incorporate exercise, prayer, and/or positive visualization into your daily habits to prevent and reduce anxiety. Deep breathing is important to calm the nervous system. Take time out during the day to take long deep breaths, especially when you feel anxious.

Kava

Kava has a history as a drink used by inhabitants of some Pacific islands. It has been shown to have anti-anxiety and muscle-relaxing effects without impairing reaction time when used at normal dosages. There is good evidence that kava supplements are effective in the treatment of anxiety. A meta-analysis of six studies using the total score on the Hamilton Anxiety Scale found that compared with placebo, kava extract appeared to be an effective symptomatic treatment option for anxiety. Kava has been shown to be similar in effectiveness to low-dose benzodiazepines (e.g., Valium).

DOSAGE

Take 200 to 250 mg of a product standardized to 30 percent kavalactones.

SAFETY

The most common side effect is digestive upset. Temporary yellowing of the skin may occur. Rarely, an allergic rash can occur. There have been reports of liver toxicity from kava use. These reports are difficult to evaluate. While we have never seen liver problems with patients using kava, it should be used under the supervision of a doctor. It should not be combined with alcohol, antidepressants, anti-anxiety pharmaceuticals, other psychotic drugs, or other pharmaceuticals. It should be avoided in those with liver disease or Parkinson's disease. It should not be taken in conjunction with alcohol.

Passionflower

This herb has mild sedative properties and is effective for mild to moderate anxiety. A study in the *Journal of Clinical Pharmacology Therapeutics* looked at the effect of passionflower on 36 people with generalized anxiety disorder. In a four-week trial, 18 people took passionflower extract at a dose of 45 drops per day plus a placebo tablet, and 18 took oxazepam (Serax) at 30 mg per day plus placebo drops. Researchers found that passionflower extract and oxazepam (Serax) were both effective in the treatment of generalized anxiety disorder. No significant difference was observed between the two compounds at the end of trial. While oxazepam (Serax) showed a rapid onset of action, it also had more side effects such as significantly more problems relating to impairment of job performance.

DOSAGE

Take 0.5 ml or 250 mg of the extract three times daily.

SAFETY

Passionflower is quite safe. It is probably best to not combine it with pharmaceutical anti-anxiety or antidepressant medications.

Inositol

This nutrient is related to B vitamins. It has been shown in studies to reduce anxiety and the frequency of panic attacks. A double-blind, controlled, crossover trial published in the *Journal of Clinical Psychopharmacology* demonstrated that 18 grams of inositol daily for one month reduced the number of panic attacks from six or seven per week to two or three per week. This is significant, since only 70 percent of patients with panic attacks respond to conventional therapies.

Another double-blind, placebo controlled, crossover trial published in the *American Journal of Psychiatry* found inositol to be effective for reducing the frequency and severity of panic attacks. After one month of supplementation, the number of panic attacks decreased from an average of ten per week to approximately three and a half per week.

DOSAGE

Take 12 to 18 grams daily in divided doses. Benefits may also be noticed at lower dosages such as 6 grams daily when combined with other supplements used to treat anxiety.

SAFETY

This supplement is quite safe. It should be avoided by those with kidney disease and by pregnant women.

5-hydroxytryptophan (5-HTP)

This amino acid increases the brain's production of serotonin, which promotes relaxation. The body manufactures 5-HTP from L-tryptophan, an amino acid found in food. The supplement 5-HTP is derived from the seeds of *Griffonia simplicifolia*, a West African plant, and it readily crosses the blood-brain barrier and increases synthesis of serotonin. It has been shown to improve the symptoms of anxiety.

SARAH'S STORY

Sarah, a 40-year-old receptionist, had been experiencing moderate anxiety for two months. Concerned about potential side effects from anxiety medications, she sought a more natural approach. Our recommendation was 100 mg of 5-HTP three times daily. She noticed improvement within two days. With the help of a job change two months later, she required 5-HTP only occasionally.

DOSAGE

Take 150 to 300 mg daily in divided doses. 5-HTP should be taken on an empty stomach for best results.

SAFETY

5-HTP should not be combined with antidepressant or other serotonin-enhancing medications. It may cause digestive upset. 5-HTP should be avoided by those with Down's syndrome.

L-theanine

This amino acid is used for its relaxing and anti-anxiety effects. It's thought to increase the levels of the neurotransmitters GABA and serotonin. L-theanine has been shown to exert a relaxing effect on healthy volunteers. We are unaware of research done with individuals diagnosed with anxiety disorder. Our experience is that it is helpful for those with mild to moderate anxiety.

DOSAGE

Take 200 mg two to three times daily on an empty stomach.

SAFETY

There are no known adverse reactions.

GABA

This amino acid has a relaxing effect on the brain. It has anti-anxiety and mild sedative properties. We find it helpful for those with mild to moderate anxiety.

DOSAGE

Take 500 mg two to three times daily on an empty stomach.

SAFETY

There are no known adverse reactions.

Alpha-casein Hydrolysate

This natural, dairy-derived protein has a calming effect on the nervous system. At a dose of 150 mg per day, it has been shown to reduce the effects of stress such as mood swings and tension. The *European Journal of Clinical Nutrition* reported a double-blind, randomized, crossover, placebo-controlled trial involving this protein derivative. It included 63 female volunteers who suffered from at least one disorder related to stress such as anxiety,

Amino Acids

One of the growing fields of holistic medicine is the use of amino acids to balance neurotransmitter levels. Amino acids are used by the brain to produce neurotransmitters. This allows one to influence brain chemistry with specific amino acid use. Laboratory tests are available that measure amino acid levels in the body. In addition, newer urinary tests allow for the testing of body neurotransmitter levels. This type of testing helps guide doctors in the most effective treatments involving amino acids.

sleep problems, and general fatigue. Those who took alpha-casein hydrolysate for 30 days had decreased stress-related symptoms.

References

Akhondzadeh, S, et al. 2001. Passionflower in the treatment of generalized anxiety: A pilot double-blind randomized controlled trial with oxazepam. *Journal of Clinical Pharmacology and Therapeutics*. October;26(5):363–7.

Benjamin, J, et al. 1995. Double-blind, placebo-controlled, crossover trial of inositol treatment for panic disorder. *American Journal of Psychiatry*. July;152(7):1084–6.

Childs, PA, et al. 1995. Effect of fluoxetine on melatonin in patients with seasonal affective disorder and matched controls. *British Journal of Psychiatry*. 166:196–8.

Cohen, AJ, B Bartlik. 1998. Ginkgo biloba for antidepressant-induced sexual dysfunction. *Journal of Sex and Marital Therapy*. 24:139–45.

Coppen, A, J Bailey. 2000. Enhancement of the antidepressant action of fluoxetine by folic acid: A randomised, placebo controlled trial. *Journal of Affective Disorders*. November;60(2):121–30.

Kim, JH, et al. 2007. Efficacy of alpha1-casein hydrolysate on stress-related symptoms in women. *European Journal of Clinical Nutrition*. 61(4):536–41.

Lu, K, et al. 2004. The acute effects of L-theanine in comparison with alprazolam on anticipatory anxiety in humans. *Human Psychopharmacology: Clinical and Experimental*. 19:457–65.

Palatnik, A, et al. 2001. Double-blind, controlled, crossover trial of inositol versus fluvoxamine for the treatment of panic disorder. *Journal of Clinical Psychopharmacology*. June;21(3):335–9.

Pittler, MH, E Ernst. 2003. Kava extract for treating anxiety. *Cochrane Database of Systematic Reviews*. (1):CD003383.

Woelk, H, et al. 1993. Comparison of kava special extract WS 1490 and benzodiazepines in patients with anxiety. *Zeitschrift für Allgemeinemedizin*. 69:271–7.

7

Atherosclerosis and Coronary Artery Disease Drugs and Their Natural Alternatives

What Is Atherosclerosis?

The medical term "atherosclerosis" comes from the Greek words "*athero*" (meaning gruel or paste) and "*sclerosis*" (hardness). This refers to the name of the process in which deposits of fatty substances, cholesterol, cellular waste products, calcium, and other substances build up in the inner lining of an artery, forming a substance called plaque. Plaque deposits can accumulate and significantly reduce the blood's flow through an artery. They can also become dislodged and block blood flow to the brain, heart, or another body part. When plaque blocks a blood vessel that supplies the brain, the result is a stroke. Blockages in vessels that supply blood to the heart result in heart attacks. Atherosclerosis has been shown to start in childhood for some individuals. Coronary artery disease (CAD) occurs when plaque builds up and inhibits blood flow to the coronary arteries. Underlying atherosclerosis and CAD is chronic inflammation. Chronic inflammation is a known cause of heart disease that contributes to blood vessel damage and plaque formation. Causes of atherosclerosis and CAD include:

- Elevated levels of cholesterol and triglycerides in the blood
- Elevated homocysteine levels
- High blood pressure
- Tobacco smoke

- Diabetes
- Obesity
- Stress
- Heavy metal toxicity (e.g., lead)
- Low-grade, chronic infections
- Physical inactivity
- Antioxidant deficiencies
- Obstructive sleep apnea

Atherosclerosis and Coronary Artery Disease Drugs

Antiplatelets

Clopidogrel (Plavix)

Ticlopidine (Ticlid)

Salicylates: aspirin, acetylsalicylic acid, Acuprin, Alka-Seltzer, Ascriptin A/D, Bayer, Bufferin, Easprin, Ecotrin, Empirin, Zorprin, aspirin gum (Aspergum)

HOW DO THESE DRUGS WORK?

These medications work by preventing platelets from sticking together to form blood clots. These drugs are often used in people with a history of heart attack, stroke, or blood clots.

WHAT ARE THE BENEFITS?

Reduction in heart attack and stroke and blood clots that can cause these cardiovascular conditions.

POTENTIAL SIDE EFFECTS

- Diarrhea
- Itchy rash
- Abdominal pain
- Vomiting

The most common side effects of aspirin involve the digestive system (ulcerations, abdominal burning, pain, cramping, nausea, gastritis, and even serious gastrointestinal bleeding and liver toxicity) and ringing in the ears. Rash, kidney impairment, vertigo, and light-headedness can also occur. Aspirin should be avoided by patients with peptic ulcer disease or kidney disease. Aspirin can increase blood uric acid levels and should be avoided in patients with hyperuricemia (high blood uric acid levels) and gout. Talk with your doctor about discontinuing aspirin therapy before surgery due to its blood-thinning properties.

MAJOR CAUTIONS

Clopidogrel (Plavix) and ticlopidine (Ticlid) rarely cause a condition called thrombotic thrombocytopenic purpura (TTP). This is a serious condition in which blood clots form throughout the body.

Aspirin may cause gastrointestinal bleeding. It can also cause kidney and liver toxicity.

Ticlopidine (Ticlid) may lower white blood cell count.

KNOWN DRUG INTERACTIONS

Clopidogrel (Plavix) or ticlopidine (Ticlid) should not be combined with non-steroidal anti-inflammatory drugs (NSAIDs), as this may cause bleeding of the digestive tract. Examples of NSAIDs include ibuprofen (Motrin, Advil, Nuprin), naproxen (Naprosyn, Aleve), diclofenac (Voltaren), etodolac (Lodine), nabumetone (Relafen), fenoprofen (Nalfon), flurbiprofen (Ansaid), indomethacin (Indocin), ketoprofen (Orudis, Oruvail), oxaprozin, piroxicam (Feldene), sulindac (Clinoril), tolmetin (Tolectin), and mefenamic acid (Ponstel). It should also not be combined with warfarin (Coumadin).

Salicylates such as aspirin should be avoided in patients taking blood-thinning medications such as warfarin (Coumadin), because of an increased risk of bleeding. Asthma patients can have worsening of breathing while taking aspirin. It can also increase the effect of diabetic medications, resulting in abnormally low blood sugar levels.

FOOD OR SUPPLEMENT INTERACTIONS

The use of ginkgo biloba, vitamin E, fish oil, or coleus forskoli may increase the risk of bleeding while on aspirin therapy. Alcohol acts as a blood thinner and can erode the stomach lining, and should be avoided while using aspirin.

NUTRIENT DEPLETION/IMBALANCE

The following can become deficient from aspirin use:

- Folic acid—take 400 micrograms daily.
- Vitamin C—take 500 mg daily.
- Vitamin B12—take 50 to 100 micrograms daily.
- Zinc—take 15 to 30 mg daily.

The use of DGL (deglycyrrhizinated licorice) and zinc carnosine while using aspirin may prevent ulceration and bleeding of the lining of the digestive tract.

- DGL—chew a 300- to 400-mg tablet twice daily before meals.
- Zinc carnosine—take 75 mg twice daily.

Nitrates

Isosorbide dinitrate, sublingual and chewable (Isordil, Sorbitrate)

Isosorbide mononitrate (Imdur, Ismo, Isotrate ER, Monoket)

Nitroglycerin ER (Nitroglyn)

Nitroglycerin ointment (Nitro-Bid ointment, Nitrol)

Nitroglycerin skin patches (Deponit, Minitran, Nitro-Dur, Nitrodisc, Transderm-Nitro)

Nitroglycerin spray (Nitrolingual)

HOW DO THESE DRUGS WORK?

This class of medications dilates the veins returning blood to the heart as well as the heart arteries, increasing oxygenation of the heart cells.

WHAT ARE THE BENEFITS?

Quick relief of heart pain (angina)

POTENTIAL SIDE EFFECTS

- Constant throbbing headache
- Flushing of the head and neck
- Increased heart rate or heart palpitations
- Nausea, vomiting

MAJOR CAUTIONS

Drop in blood pressure, causing dizziness and weakness

KNOWN DRUG INTERACTIONS

Medications that reduce blood pressure (see chapter 9 on blood pressure) combined with nitroglycerin may cause too much of a reduction in blood pressure.

Caution with medications that have a vasoconstriction effect, the opposite of nitroglycerin, such as ergot alkaloids (e.g., Cafergot) and sumatriptan (Imitrex), and decongestants such as pseudoephedrine (Sudafed).

FOOD OR SUPPLEMENT INTERACTIONS

Avoid alcohol, since it can increase the blood-pressure-lowering effects of nitroglycerin. Vitamin C at a dose of 1,500 to 2,000 mg daily in divided doses may help prevent tolerance to nitroglycerin.

Oral Anticoagulants

These are medications that dissolve blood clots; for example, warfarin (Coumadin, Jantoven).

HOW DO THESE DRUGS WORK?

These medications dissolve blood clots present in blood vessels.

WHAT ARE THE BENEFITS?

Blood clots that form in the blood vessels can block blood flow to the heart or brain, causing a heart attack or stroke. By dissolving blood clots, anticoagulants can lower the risk for heart attack and stroke.

POTENTIAL SIDE EFFECTS

Painful, purple toes; rash; hair loss; bloating; diarrhea; jaundice; bleeding gums; bruising; nosebleeds; heavy menstrual bleeding; cuts that bleed too long; hematuria—bleeding from the urinary tract.

MAJOR CAUTIONS

Bleeding and gangrene (death of tissue) of the skin. Bleeding can also occur in any organ or tissue.

KNOWN DRUG INTERACTIONS

Drugs with potential interactions include:

- Acetaminophen
- Allopurinol
- Amiodarone
- Antibiotics
- Anti-inflammatory drugs, NSAIDs such as ibuprofen
- Aprepitant
- Aspirin
- Azathioprine
- Barbiturate medicines for inducing sleep or treating seizures
- Bosentan
- Cimetidine (Tagamet)
- Cyclosporine
- Disulfiram
- Hormones, including testosterone, estrogen, and contraceptive or birth control pills, thyroid medication
- Certain medicines for heart arrhythmias
- Quinidine, quinine
- Seizure or epilepsy medicine such as carbamazepine, phenytoin, and valproic acid
- Thyroid medicine
- Tolterodine

FOOD OR SUPPLEMENT INTERACTIONS

The following supplements enhance with blood-thinning medications:

- American ginseng
- Panax (Asian) ginseng
- Cranberry
- Dan shen
- Devil's claw
- Dong quai
- Fenugreek
- Ginkgo
- Goji berry
- Grapefruit seed extract
- Garlic
- Ginger
- Horse chestnut
- Papain
- Red clover
- Reishi
- Pycnogenol
- Coenzyme Q10
- Green tea
- Iron
- Magnesium
- St. John's wort
- Vitamin C
- Zinc
- Vitamin E
- Vitamin K
- High amounts of foods rich in vitamin K such as broccoli, spinach, or kale
- Alcohol

NUTRIENT DEPLETION/IMBALANCE

Since most patients on Coumadin are advised to avoid or limit vitamin K–rich foods, they are susceptible to vitamin K deficiency. Vitamin K is important for bone formation and healthy arteries. Vitamin K supplementation is possible but only under the supervision of a doctor. Consult with your doctor first before supplementing vitamin K at a dose of 500 micrograms daily.

Statins

HMG-CoA reductase inhibitors (statins) include:

Rosuvastatin (Crestor)

Fluvastatin (Lescol)

Atorvastatin (Lipitor)

Lovastatin (Mevacor)

Pravastatin (Pravachol)

Simvastatin (Zocor)

HOW DO THESE DRUGS WORK?

Statins are a class of cholesterol-lowering drugs that inhibit the enzyme called hydroxy-methylglutaryl-coenzyme A reductase (HMG-CoA reductase), which is involved in the manufacturing of cholesterol in the liver. They also reduce arterial inflammation associated with atherosclerosis.

WHAT ARE THE BENEFITS?

LDL cholesterol reduced 18 to 55 percent

HDL cholesterol increased 5 to 15 percent

Triglycerides reduced 7 to 30 percent

There is a decreased risk of dying when statins are given in the hospital after a heart attack, and a reduction in the long-term death rate. These medications have also been shown to reduce inflammation.

POTENTIAL SIDE EFFECTS?

The most common side effects are headache, nausea, vomiting, constipation, diarrhea, rash, weakness, muscle and joint pain, and increased liver enzymes. The most serious (but fortunately rare) side effects are liver failure and rhabdomyolysis, a serious side effect in which there is damage to muscles.

Statins should not be used by pregnant women or nursing mothers.

MAJOR CAUTIONS

A rare but serious side effect is liver failure. Therefore it is recommended that liver enzyme levels be checked prior to and at 12 weeks after starting a statin drug.

Rhabdomyolysis, with muscle damage, is another rare side effect that could pose a danger. It often begins as muscle pain and can progress to the destruction of muscle tissue, kidney failure, and death. Rhabdomyolysis occurs more often when statins are used in combination with other drugs, including protease inhibitors (drugs used for AIDS), erythromycin, itraconazole, clarithromycin, diltiazem, verapamil, niacin, or fibric acids—e.g., gemfibrozil (Lopid), clofibrate (Atromid-S), and fenofibrate (Tricor). Any of these drugs should be used with caution if combined with statins.

KNOWN DRUG INTERACTIONS

Cholestyramine (Questran) as well as colestipol (Colestid) bind statins in the intestine and reduce their absorption. Statins therefore should be taken one hour before or four hours after taking either of these cholesterol-lowering medications.

FOOD OR SUPPLEMENT INTERACTIONS

Avoid grapefruit or grapefruit juice while on a statin drug.

One study found that blood vitamin A levels increased over two years among people who were on a statin drug, so you don't want to take large doses of vitamin A supplements while taking a statin. Avoid supplementing vitamin A above 5,000 IU daily and have blood vitamin A levels checked yearly by your doctor. Caution should be used when combining vitamin B3 (niacin) with a statin drug. Check with your doctor before starting this combination.

NUTRIENT DEPLETION/IMBALANCE

Statin drugs have been shown to deplete the body of coenzyme Q10 (CoQ10), which your body needs to create energy in cells, particularly heart cells. One study found that people taking atorvastatin (Lipitor) had blood CoQ10 levels reduced by 50 percent after 30 days. We recommend 100 to 200 mg daily of CoQ10 supplements to prevent deficiency for those using statin drugs.

Note that there are other classes of cholesterol-lowering drugs that cardiologists may prescribe. For an overview of these, see chapter 10.

Natural Alternatives to Atherosclerosis Drugs

Diet and Lifestyle

Dean Ornish, M.D., a leader in promoting lifestyle changes to reduce cardiovascular risk, emphasizes the importance of a restricted diet for patients with cardiac disease. In a study published in 1990 in the journal *Lancet*, Dr. Ornish reported that 23 of the 28 participants who followed his special diet for one year showed "measurable reversal of coronary artery blockages." The participants also quit smoking, had stress-management training, and followed moderate exercise. Among the 20 patients in the control group, who reportedly followed standard medical advice regarding a low-fat diet, coronary artery plaque more than doubled after one year.

This demonstrated to Dr. Ornish that atherosclerosis patients needed to do more than just reduce dietary fats to improve their condition. As a result, he developed the Ornish Reversal Diet, which recommends:

- 10 percent of daily calories from polyunsaturated or monounsaturated fats (no saturated fats).
- 70 to 75 percent of calories from carbohydrates.
- 15 to 20 percent of calories from protein.
- No more than 5 milligrams of dietary cholesterol.

Dr. Ornish's limited protein diet calls for a near-vegetarian approach. Recommended foods include egg whites, fat-free milk or yogurt, grains, legumes, vegetables and fruits, juices, herb teas, and mineral water. Dr. Ornish's diet is good with a few modifications. First, it is important to add moderate amounts of heart-healthy omega-3 fatty acids, found in cold-water fish such as wild salmon and sardines, as well fish oil supplements. Second, we suggest supplementing daily with calcium (500 mg twice daily), vitamin B12 (50 to 100 micrograms), and iron (supplement only if blood tests show anemia).

Another great option we recommend is the Mediterranean diet, with its emphasis on heart-healthy olive oil, fruits, vegetables, and fish. While there is no one specific Mediterranean diet (since 16 countries border the Mediterranean Sea), they do have the following in common:

- They have a high consumption of fruits, vegetables, bread and other cereals, potatoes, beans, nuts, and seeds.
- Olive oil is an important monounsaturated fat source.
- Dairy products, fish, and poultry are consumed in low to moderate amounts, and little red meat is eaten.
- Eggs are consumed zero to four times a week.
- Wine is consumed in low to moderate amounts.

The Mediterranean diet is associated with a lower incidence of coronary heart disease, and two randomized trials indicated that it improves the prognosis for coronary patients. A more recent study evaluated the results of following a modified Mediterranean diet, in which unsaturated fats were substituted for monounsaturated fats. Researchers then looked at survival among elderly working people with a previous history of heart attack. The study involved 2,671 EPIC participants from nine countries who were 60 years or older. The median follow-up was 6.7 years. Researchers found that an increased adherence to a modified Mediterranean diet was associated with an 18 percent lower overall mortality rate.

Adequate vitamin K in the diet is important as well to prevent calcium deposition in the arteries. Forms of vitamin K include phylloquinone (K1) and menaquinone (K2). Vitamin K1 is abundant in the diet in dark green leafy vegetables such as lettuce, spinach, and broccoli. However, vitamin K2 is better absorbed and remains active in the body longer than vitamin K1. The best food source of vitamin K2 is natto (fermented soybeans) and, to a lesser degree, fermented cheeses (the type with holes, such as Swiss and Jarlsberg), butter, beef liver, chicken, and egg yolks.

Pomegranate Juice and Its Effect on Plaque

Pomegranate juice has proven to be a powerful food for arterial health. It is loaded with antioxidants called polyphenols that prevent cholesterol oxidation and improve blood flow. Israeli researchers discovered its effectiveness in a three-year study of patients with carotid artery plaque. The study included 19 men and women, 65 to 75 years old, who had severe carotid artery blockage. Ten participants received 1.7 ounces (50 ml) of 100 percent pomegranate juice daily and nine participants drank a placebo. Results: Among juice drinkers, plaque thickness decreased an average of 13 percent in the first three months and 35 percent after one year. Systolic blood pressure was also reduced. Participants who did not drink pomegranate juice had a 9 percent increase in plaque thickness after one year.

Tocotrienols

Vitamin E is not just one vitamin, but rather a family of eight slightly different molecular structures that function differently in the body. There are two principal categories of vitamin E: tocopherols and tocotrienols. Each of these has four subcategories: alpha, beta, gamma, and delta. Tocotrienols reduce triglycerides and inflammation of arterial walls, promote dilation and flexibility of arteries, improve blood flow, change LDL cholesterol to a form that does not promote plaque formation, and lower blood pressure. They also help to reduce plaque in the arteries, particularly delta tocotrienols. A four-year study from Elmhurst Medical Center in Queens, New York, involved 50 participants who had plaque in their carotid arteries (the main arteries that carry blood to the brain). This dangerous condition can lead to a stroke if plaque breaks off and lodges in the brain arteries. Among the participants who took 240 mg a day of tocotrienols along with 60 mg of alpha-tocopherol, 88 percent experienced stabilization or actual reduction of plaque. Among participants taking a placebo, 60 percent experienced a worsening of their condition and only 8 percent stabilized or improved.

Tocotrienols also combat cholesterol. According to a review published in the *Journal of the American Nutraceutical Association*, supplementation with gamma and delta tocotrienols at 75 mg to 100 mg per day for two months reduced total cholesterol levels by 13 to 22 percent and cut LDL "bad" cholesterol by 9 to 20 percent.

Cholesterol levels alone are not predictive of heart attacks—in fact, about half of people who suffer heart attacks do not have high cholesterol. However, tocotrienols may contribute to heart and arterial health in several other ways.

LDL cholesterol molecules in their natural state are soft, large, and fluffy. They become a problem only if they oxidize (get damaged by negatively charged molecules known as free radicals), which makes them dense and more likely to cling to artery walls. Tocotrienols are powerful antioxidants that protect LDL against harmful oxidation.

In addition, tocotrienols

- Change LDL cholesterol to a form that does not promote plaque formation.
- Reduce triglycerides (blood fat) that can contribute to cardiovascular disease.
- Inhibit the biochemical process that triggers damaging inflammation of arterial walls.
- Promote dilation and flexibility of arteries, increasing blood flow.
- Lower blood pressure, further protecting arteries.

DOSAGE

Take 240 to 300 mg daily.

SAFETY

Discontinue tocotrienol supplementation 10 to 14 days prior to scheduled surgery to reduce the risk of excess bleeding.

Vitamin K

Vitamin K not only helps with regulating bone calcification but also protects against harmful arterial calcification. Vitamin K is required for normal function of the protein osteocalcin. When vitamin K is deficient, blood calcium accumulates in the arteries.

The Rotterdam Study, an ongoing European clinical trial started in 1990, evaluated (among many other things) how vitamin K intake affected 4,807 subjects over a period of 7 to 10 years. Results published in the *Journal of Nutrition* showed that a diet providing 45 mcg per day of vitamin K2 was associated with 50 percent less arterial calcification, a 50 percent decreased cardiovascular mortality risk, and a 25 percent reduction in risk of dying from any cause.

Clinical trials also have demonstrated that vitamin K2 improves elasticity of the carotid arteries, thereby promoting better blood flow.

Warfarin and Vitamin K

People taking warfarin (Coumadin) are at higher risk for atherosclerosis and osteoporosis (brittle bones) because the drug increases arterial calcification and decreases bone calcification. A study in the journal *Pharmacotherapy* demonstrated the safety and benefit of low-dose vitamin K supplementation in patients taking warfarin. However, it is imperative that a person who takes blood thinners use vitamin K2 only under the close supervision of a doctor.

DOSAGE

Take 150 to 200 micrograms of vitamin K2 daily.

SAFETY

If you are on a blood-thinning medication, consult with your doctor first before supplementing vitamin K.

Garlic

Garlic has been shown to have many medicinal benefits for the cardiovascular system and arteries. It has been shown to reduce cholesterol (total and LDL), increase HDL cholesterol, and lower homocysteine. In addition, it prevents the oxidative damage of LDL cholesterol and reduces pressure in the blood vessel walls, both of which are initiating factors for plaque formation in the arteries. Garlic also has anticlotting properties.

The most well researched garlic for benefiting cardiovascular health is aged garlic extract (AGE).

A study at the University of California, Los Angeles, involved 19 cardiac patients who were taking statin drugs and aspirin daily. Participants took either a placebo or 4 milliliters (ml) of liquid aged garlic extract for one year. Participants who took AGE had a 66 percent reduction in new plaque formation compared to those who took a placebo.

DOSAGE

Take 4 ml to 6 ml of liquid AGE or 400 to 600 mg in capsule or tablet form daily.

SAFETY

Stop taking garlic 10 to 14 days prior to scheduled surgery and resume use according to your doctor's instructions.

References

Aviram, M, et al. 2004. Pomegranate juice consumption for 3 years by patients with carotid artery stenosis reduces common carotid intima-media thickness, blood pressure and LDL oxidation. *Clinical Nutrition.* June;23(3):423–33.

Bassenge, E, et al. 1998. Dietary supplement with vitamin C prevents nitrate tolerance. *Journal of Clinical Investigations.* 102:67–71.

Geleijnse, JM, et al. 2004. Dietary intake of menaquinone is associated with a reduced risk of coronary heart disease: The Rotterdam Study. *Journal of Nutrition.* November;134(11):3100–5.

Kooyenga, DK, et al. 2001. Micronutrients and health: Antioxidants modulate the course of carotid atherosclerosis: A four-year report. Nesaretnam K, L Packer (Eds). Illinois: *AOCS Press.* 366–375.

Ornish, D, et al. 1990. Can lifestyle changes reverse coronary heart disease? The Lifestyle Heart Trial. *Lancet.* July 21;336(8708):129–33.

Trichopoulou, A, et al. 2007. Modified Mediterranean diet and survival after myocardial infarction: The EPIC-Elderly study. *European Journal of Epidemiology.* October 10; (Epub).

Watanabe, H, et al. 1998. Randomized, double-blind, placebo-controlled study of the preventive effect of supplemental oral vitamin C on attenuation of development of nitrate tolerance. *Journal of the American College of Cardiology.* 31:1323–9.

8

Attention Deficit Hyperactivity Disorder Drugs and Their Natural Alternatives

What Is ADHD?

Attention deficit hyperactivity disorder (ADHD) is a condition that typically manifests in children of early school years, and is more often seen in boys. These children generally have long-standing and ongoing difficulty controlling their behaviors and/or paying attention. It's estimated that between 3 and 5 percent of children have ADHD, or approximately 2 million children in the United States. In fact, ADHD is the most commonly diagnosed behavior disorder of childhood. ADHD has been shown to have long-term adverse effects on social-emotional development and school performance, as well as on vocational success when it continues into adulthood.

How Is ADHD Diagnosed?

According to some of the most recent diagnostic data, there are three patterns of behavior that indicate ADHD. People with ADHD may: (1) show several signs of being consistently inattentive, (2) have a pattern of being more hyperactive than others their age, and (3) be impulsive far more than others their age. It should also be noted that one or another of these three patterns can be predominant. When these behaviors begin to interfere with school, social relationships, or home life, ADHD may be suspected. It is crucial that each child have thorough testing by a trained professional before any diagnosis can be made because such patterns may be caused by another disorder (e.g., severe mood disorder or other mental illness), and because all children display these diagnostic patterns at some point (but usually at lower levels). Individuals with ADHD may show the following signs:

Signs of hyperactivity:

- Is restless/squirmy, fidgety with hands and feet
- Is unable to sit quietly
- Runs, climbs, or leaves in situations when inappropriate
- Talks excessively

Signs of impulsivity:

- Blurts out answers
- Has difficulty waiting in line/taking turns
- Interrupts and/or intrudes on others

Signs of inattention:

- Is easily distracted
- Gives little attention to detail, makes careless mistakes
- Has difficulty sustaining attention to tasks or at play
- Doesn't follow instructions carefully
- Has difficulty organizing tasks and activities
- Loses or forgets things consistently
- Skips from one incomplete task to another

According to the American Psychiatric Association's *Diagnostic and Statistical Manual of Mental Disorders*, fourth edition, symptoms of inattention, hyperactivity, and impulsivity must have persisted for at least six months to a level that indicates poor adaptation and is inconsistent with the child's developmental level.

What Causes ADHD?

Different brain activity, different brain chemistry, and genetic predisposition are some clear findings in the search for the cause of ADHD. Different brain structure may also be an important aspect of ADHD. In fact, recent research into brain anatomy using MRI (magnetic resonance imaging) and PET (positron emission tomography) suggests that children with ADHD showed 3 to 4 percent smaller brain volume in all parts of the brain studied than their control (non-ADHD) counterparts. Even with all that is known, no single cause applies to everyone. Researchers are exploring other possible causes and contributing factors. Over the past several decades, scientists have investigated many theories, which include, but are not limited to, environmental toxins, food additives, nutritional deficiencies, and food allergies.

Environmental Toxins

The rapid development of the brain during pregnancy and the first year of life have necessitated a look at the negative effects of environmental agents such as cigarettes, alcohol, drugs, pesticides, xenoestrogens such as bisphenol (found in many plastics) and lead exposure in pregnancy and early childhood. Such substances can be damaging to the developing brain and nerve cells.

Food Additives

Some food additives are thought to play a contributing role in and/or be associated with ADHD. Most specifically, research has been focused on a link between sodium benzoate found in some carbonated beverages and fruit juices, and food colorings found in processed foods, juices, candy, jams, carbonated drinks, and many other food items.

Nutritional Deficiencies and Food Allergies

The human body requires good nutrition to function properly and optimally. When children (and adults) consume foods laden with refined carbohydrates (e.g., white flour, sugars) and devoid of natural vitamins, minerals, fats, and fiber, the body and brain may respond negatively. Diets high in sugars can also deplete the body of the very nutrients critical to neurological health such as the B vitamins, magnesium, and zinc. Furthermore, hypersensitivity reactions to certain foods or food components share some of the physical and behavioral symptoms seen in ADHD.

While many aspects of ADHD etiology are controversial, it is generally agreed that purely social factors and/or child-rearing methods do not cause ADHD—but they may indeed affect its severity.

Treatment

Treatment of ADHD often requires behavioral therapy that focuses on increasing the child's interest in pleasing parents and providing positive consequences for desirable behaviors. Conventional medicine often employs behavioral therapy and drug therapy. We find that holistic therapies are quite effective for most children with ADHD. The three major classes of drugs used to treat ADHD include stimulants, nonstimulants, and antidepressants.

ADHD Drugs

Stimulants

Methylphenidate (Ritalin, Concerta, Metadate)

Pemoline (Cylert)

Dextroamphetamine (Dexedrine)

Mixed amphetamines (Adderall)

HOW DO THESE DRUGS WORK?

Central nervous system stimulants help to balance the activity of neurotransmitters (chemical messengers) in the brain. Through this mechanism, they tend to increase attention span, improve focus, and decrease distractibility in people with ADHD. Although these medicines have a stimulating effect in most people, they tend to have a calming effect in children and adults with ADHD.

WHAT ARE THE BENEFITS?

Symptoms are improved in about 70 percent of people with ADHD. In children specifically, 75 to 80 percent improve after starting a stimulant medication.

POTENTIAL SIDE EFFECTS

Loss of appetite, difficulty sleeping, dry mouth, weight loss, stomachache, headache, overstimulation/anxiety, dizziness, tics, listlessness/lethargy, angina, and mood changes are the more common side effects associated with stimulants. In higher doses, paranoid psychotic reactions may be seen. In typical doses, clinically insignificant elevation of blood pressure and increased heart rate may occur.

MAJOR CAUTIONS

In February 2007, the United States Food and Drug Administration (FDA) ordered that all companies making stimulant drugs for ADHD add warning labels to their products. These new labeling regulations addressed two major concerns. First, heart-related problems, including risk of sudden death in children with heart problems; risk of stroke, heart attacks; and sudden death in adults with a history of heart disease. Second, psychiatric problems: these drugs may trigger or exacerbate negative behaviors and emotions, especially in those with any family history of mental illness. Suppression of growth is also a major concern with long-term use of stimulants in children. Psychological and/or physical dependence on stimulants can occur.

MEDICAL PRECAUTIONS

People with the following conditions or disorders should discuss their risks with their physician:

- Personal or family history of high blood pressure, heart problems, or sudden death
- Heart defects
- Heart rhythm irregularities or other heart problems
- Personal or family history of mental illness
- Hyperthyroidism
- Impaired hepatic function
- Glaucoma
- Anxiety
- History of drug abuse
- Pregnancy
- Breast-feeding

KNOWN DRUG INTERACTIONS

Stimulants should not be used concurrently with monoamine oxidase (MAO) inhibitors, or within two weeks before using them. Caution should be used when combining them with pressor agents (used to increase blood pressure). Methylphenidate may decrease the effectiveness of drugs used to treat hypertension, and it may inhibit the metabolism of coumarin anticoagulants, anticonvulsants (e.g., phenobarbital, phenytoin, primidone), and tricyclic drugs (e.g., imipramine, clomipramine, desipramine), so downward dose adjustments of these drugs may be required. Serious adverse events have been reported in concomitant use of Ritalin with clonidine.

Excessive serotonin activity may result when amphetamine is combined with SSRIs (selective serotonin reuptake inhibitors) such as fluoxetine, citalopram, and paroxetine. When amphetamine is combined with NRIs (norepinephrine reuptake inhibitors), such as Strattera, there may be a potentiation of its effects. Bupropion (Wellbutrin) has pro-convulsant properties that may be enhanced by amphetamine. Concomitant use of amphetamine and tricyclic antidepressants may increase serotonin-, dopamine-, and norepinephrine-related drug effects.

FOOD OR SUPPLEMENT INTERACTIONS

Alcohol should be avoided with use of stimulants, and fruit juices may inhibit their absorption. Supplements of magnesium hydroxide are known to cause retention of amphetamines in the body, and may therefore increase blood levels of amphetamine. Vitamin C supplementation may decrease absorption of amphetamines. Tyrosine deficiency (usually seen with protein deficiency) may reduce amphetamine effectiveness because tyrosine is needed to produce the brain chemicals stimulated by amphetamines. Concurrent use of lithium with amphetamines may reduce amphetamine effectiveness. The use of amphetamines with stimulant herbs such as *Ephedra sinica* may cause excessive stimulation of the heart and nervous system. Vitamin B6 and L-tryptophan may have beneficial effects on some adverse symptoms associated with stimulant use.

NUTRIENT DEPLETION/IMBALANCE

Dextroamphetamine can enhance magnesium blood levels, causing a significant lowering of the calcium-to-magnesium ratio in the blood.

Nonstimulants

The only currently existing, approved nonstimulant ADHD medication is atomoxetine (Strattera).

HOW DOES THIS DRUG WORK?

Strattera is a selective norepinephrine reuptake inhibitor, which essentially means it increases the activity of the brain chemical (or neurotransmitter) norepinephrine. More norepinehrine is thought to increase attention and control hyperactivity and impulsivity in ADHD.

WHAT ARE THE BENEFITS?

The effectiveness of Strattera in the treatment of ADHD was established in four studies of pediatric patients ages 6 to 18. Compared with placebo, Strattera proved to be superior with respect to reducing impulsiveness, hyperactivity, and inattention. The effectiveness of Strattera for long-term use (for more than nine weeks) in child and adolescent patients has not been thoroughly evaluated.

POTENTIAL SIDE EFFECTS

Common side effects are loss of appetite, drowsiness, headache, stomachache, nausea, vomiting, dizziness, dry mouth, diarrhea, constipation, difficulty sleeping, sexual dysfunction, agitation, irritability, and difficulty urinating.

MAJOR CAUTIONS

The foremost warning associated with use of Strattera is an increase in suicidal thoughts and actions in some children and teenagers, particularly those with bipolar disorder or depression in addition to ADHD. Psychotic symptoms (hearing voices, believing things that are not true, being suspicious), manic symptoms, heart-related problems such as stroke or heart attack, and liver problems have also been reported. Like stimulants, Strattera may also cause slowing of growth in children.

MEDICAL PRECAUTIONS

People with the following conditions, disorders, or family history should discuss their risks with their physician:

- Suicidal thoughts or actions

- Heart problems, heart defects, irregular heartbeat, high blood pressure, or low blood pressure
- Mental problems, psychosis, mania, bipolar illness, or depression
- Liver problems
- Narrow-angle glaucoma
- Allergy to anything in Strattera
- Pregnant or planning to become pregnant
- Breast-feeding

KNOWN DRUG INTERACTIONS

Concurrent use of Strattera and MAOIs such as Nardil, Parnate, and Emsam may cause a serious, sometimes fatal reaction.

Use with CYP2D6 inhibitors such as paroxetine (Paxil), fluoxetine (Prozac), and quinidine (Quinidex) may increase Strattera plasma concentrations. Due to the possibility of boosted effects, you should check with your doctor before combining Strattera with Proventil and similar asthma medications, and with drugs that raise blood pressure such as the phenylephrine in some over-the-counter cold medications. Use with albuterol (or other beta-agonists) may potentiate the action of albuterol on the cardiovascular system.

FOOD OR SUPPLEMENT INTERACTIONS

In conjunction with heavy alcohol drinking, Strattera may cause liver damage. Alcohol may also contribute to mood problems.

NUTRIENT DEPLETION/IMBALANCE

None known.

Antidepressants

Tricyclic antidepressants approved for ADHD include imipramine (Tofranil, Janimine) and desipramine (Norpramin, Pertofrane).

Other antidepressants prescribed for ADHD, but not officially approved for ADHD, include bupropion (Wellbutrin), reboxetine (Edronax), and venlafaxine (Effexor). It should be noted that the exact effects of Wellbutrin are not known with certainty; it may act on the neurotransmitters dopamine and norepinephrine, and have a stimulant effect.

HOW DO THESE DRUGS WORK?

Antidepressants are considered second-line therapy for ADHD because they are typically used in patients who have both ADHD and depression, or when stimulants are not working. Generally speaking, antidepressants are believed to work by increasing levels of three neurotransmitters: serotonin, dopamine, and norepinephrine. These neurotransmitters are believed to be low in the ADHD patient's brain. Antidepressants increase the levels of these neurotransmitters in the brain by blocking their reabsorption, thereby allowing them to stay around longer in the blood and be used by the body more productively.

It should be noted that the exact effects of Wellbutrin are not known with certainty; it may act on the neurotransmitters dopamine and norepinephrine, and have a stimulant effect.

To learn more about antidepressants, please refer to chapter 12 on depression drugs.

Natural Alternatives to ADHD Drugs

Diet and Lifestyle Changes

Proper nutrition is very important to help children and adults with attention and behavior problems. Regular meals and snacks that are low in refined carbohydrates and balanced with whole foods can be essential for proper brain function.

In addition, foods rich in essential fatty acids promote better brain function. Examples include fish such as salmon and sardines. Walnuts, almonds, pumpkin seeds, and flaxseeds are great sources as well.

An area of controversy is the effect that artificial food additives have on behavior, particularly in children. A 2007 randomized, double-blind, placebo-controlled, crossover trial published in the *Lancet* tested whether the intake of artificial food color and additives affected childhood behavior. In the six-week trial, researchers gave a randomly selected group of 153 3-year-old and 144 8- to 9-year-old children drinks with additives, colors, and a common preservative. These included sunset yellow, carmoisine, tartrazine, and ponceau, quinoline yellow (E104), allura red (E129), and sodium benzoate. This combination was chosen to mimic the mix of commercially available children's drinks. The dose of additives consumed was equivalent to that in one or two servings of candy a day. Those children in the placebo group received an additive-free placebo drink that looked and tasted the same. The children were evaluated by parents and teachers, and through a computer test. Neither the researchers nor the children knew which drink was being consumed. Children in both age groups were significantly more hyperactive and had shorter attention spans from consuming the drink containing the additives. Hyperactivity was found to increase for some children in as little as an hour after artificial additives were consumed.

For children, adequate parental or guardian support, discipline, and quality parental time are important components of a holistic treatment.

Fish Oil

Fish oil is a rich source of essential fatty acids that are required for optimal brain function including focus and mood. An emerging body of research is demonstrating that essential fatty acids such as fish oil are helpful for those with ADHD.

An eight-week study of nine children with ADHD, ages 8 to 16, evaluated the effects of taking high daily doses (8 g to 16 g) of the omega-3 fatty acids found in fish oil—eicosapentaenoic acid (EPA) and docosahexaenoic acid (DHA). The study was published in the *Nutritional Journal*. The children demonstrated significant improvement in behavior, including inattention, hyperactivity, and defiance, as rated by both their parents and a psychiatrist.

Other research conducted at Oxford University in England studied 41 children ages 8 to 12 years with both specific learning difficulties and above-average ADHD ratings. The children took fish oil or a placebo for 12 weeks. The mean scores for cognitive problems and general behavior problems were significantly lower for the group treated with fish oil than for the placebo group. Also, there were significant improvements from baseline on 7 out of 14 scales for active treatment compared with none for placebo.

DOSAGE

Take 2,000 mg or higher of combined EPA and DHA daily for symptom improvement.

SAFETY

Fish oil is quite safe. At higher doses it may cause digestive upset such as diarrhea. Those on blood-thinning medications should consult with their doctor before using, since it has a blood-thinning effect.

The parents of Barry, an 11-year-old with ADHD, had a difficult decision. They were told by school administrators that Barry needed to be on ADHD pharmaceutical medication or he would have to leave the school. His restlessness, impulsivity, and inattentiveness were too much of a class distraction. His parents brought him to our clinic for a nondrug approach, since the family was concerned about the many potential side effects associated with ADHD medications. Barry was put on a healthy diet that eliminated the food sensitivities he tested positive for. In addition, he was put on supplements such as fish oil and phosphatidylserine, and a homeopathic remedy that matched up to his symptom profile. For the next two months Barry's teachers, family, and family friends watched in amazement as his symptoms and grades dramatically improved. The school administration lifted its requirements for drug therapy.

BARRY'S STORY

Phosphatidylserine (PS)

Phosphatidylserine (PS) is a phospholipid that is a normal component of brain cells. A study in *Alternative Medicine Review* involved 21 cases of youths ages 4 to 19 with ADHD. Participants were given daily supplementation of PS at dosages between 200 and 300 mg daily for four months. Supplementation was found to benefit greater than 90 percent of cases. The symptoms that most improved were attention and learning.

DOSAGE

Take 300 mg daily.

SAFETY

Phosphatidylserine is quite safe without any notable side effects.

Zinc

Studies suggest that children with ADHD are more likely to have zinc deficiency. A study published in *Progress in Neuropsychopharmacology and Biological Psychiatry* looked at the effect of zinc supplementation on 9-year-old boys and girls with ADHD. This was a 12-week double-blind treatment with zinc sulfate (150 mg per day) or placebo. Researchers found zinc supplementation superior to placebo in reducing symptoms of hyperactivity, impulsivity, and impaired socialization in patients with ADHD. Zinc may be most effective in those diagnosed with a zinc deficiency.

DOSAGE

Give 10 to 15 mg for younger children under age 5. Higher doses such as 50 to 150 mg can be used for older children under the supervision of a doctor.

SAFETY

Too much zinc can cause digestive upset such as diarrhea. It may also suppress immunity at doses beyond 150 mg daily. A few milligrams of copper should be taken along with zinc supplementation.

Multivitamin

The brain requires a vast array of nutrients for optimal functioning. A study in the *Journal of Alternative and Complementary Medicine* demonstrated that vitamin-mineral supplementation modestly raised the nonverbal intelligence of some groups of schoolchildren. The study involved 245 U.S. schoolchildren ages 6 to 12 years.

DOSAGE

Take as directed on children's multivitamin/mineral supplement labels with a meal.

SAFETY

Multivitamins are very safe. They occasionally cause digestive upset.

L-carnitine

This aminolike substance can be effective for boys with ADHD. An eight-week double-blind study resulted in improvement in 54 percent of boys compared to 13 percent for those taking placebo. L-carnitine significantly decreased the attention problems and aggressive behavior in boys with ADHD.

DOSAGE

Take 100 mg per 2.2 pounds of body weight daily.

SAFETY

L-carnitine is quite safe.

Calcium/Magnesium

Calcium and magnesium both have a relaxant effect on the nervous system. One controlled trial looked at children with ADHD and low magnesium levels. Researchers found that 200 mg daily of magnesium led to a significant decrease in hyperactive behavior.

DOSAGE

Take 500 mg of calcium and 200 mg of magnesium daily.

Amino Acids

The use of individual amino acids is becoming more common among nutrition-oriented doctors in helping kids and adults with ADHD. Consult with a holistic doctor for individualized amino acid therapy.

References

Bilici, M, et al. 2004. Double-blind, placebo-controlled study of zinc sulfate in the treatment of attention deficit hyperactivity disorder. *Progress in Neuropsychopharmacology and Biological Psychiatry*. January;28(1):181–90.

Kidd, P. 2000. Attention deficit/hyperactivity disorder (ADHD) in children: Rationale for its integrative management. *Alternative Medicine Review*. 5(5):402–28.

McCann, D, et al. 2007. Food additives and hyperactive behaviour in 3-year-old and 8/9-year-old children in the community: A randomised, double-blind, placebo-controlled trial. *Lancet*. November 3;370(9598):1560–7.

Richardson, AJ, BK Puri. 2002. A randomized double-blind, placebo-controlled study of the effects of supplementation with highly unsaturated fatty acids on

ADHD-related symptoms in children with specific learning difficulties. *Progress in Neuropsychopharmacology and Biological Psychiatry.* February;26(2):233–9.

Schoenthaler, SJ, et al. 2000. The effect of vitamin-mineral supplementation on the intelligence of American schoolchildren: A randomized, double-blind placebo-controlled trial. *Journal of Alternative and Complementary Medicine.* February;6(1):19–29.

Starobrat-Hermelin, B, T Kozielec. 1997. The effects of magnesium physiological supplementation on hyperactivity in children with attention deficit hyperactivity disorder (ADHD). Positive response to magnesium oral loading test. *Magnesium Research.* 10:149–56.

Van Oudheusden, LJ, and HR Scholte. 2002. Efficacy of carnitine in the treatment of children with attention-deficit hyperactivity disorder. *Prostaglandins, Leukotrienes, and Essential Fatty Acids.* 67:33–8.

9

Blood Pressure Drugs and Their Natural Alternatives

What Is Blood Pressure?

Blood pressure can be defined as the force of blood pushing against blood vessel walls as it circulates through the body. The more blood your heart pumps and the narrower your arteries, the higher the pressure. When pressure is too high, it negatively affects the arterial wall and the heart must work harder. Though it's normal for blood pressure to rise temporarily from such things as exercise, stress, or emotions, in most people this rise is temporary. But in others, high blood pressure is chronic; and if left untreated, it can lead to serious medical problems.

High blood pressure, or hypertension, can carry such symptoms as headaches, nosebleeds, and episodes of dizziness or sweating. But in most cases, patients are asymptomatic; for this reason, hypertension is often referred to as the "silent killer." You could be symptom-free until you experience a heart attack or stroke, or suffer brain, kidney, or vision problems!

It is estimated that one in three adults in the United States has hypertension. Although this disorder can affect anyone, you are at higher risk if you:

- Are overweight
- Are a man over the age of 45
- Are a woman over the age of 55
- Have a family history of hypertension
- Are African American

What Do Blood Pressure Numbers Mean?

Blood pressure has two measurements: systolic and diastolic. These measures are represented as a fraction (e.g., 120/80). Systolic is the top, or first, number (120) and is the amount of blood pressure when the heart is beating. The bottom, or second number, (80) is the level of blood pressure when the heart is at rest—in between beats. Readings are broken down into several categories:

- Normal: Less than 120/80
- Prehypertension: 120 to 139/80 to 89
- Stage 1 hypertension: 140 to 159/90 to 99
- Stage 2 hypertension: 160 and above/100 and above

It is important to note that hypertension is classified into one of two groups: essential or secondary. Essential, or primary, hypertension is the most common type—accounting for about 90 percent of all cases. A single, specific cause is not known. However, many risk factors have been identified:

- Eating too much salt, fat, or sugar
- Drinking too much alcohol or caffeine
- Using stimulants
- Eating a low-potassium diet
- Not doing enough physical activity
- Taking certain medicines (e.g., birth control pills)
- Smoking (causes a temporary rise in blood pressure)
- Having an underlying medical disorder
- Chronic stress
- Heavy metal poisoning such as lead

Secondary hypertension is elevated blood pressure that results from an underlying, identifiable, and often correctable cause. Only about 5 to 10 percent of hypertension cases are thought to result from secondary causes. Patients with secondary hypertension are treated by controlling or removing the underlying disease or pathology, although they may still require antihypertensive medication.

Blood Pressure Drugs

Medicines can control hypertension, but they cannot cure it. Once started, these medications need to be taken for the rest of your life; although in many cases, the dosage can be reduced over time if there are concurrent and adequate positive changes in diet and lifestyle. What are the benefits of high blood pressure medications? A target blood pressure of less than 140/90 mm Hg is achieved in about 50 percent of patients treated with one medication; two or more agents from different pharmacologic classes are often needed to achieve adequate blood pressure control. There are several classes of drugs commonly prescribed for hypertension.

Diuretics

There are three main types of diuretics: potassium-sparing, thiazide, and loop.

Potassium-sparing: amiloride (Midamor)

Thiazide: hydrochlorothiazide (Esidrix, HydroDIURIL)

Loop: furosemide/frusemide (Lasix), torsemide (Demadex, Torem, Bumex)

Combination: valsartan (Diovan HCT)

HOW DO THESE DRUGS WORK?

Diuretics essentially work by increasing the amount of urine the kidneys produce. This action decreases overall body fluid levels, including blood volume, thereby reducing pressure. Diuretics are the oldest antihypertensive therapy and often are the first treatment option for people with hypertension. They are frequently used along with other antihypertensive drugs, and more recently can be found in new combination drugs (e.g., Diovan HCT).

WHAT ARE THE BENEFITS?

Diuretics are a common first choice of drug therapy because they consistently lower blood pressure.

POTENTIAL SIDE EFFECTS

Potassium depletion is common with loop and thiazide diuretics, while elevated blood potassium can be problematic with potassium-sparing diuretics. Other common side effects are dry mouth, headaches, dizziness, fatigue, depression, irritability, reduced sex drive, excessive urination, and electrolyte imbalance. Less common adverse reactions include elevated blood triglycerides, elevated blood uric acid, and elevated blood glucose.

MAJOR CAUTIONS

In rare cases, severe allergic reaction causing photosensitivity dermatitis, generalized dermatitis, or even necrotizing vasculitis may occur. Other rare and very serious side effects include ear damage, severe injury to the pancreas, and acute allergic kidney inflammation with fever, rash, and increased white blood cells, which may result in permanent renal failure if the drug exposure is prolonged.

MEDICAL PRECAUTIONS

People with liver or kidney problems should discuss their risks with their doctor, and pregnant women should not use diuretics.

KNOWN DRUG INTERACTIONS

- Potassium-sparing diuretics and angiotensin-converting-enzyme (ACE) inhibitors: risk of elevated blood potassium, which can lead to cardiac problems.
- Loop diuretics and aminoglycoside antibiotics: interaction can lead to ear and kidney toxicity.
- Loop diuretics/thiazide diuretics and digoxin: risk of low potassium and digoxin toxicity.
- Loop diuretics/thiazide diuretics and steroids: risk of low potassium.
- Thiazide diuretics and beta-blockers: may elevate blood sugar, lipids, and uric acid.
- Thiazide diuretics and carbamazepine (Tegretol) or chlorpropamide (Diabinese): risk of low sodium.

FOOD OR SUPPLEMENT INTERACTIONS

Because potassium-sparing diuretics can increase blood potassium levels, avoid eating large quantities of potassium-rich foods such as bananas, oranges, and green leafy vegetables; also avoid salt substitutes that contain potassium. Excess potassium may result in irregular heartbeat and heart palpitations. Consuming foods high in sodium may decrease the effectiveness of some diuretics.

The following herbs should be avoided, as they may interfere with potassium metabolism: buckthorn or alder buckthorn, buchu, cleavers, dandelion, digitalis, ginkgo biloba, gravel root, horsetail, juniper, licorice, and uva ursi.

NUTRIENT DEPLETION/IMBALANCE

Various diuretics may deplete calcium, magnesium, potassium, zinc, iron, folic acid, thiamin, vitamin B6, and vitamin C. We recommend the following supplementation:

- Calcium—take 500 to 1,200 mg daily.
- Magnesium—take 200 to 250 mg twice daily.
- Potassium—check with your doctor before supplementation.
- Zinc—take 15 mg daily.
- Folic acid, thiamin, vitamin B6—take a multivitamin or B complex daily.
- Vitamin C—take 500 mg daily.

Calcium Channel Blockers (CCBs)

Diltiazem (Cardizem, Dilacor XR, Tiazac)

Amlodipine (Norvasc)

Nifedipine (Adalat, Procardia)

Nicardipine (Cardene)

Verapamil (Calan, Isoptin, Verelan)

Combination: amlodipine and benazepril (Lotrel)

HOW DO THESE DRUGS WORK?

Calcium channel blockers (CCBs) work by preventing calcium from entering specific muscle cells of the heart and blood vessels. (Calcium is needed for muscle contraction.) This in turn helps relax those muscle cells and widen vessels, which improves blood flow and heartbeat efficiency.

WHAT ARE THE BENEFITS?

Calcium channel blockers effectively lower blood pressure for most users.

POTENTIAL SIDE EFFECTS

The most common side effects associated with CCBs are constipation, nausea, headache, rash, breathing problems, coughing, edema (swelling of the legs with fluid), low blood pressure, drowsiness, and dizziness.

MAJOR CAUTIONS

People with the following conditions or disorders should discuss their risks with their physician:

- Pregnancy
- Breast-feeding
- Heart and blood vessel disease
- Known allergy to CCBs
- Kidney or liver disease
- History of heart rhythm problems or depression
- Parkinson's disease

KNOWN DRUG INTERACTIONS

Most interactions with CCBs relate to increasing the activity of other drugs taken concomitantly. This may result from decreased elimination of other drugs by the liver. Examples include, but may not be limited to, beta-blockers,

---

A Rise in Calcium Channel Blocker Overdose

In an article titled "Toxicity, Calcium Channel Blockers," B. Zane Horowitz, M.D., states that "calcium channel blocker overdose is rapidly emerging as the most lethal prescription drug ingestion. Overdose by short-acting agents is characterized by rapid progression to cardiac arrest. Overdose by extended-relief formulations results in delayed onset of arrhythmias, shock, sudden cardiac collapse, and bowel ischemia."
The article can be found at www.emedicine.com/emerg/TOPIC75.htm.

medicines that affect heart rhythms, antiseizure medicines, digitalis heart medicines, and certain immune-suppressing drugs. In addition, diuretics that lower body potassium may increase the unwanted side effects of CCBs.

FOOD OR SUPPLEMENT INTERACTIONS

Ingestion of grapefruit, grapefruit juice, and grapefruit products may increase the adverse effects associated with CCBs, as it keeps these drugs in the body longer, and supplementation with calcium, vitamin D, and St. John's wort may reverse or interfere with the effectiveness of certain CCBs. Furthermore, pleurisy root should be avoided because it contains cardiac glycosides that slow the heart rate, but increase its force of contraction.

NUTRIENT DEPLETION/IMBALANCE

Some CCBs may deplete the body of potassium. Check with your doctor first before supplementing potassium.

Angiotensin-Converting Enzyme (ACE) Inhibitors

Captopril (Capoten)

Benazepril (Lotensin)

Enalapril (Vasotec)

Lisinopril (Prinivil, Zestril)

Combination drug: benazepril and hydrochlorothiazide (Lotensin HCT)

HOW DO THESE DRUGS WORK?

ACE inhibitors lower the levels of angiotensin II—a hormone made by the body that normally causes blood vessels to constrict. When blood vessels constrict, blood flow is hampered and pressure increases. By inhibiting angiotensin II formation, these drugs help arteries and veins to widen and blood flow to improve. ACE inhibitors also help the kidneys eliminate excess water.

WHAT ARE THE BENEFITS?

Reduced moderate to severe blood pressure.

POTENTIAL SIDE EFFECTS

Various ACE inhibitors produce these common adverse effects: elevated blood potassium levels, low blood pressure, dry and persistent cough, headache, dizziness, drowsiness, weakness, and abnormal taste sensation (e.g., metallic, salty).

MAJOR CAUTIONS

Rare, but serious, side effects of various ACE inhibitors are kidney failure, severe allergic reactions, decreased white blood cell count, and tissue swelling (or angioedema). In addition, ACE inhibitors may cause birth defects.

People with the following conditions or disorders should discuss their risks with their doctor:

- Pregnancy
- Severe kidney problems
- Known allergy to ACE inhibitors

KNOWN DRUG INTERACTIONS

Because ACE inhibitors may increase blood potassium levels, drugs that increase the body's potassium—such as potassium-sparing diuretiucs—should be avoided. In addition, ACE inhibitors may increase the effects of lithium (Eskalith) by causing blood levels to rise. Rifampin (Rifadin, Rimactane) can reduce blood levels of the ACE-inhibitor losartan (Cozaar), and fluconazole (Diflucan) reduces conversion of losartan to its active form.

FOOD OR SUPPLEMENT INTERACTIONS

Avoid salt substitutes and supplements containing potassium, as well as large amounts of foods high in potassium such as bananas, green leafy vegetables, and oranges, due to hyperkalemia (elevated blood potassium) risk.

In a double-blind study of patients who had developed a cough attributed to an ACE inhibitor, four weeks of iron (256 mg a day) reduced the severity of the cough by 45 percent, compared with only 8 percent improvement in the placebo group.

NUTRIENT DEPLETION/IMBALANCE

Zinc, sodium, and iron may be depleted with use of some ACE inhibitors.

- Zinc—take 30 mg daily.
- Sodium—take as part of a balanced diet. Check with your physician.
- Iron—have your doctor check your level.

Angiotensin II Receptor Blockers (ARBs)

Candesartan (Atacand)

Ibesartan (Avapro)

Losartan (Cozaar)

Telmisartan (Micardis)

Valsartan (Diovan)

Combination drug: losartan and hydrochlorothiazide (Hyzaar)

HOW DO THESE DRUGS WORK?

Angiotensin II (as discussed under ACE inhibitors) is a powerful vasoconstrictor. ARBs essentially shield blood vessels so that angiotensin's ability to tighten them is reduced and blood vessels remain relaxed. This action helps lower blood pressure.

POTENTIAL SIDE EFFECTS

ARBs are similar to ACE inhibitors but may have fewer side effects, especially coughing. ARBs are sometimes prescribed as an alternative to ACE inhibitors. Nonetheless, various ARBs produce cough, elevated potassium levels, low blood pressure, dizziness, headache, drowsiness, diarrhea, rash, and abnormal taste sensation (metallic or salty taste).

MAJOR CAUTIONS

Serious, but rare, side effects can include kidney failure, liver failure, allergic reactions, a decrease in white blood cells, and swelling of tissues (angioedema).

People with the following conditions or disorders should discuss their risks with their doctor:

- Pregnancy
- Severe kidney problems
- Known allergy to ARBs

KNOWN DRUG INTERACTIONS

Avoid potassium-sparing drugs, and drugs containing potassium or lithium due to risk of elevated blood levels when taken in conjunction with ARBs.

FOOD OR SUPPLEMENT INTERACTIONS

Avoid salt substitutes and supplements containing potassium, as well as large quantities of foods high in potassium, such as bananas, green leafy vegetables, and oranges, due to risk of hyperkalemia (elevated blood potassium).

NUTRIENT DEPLETION/IMBALANCE

None known.

Beta-Blockers

Propranolol (Inderal)

Metoprolol (Lopressor, Toprol XL)

Acebutolol (Sectral)

Atenolol (Tenormin)

Bisoprolol/hydrochlorothiazide (Ziac)

Combination drug: propranolol and hydrochlorothiazide (Inderide)

HOW DO THESE DRUGS WORK?

Beta-blockers work at the sympathetic nervous system level by blocking the effect of adrenaline at special sites (receptors) in arteries and the heart muscle. Adrenaline is a hormone that mediates the "fight or flight" response. Blocking adrenaline slows the nerve impulses that travel through the heart. As a result, the heart beats more slowly and with less force, thereby reducing blood pressure. Beta-blockers also help blood vessels relax and open up to improve blood flow.

WHAT ARE THE BENEFITS?

Reduces blood pressure for most users.

POTENTIAL SIDE EFFECTS

Common side effects associated with various beta-blockers are fatigue, cold hands and feet, tiredness, and sleep disturbances. Less common side effects include impotence, dizziness, wheezing, digestive tract problems, skin rashes, and dry eyes.

MAJOR CAUTIONS

There is increasing evidence that the most frequently used beta-blockers, especially in combination with thiazide-type diuretics, carry an unacceptable risk of provoking type 2 diabetes. Furthermore, recent research indicates that compared to use of other antihypertensive drugs, first-line therapy with beta-blockers has been associated with elevated risk of stroke, lack of efficacy, and numerous adverse effects in patients with uncomplicated hypertension.

People with the following conditions or disorders should discuss their risks with their doctor:

- Breathing difficulties (e.g., asthma, chronic bronchitis)
- Worsening or severe heart failure
- Disease of arm and leg arteries
- Pregnancy
- Poor blood circulation/Raynaud's disease
- Diabetes
- Liver or kidney problems

KNOWN DRUG INTERACTIONS

Certain cough and cold remedies and appetite suppressants can cause a dramatic rise in blood pressure when taken concomitantly with a beta-blocker. Anesthetics, nonsteroidal anti-inflammatory drugs, and other blood pressure–lowering drugs can intensify the blood pressure–lowering effects of beta-blockers. In addition, drugs that affect the heart's rhythm can increase the heart-slowing effects of beta-blockers.

FOOD OR SUPPLEMENT INTERACTIONS

Avoid drinking alcohol with propranolol (Inderal)—the combination lowers blood pressure too much. One study showed that piperine, a chemical found in black pepper and long pepper, increased blood levels of propranolol; this can potentiate the drug's activity and its side effects. In another study, when antacids were taken concomitantly with sotalol (Betapace), absorption of the drug was reduced.

Because some beta-blockers decrease the uptake of potassium from the blood, avoid high-potassium foods, salt substitutes, and potassium supplements. Chromium supplements taken with beta-blockers may raise HDL cholesterol levels. Calcium supplements might interfere with the absorption of the beta-blocker atenolol and possibly with other beta-blockers as well. Pleurisy root should be avoided because it contains cardiac glycosides, which can affect heart rhythm.

NUTRIENT DEPLETION/IMBALANCE

Research suggests that beta-blockers (specifically propranolol, metoprolol, and alprenolol) might impair the body's ability to utilize coenzyme Q10 (CoQ10). Because CoQ10 appears to play a significant role in normal heart function, this is particularly troublesome. In fact, depletion of CoQ10 might be responsible for some of the side effects of beta-blockers.

- Coenzyme Q10—take 100 to 200 mg daily.

Natural Alternatives to Blood Pressure Drugs

Diet and Lifestyle Changes

Consuming a diet rich in plant foods is one of the best ways to reduce blood pressure. There are a few reasons for this. First, plant foods are generally richer in blood pressure–lowering potassium than animal products. Second, they are not loaded with sodium, as many packaged foods are. Societies that consume little salt (sodium chloride) have little problem with hypertension. You can reduce salt intake by not adding salt to your meals. Salt substitutes that contain potassium chloride can be helpful to reduce added amounts to food. However, most sodium comes from eating packaged foods or dining out. One teaspoon of salt contains 2,325 mg of sodium. Limiting sodium intake to 1,500 to 2,000 mg daily can help some individuals lower their blood pressure. Consult with your doctor on the optimal intake for you depending on your medical status.

The DASH diet, which stands for "Dietary Approaches to Stop Hypertension," has been shown to reduce blood pressure. The DASH eating plan includes whole grains, poultry, fish, and nuts, and has low amounts of fats, red meats, sweets, and sugary beverages. It is high in potassium, calcium, and magnesium which help lower blood pressure. Potassium is particularly important in reducing blood pressure.

SUGGESTED MENU PLAN FOR DASH DIET

Food	Amount of Sodium (mg)
Breakfast	
Scrambled eggs, 2 large	342
Bacon, 1 slice	192
Whole-wheat bread, 1 slice	148
Butter, 2 teaspoons	54
Total sodium for meal	736
Lunch	
Whole-wheat bread, 2 slices	296
Ham, luncheon meat, 1 slice	350
Mayonnaise, 1 tablespoon	105
Dill pickle, 1 spear	385
Pretzels, 1 ounce	486
Orange, 1 large	0
Total sodium for meal	1,622
Dinner	
Spaghetti, 1 cup	179
Spaghetti sauce, ½ cup	601
Parmesan cheese, 1 tablespoon	76
Green beans, canned, ½ cup	177
Garlic bread, 1 slice	200
Total sodium for meal	1,233
Total sodium for the day	**3,591**

Source: Department of Agriculture, Nutrient Data Laboratory, 2005

Other foods that can help reduce blood pressure are celery, onions, and garlic. Include these often in your diet. Lastly, a number of clinical studies show that consuming dark chocolate (46 to 105 grams per day, providing 213 to 500 mg of cocoa polyphenols) modestly lowers systolic blood pressure; and that pomegranate juice has been shown to reduce blood pressure. Consume 4 to 8 ounces daily.

POTASSIUM-RICH FOODS

Food, Standard Amount	Potassium (mg)
Sweet potato, baked, 1 potato (146 g)	694
Tomato paste, ¼ cup	664
Beet greens, cooked, ½ cup	655
Potato, baked, 1 potato (156 g)	610
White beans, canned, ½ cup	595
Yogurt, plain, nonfat, 8-oz container	579
Tomato puree, ½ cup	549
Clams, canned, 3 oz	534
Yogurt, plain, low-fat, 8-oz container	531
Prune juice, ¾ cup	530
Carrot juice, ¾ cup	517
Blackstrap molasses, 1 tbsp	498
Halibut, cooked, 3 oz	490
Soybeans, green, cooked, ½ cup	485
Tuna, yellowfin, cooked, 3 oz	484
Lima beans, cooked, ½ cup	484
Winter squash, cooked, ½ cup	448
Soybeans, mature, cooked, ½ cup	443
Rockfish, Pacific, cooked, 3 oz	442
Cod, Pacific, cooked, 3 oz	439
Banana, 1 medium	422
Spinach, cooked, ½ cup	419
Tomato juice, ¾ cup	417
Tomato sauce, ½ cup	405
Peaches, dried, uncooked, ¼ cup	398
Prunes, stewed, ½ cup	398
Milk, nonfat, 1 cup	382
Pork chop, center loin, cooked, 3 oz	382
Apricots, dried, uncooked, ¼ cup	378
Rainbow trout, farmed, cooked, 3 oz	375
Pork loin, center rib (roasts), lean, roasted, 3 oz	371
Buttermilk, cultured, low-fat, 1 cup	370
Cantaloupe, ¼ medium	368
1 percent/2 percent milk, 1 cup	366
Honeydew melon, ⅛ medium	365
Lentils, cooked, ½ cup	365
Plantains, cooked, ½ cup slices	358

Food, Standard Amount	Potassium (mg)
Kidney beans, cooked, ½ cup	358
Orange juice, ¾ cup	355
Split peas, cooked, ½ cup	355
Yogurt, plain, whole milk, 8 oz container	352

Source: Nutrient values from Agricultural Research Service (ARS) Nutrient Database for Standard Reference, Release 17.

Reduce or avoid the intake of caffeine-containing foods such as coffee, tea, chocolate, or soda pop, as they can elevate blood pressure in some individuals.

Stop smoking, as it acts as a vasoconstrictor to elevate blood pressure; and do not consume more than one alcohol drink a day. Regular exercise and weight loss will also help to lower blood pressure effectively.

It has been our experience that many patients with mild to moderate hypertension can avoid pharmaceutical use with the recommendations in this chapter. Those with moderate to severe high blood pressure may be able to reduce their medication dosage with the use of the diet, lifestyle, and supplements discussed in this chapter. It is important that you do not discontinue any medications or change dosages without your physician's knowledge.

Hawthorn

Hawthorn extract has been used for centuries by European and American herbalists for improving circulation and reducing blood pressure. It has a mild benefit for those with hypertension and works well with the other supplements described in this chapter.

DOSAGE

We recommend 250 mg of a standardized extract to be taken three times daily.

SAFETY

People taking prescription cardiac or blood-thinning medications should consult with their doctor before using hawthorn.

Magnesium

This mineral has a relaxant effect on the nervous system and blood vessel walls. It is commonly deficient in the U.S. diet and is commonly depleted by alcohol and caffeine consumption. It is also thought that high stress levels deplete the body's magnesium. Lastly, some pharmaceutical medications cause this nutrient to be depleted. Our experience is that higher doses are effective for some but not all patients with hypertension.

A variety of studies have shown that dosages of magnesium between 350 to 1,000 mg daily help to reduce blood pressure, especially diastolic pressure.

DOSAGE

A therapeutic dosage is 250 to 500 mg taken twice daily. We also advise that calcium be taken at a dose of 500 mg twice daily, which has mild blood pressure–lowering effects.

SAFETY

For some individuals, more than 400 mg of magnesium daily causes loose stools. This is less likely with one type of magnesium known as magnesium glycinate. People with kidney disease should not supplement magnesium without consulting a doctor.

Fish Oil

Fish oil has several benefits for the cardiovascular system. In particular it reduces the inflammatory response common to many cardiovascular conditions. It also has a blood-thinning effect, which reduces pressure inside the artery walls. An analysis of 31 trials demonstrates that fish oil lowers blood pressure.

Resperate

Resperate is an effective device to lower blood pressure through proper breathing. This small computer unit looks like a portable CD player with a headphone set and a sensor belt to wrap around the chest or upper abdomen. Resperate is designed to slow your respiration rate from an average of 12 to 19 breaths per minute to the hypertension-lowering rate of 10 or fewer breaths per minute. You listen to tones that guide your breathing rate. An average reduction is 10 points for systolic pressure and five points for diastolic pressure. So far, eight clinical trials published in medical journals have confirmed its benefits. The first such study appeared in the *Journal of Human Hypertension* in 2001. It involved 61 men and women whose blood pressure was around 155/95 on average. For 10 minutes each day, one group of participants used the Resperate device and the other group listened to a Walkman playing quiet music. After eight weeks, the average decrease in the Resperate group was 15.2 points for systolic pressure (the top number) and 10 points for diastolic pressure (the bottom number) compared with the Walkman group's average reduction of 11.3 points (systolic) and 5.6 points (diastolic). Furthermore, six months after treatment stopped, the Resperate group's average diastolic pressure remained lower than the Walkman group's. See www.resperate.com.

DOSAGE

A relatively high dosage of fish oil is generally required for a blood pressure–lowering effect. Based on the studies mentioned above, we recommend 4 grams of combined eicosapentaenoic acid (EPA) and docosahexaenoic acid (DHA) daily.

SAFETY

Consult with a doctor if you are on blood-thinning medications before using fish oil.

Coenzyme Q10

Coenzyme Q10 is a vitaminlike compound that has many benefits for the cardiovascular system.

Several studies have shown that coenzyme Q10 reduces blood pressure. In one study, researchers followed 109 patients with essential hypertension who were given an average of 225 mg of CoQ10 in addition to their existing drug regimen. Participants had significantly improved systolic and diastolic blood pressure, and 51 percent of patients came completely off of between one and three antihypertensive drugs at an average of 4.4 months after starting CoQ10.

A study published in the *European Journal of Clinical Nutrition* involved a randomized, double-blind, placebo-controlled study of 74 people with type 2 diabetes. Subjects were randomly assigned to receive an oral dose of 100 mg CoQ twice daily (200 mg per day), 200 mg fenofibrate each morning, both, or neither for 12 weeks. CoQ was found to significantly decrease systolic (-6.1 mm Hg) and diastolic (-2.9 mm Hg) blood pressure.

Coenzyme Q10 and Your Heart

Coenzyme Q10 is a super-nutrient for the cardiovascular system. It not only can help lower blood pressure but also is involved in normal heart contraction and rhythm. We recommend that all adults supplement 50 to 100 mg of coenzyme Q10 daily. For those who have cardiovascular conditions, it is even more important to regularly supplement this vital nutrient.

DOSAGE

Take 100 mg three times daily.

SAFETY

Coenzyme Q10 is very safe. Those on blood-thinning medications should consult with their doctor before using it.

Melatonin

This over-the-counter hormone is commonly used to help with insomnia. Research has also shown it to be beneficial for nighttime hypertension. This is important, since elevated blood pressure at night injures the heart and blood vessels just as it does during the day.

A study published in the *American Journal of Hypertension* found that melatonin reduces nighttime blood pressure in women with hypertension. This randomized, double-blind study involved 18 women, ages 47 to 63, half with hypertension being successfully controlled with ACE inhibitor medication and half who had normal blood pressure. For three weeks, participants took either 3 mg of time-released melatonin or a placebo one hour before going to bed. They were then switched to the other treatment for another three weeks. After taking melatonin for three weeks, 84 percent of the women had at least a 10 mm Hg (systolic and diastolic) decrease in nocturnal (nighttime) blood pressure, while only 39 percent experienced a decrease in nocturnal blood pressure after taking the placebo. No change was found in daytime blood pressure readings. The reduction in nighttime blood pressure was the greatest in the women with controlled hypertension. Previous studies have found similar results when men with untreated hypertension took melatonin.

DOSAGE

Take 0.5 to 3 mg 30 to 60 minutes before bedtime.

SAFETY

Melatonin should not be used by pregnant or breast-feeding women.

Potassium

As described in the diet section, potassium is a key mineral for the reduction of blood pressure. It must be maintained in good balance with sodium. More than 33 trials have demonstrated that potassium lowers blood pressure. Potassium is most effective for people with low potassium levels and high daily sodium intake, and for African Americans.

TIMOTHY'S STORY

Timothy, a 49-year-old office worker and beach volleyball enthusiast, had just been prescribed blood pressure medication by his family doctor for mild hypertension. He felt increased fatigue and mild dizziness from the medication. Looking for a natural alternative, we prescribed a natural regimen while simultaneously weaning him off his medication. His protocol consisted of a potassium-rich vegetable juice, coenzyme Q10, hawthorn, and extra calcium and magnesium. Since he was already physically fit and active, there were no exercise changes. With regular blood pressure monitoring, we confirmed normal blood pressure readings over several months without the use of pharmaceuticals.

DOSAGE

A daily dosage of around 2,400 mg of potassium is therapeutic for hypertension. The problem is that supplements cannot by law contain more than 99 mg per capsule or tablet. Therefore we recommend that you get potassium from food sources as discussed in the diet section. Tomato juices are one way to get in a high amount of potassium per serving, such as low-sodium V8 juice, with 820 mg per 8 ounces.

SAFETY

People on potassium-sparing diuretics or those with kidney disease should not take potassium supplements or eat large quantities of potassium-laden foods without consulting with a doctor. Potassium supplements can also cause stomach upset.

References

Bano, G, et al. 1991. Effect of piperine on bioavailability and pharmacokinetics of propranolol and theophylline in healthy volunteers. *European Journal of Clinical Pharmacology.* 41(6):615–7.

Cagnacci, A, et al. 2005. Prolonged melatonin administration decreases nocturnal blood pressure in women. *American Journal of Hypertension.* 18(12 Pt 1):1614–8.

Digiesi, V, et al. 1994. Coenzyme Q10 in essential hypertension. *Molecular Aspects of Medicine.* 15 Suppl.:s257–63.

Folkers, K, et al. 1981. Bioenergetics in clinical medicine. XVI. Reduction of hypertension in patients by therapy with coenzyme Q10. *Research Communications in Chemical Pathology and Pharmacology.* 31:129–40.

Hodgson, JM, et al. 2002. Coenzyme Q10 improves blood pressure and glycaemic control: A controlled trial in subjects with type 2 diabetes. *European Journal of Clinical Nutrition.* 56: 1137–42.

Laer, S, et al. 1997. Interaction between sotalol and an antacid preparation. *British Journal of Clinical Pharmacology.* 43(3):269–72.

Langsjoen, P, et al. 1994. Treatment of essential hypertension with coenzyme Q10. *Molecular Aspects of Medicine.* 15 Suppl.:s265–72.

Lee, C, et al. 2001. Iron supplementation inhibits cough associated with ACE inhibitors. *Hypertension.* 2001;38:166–70.

Morris, MC, F Sacks, B Rosner. 1993. Does fish oil lower blood pressure? A meta-analysis of controlled trials. *Circulation.* 88:523–33.

Motoyama, T, et al. 1989. Oral magnesium supplementation in patients with essential hypertension. *Hypertension.* 13:227–32.

Sanjuliani, AF, VG de Abreu Fagundes, EA Francischetti. 1996. Effects of magnesium on blood pressure and intracellular ion levels of Brazilian hypertensive patients. *International Journal of Cardiology.* 56:177–83.

Whelton, PK, et al. 1997. Effects of oral potassium on blood pressure: Meta-analysis of randomized controlled clinical trials. *Journal of the American Medical Association.* 277:1624–32.

Widman, L, et al. 1993. The dose-dependent reduction in blood pressure through administration of magnesium. A double blind placebo controlled cross-over study. *American Journal of Hypertension.* 6:41–5.

10

Cholesterol Drugs and Their Natural Alternatives

What Is Cholesterol?

Cholesterol is an essential component of every cell in your body and is needed to manufacture hormones and other life-giving substances. Although cholesterol is obtained through high-fat and/or high-cholesterol foods, approximately 85 percent of cholesterol in the body is manufactured by the liver and, to a lesser degree, by the small intestine. Cholesterol circulates in the bloodstream in carrier packages called lipoproteins, which have fat (lipid) inside and protein outside.

Two types of lipoproteins transport cholesterol in the blood:

- Low-density lipoprotein (LDL) cholesterol, considered the "bad" cholesterol, is a sticky, fat-like substance that can adhere to the walls of the arteries. When someone has a high level of LDL, the excess can be deposited onto the artery walls, creating blockages and resulting in increased risk of heart disease.

- High-density lipoprotein (HDL) cholesterol, considered the "good" cholesterol, works to remove LDL cholesterol from the arteries and transport it back to the liver to be metabolized. If you have a low level of HDL, you have increased risk of heart disease.

We all have been told, or have read, that excessive cholesterol in the blood accumulates in the artery walls. However, there appears to be more to the story. Research over the past decade has shown that much of the artery problem caused by cholesterol is the result of oxidation. Oxidation occurs when free radicals (unstable negatively charged molecules) damage cells of the body. Free radicals are the by-product of energy production by the body's cells, as well as the body's exposure to pollutants and radiation.

Oxidized cholesterol (particularly LDL cholesterol) initiates inflammation and eventual plaque buildup in the blood vessel wall, which inhibits blood flow through the arteries. This oxidation leads to inflammation and damage in the artery walls.

Your body has a defense mechanism against free radicals and oxidation. Substances called antioxidants are an integral part of that defense mechanism. Antioxidants neutralize or reduce the effects of cell-damaging free radicals. Though your body has naturally occurring antioxidant enzyme systems, you also need antioxidants from foods, particularly plant foods such as fruits, vegetables, and legumes. In addition, antioxidant supplements such as vitamins A, C, E, selenium, and many others provide antioxidant protection.

Elevated fats in the blood also help contribute to atherosclerosis and heart disease risk. These fats in the blood are known as triglycerides. Triglycerides come from the diet or are manufactured by the liver. Elevated levels are common in those with increased blood sugar levels as seen with diabetes or insulin resistance. A high level of these fats can restrict blood flow and make you more susceptible to stroke.

Cholesterol-lowering drugs are frequently prescribed by U.S. doctors. Lipitor, for example, a common cholesterol-lowering drug, was the second most prescribed drug in the United States in 2005. The purpose of these drugs is to prevent and treat heart disease by slowing or halting the buildup of plaque in the arteries. The accumulation of plaque, known as atherosclerosis, results in the blockage of blood flow, which increases the risk of a heart attack or stroke. Plaque accumulation in the heart arteries is of particular concern. It contributes to high blood pressure and reduces the amount of oxygen that reaches the heart, a dangerous situation.

Cholesterol-lowering drugs are also prescribed as a preventive measure. They can help people who have suffered from previous heart attacks. According to guidelines set by the National Institutes of Health, an estimated 65 million people have high cholesterol; and approximately 37 million, or one in five adults, are eligible for cholesterol-lowering therapy.

What Happens to the Arteries?

Atherosclerosis is a common occurrence with cardiovascular disease. This medical term refers to hardening of the arteries. In this condition, artery walls thicken and lose their flexibility, interfering with circulation. This can happen to any blood vessel in the body, including the coronary arteries that supply blood to the heart muscle.

A partial blockage of coronary arteries reduces the flow of oxygen and nutrients to heart tissues. This can cause chest pain, known as angina pectoris, often just called "angina."

Also, plaque buildups can break off and occlude blood flow in various arteries of the body, leading to blood clots and serious events such as stroke, heart attack, or a clot in the lung.

Banish the Trans Fats

In a 2006 article published in the *New England Journal of Medicine*, researchers predicted that the "near elimination of industrially produced trans fats might avert between 72,000 and 228,000 coronary heart disease events (in the United States) each year."

Cholesterol Ranges

Following is the National Institutes of Health's National Cholesterol Education Program classification of cholesterol and triglyceride values.

ATP III Classification of LDL, Total, and HDL Cholesterol (mg/dL)

LDL Cholesterol

Lower than 100 mg/dL: Optimal

100 to 129 mg/dL: Near optimal/above optimal

130 to 159 mg/dL: Borderline high

160 to 189 mg/dL: High

190 mg/dL: Very high

Total Cholesterol

<200 Desirable

200-239 Borderline high

240 High

HDL Cholesterol

<40 Low

>60 High (optimal)

Triglycerides

< 150 Normal

150-199 Borderline high

200-499 High

500 Very high

Are Statins Overprescribed?

In the July 13, 2004, issue of Circulation: *Journal of the American Heart Association*, the National Institutes of Health's National Cholesterol Education Program (NCEP) published new guidelines for LDL cholesterol levels. According to the NCEP, "These options include setting lower treatment goals for LDL ('bad') cholesterol and initiating cholesterol-lowering drug therapy at lower LDL thresholds." These new recommendations were based on the review of five major clinical trials using a group of cholesterol-lowering drugs known as "statins."

The science behind these new conclusions was challenged by more than three dozen physicians, epidemiologists, and other scientists, together with the Center for Science in the Public Interest (CSPI). In a letter that detailed their objections, physicians and scientific researchers urged the National Institutes of Health (NIH) to seek an independent panel to re-review the studies. They wrote, "There is strong evidence to suggest that an objective, independent re-evaluation of the scientific evidence from the five new studies of statin therapy would lead to different conclusions than those presented by the current NCEP. The studies cited do not demonstrate that statins benefit women of any age or men over 70 who do not already have heart disease."

In the letter, doctors from the CSPI also cited concerns that were raised after one study showed that statin therapy significantly increases the risk of cancer in the elderly. In addition, researchers noted, three of four studies involving people with diabetes showed that these patients got no significant benefit from increased statin use.

There was another alarming discovery as well. Eight of the nine authors of the new LDL recommendations had financial ties to manufacturers of statin drugs, including the pharmaceutical companies Pfizer, Merck, Bristol-Myers Squibb, and AstraZeneca. (Normal medical publishing requires the disclosure of financial ties associated with the authors of a study.) Authors of the CSPI letter summarized their suspicions about the NCEP report by stating, "The sad fact is that these lifestyle recommendations are being largely ignored, partly because the 'experts,' many of whom have conflicts of interest through their relationships with statin manufacturers, focus ever more attention on lowering cholesterol with expensive drugs." The response from the acting director of the National Institutes of Health National Heart, Lung, and Blood Institute was to declare that the scientific basis was adequate and there was no conflict of interest from panel members.

Risk Factors for High Cholesterol That You Cannot Control

- Age: 45 or older for men; 55 or older for women
- Family history of early heart disease: father or brother diagnosed before age 55, or mother or sister diagnosed before age 65

Risk Factors for High Cholesterol That You Can Change

- Smoking
- High blood pressure
- High blood cholesterol
- Overweight/obesity
- Physical inactivity
- Diabetes
- Omega-3 fatty acid level*
- Reaction to stress*
- Nutrient deficiencies such as magnesium*
- Cardiovascular blood risk factors (homocysteine, lipoprotein (a), fibrinogen, Apolipoprotein A-1 and B)*

*Represents risk factors added by authors not commonly listed by the National Institutes of Health and other medical authorities. See our book, *Prescription for Natural Cures* (Wiley, 2004), for further discussion and recommendations on these newer markers.

Cholesterol Drugs

HMG CoA Reductase Inhibitors (Statins)

Rosuvastatin (Crestor)

Fluvastatin (Lescol)

Atorvastatin(Lipitor)

Lovastatin (Mevacor)

Pravastatin (Pravachol)

Simvastatin (Zocor)

HOW DO THESE DRUGS WORK?

Statins are a class of cholesterol-lowering drugs that inhibit the enzyme called hydroxy-methylglutaryl-coenzyme A reductase (HMG-CoA reductase) that is involved in the manufacturing of cholesterol in the liver.

WHAT ARE THE BENEFITS?

LDL cholesterol reduced 18 to 55 percent

HDL cholesterol increased 5 to 15 percent

Triglycerides reduced 7 to 30 percent

These drugs decrease the risk of dying when they are given in the hospital after a heart attack, and they reduce the long-term death rate.

POTENTIAL SIDE EFFECTS?

The most common side effects are headache, nausea, vomiting, constipation, diarrhea, rash, weakness, muscle and joint pain, and increased liver enzymes. The most serious (but fortunately rare) side effects are liver failure and rhabdomyolysis, a serious side effect in which there is damage to muscles.

Statins should not be used by pregnant or nursing women.

MAJOR CAUTIONS

A rare but serious side effect is liver failure. Therefore it is recommended that liver enzyme levels be checked prior to and at 12 weeks after starting a statin drug.

Rhabdomyolysis, with muscle damage, is another rare side effect that could pose a danger. It often begins as muscle pain and can progress to the destruction of muscle tissue, kidney failure, and death. Rhabdomyolysis occurs more often when statins are used in combination with other drugs, including protease inhibitors (drugs used for AIDS), erythromycin, itraconazole, clarithromycin, diltiazem, verapamil, niacin, or fibric acids; for example, gemfibrozil (Lopid), clofibrate (Atromid-S), and fenofibrate (Tricor). Any of these drugs should be used with caution if combined with statins.

KNOWN DRUG INTERACTIONS

Cholestyramine (Questran) as well as colestipol (Colestid) bind cholesterol in the intestine and reduce absorption. Statins should be taken one hour before or four hours after cholestyramine, a drug that binds cholesterol and decreases its absorption. Similar caution should be used when taking colestipol, a medication that also binds cholesterol.

FOOD OR SUPPLEMENT INTERACTIONS

Avoid the consumption of grapefruit or grapefruit juice while on a statin drug.

One study found that blood vitamin A levels increased over two years among people who were on a statin drug, so you don't want to take large doses of vitamin A supplements while taking a statin. Avoid supplementing vitamin A above 5,000 IU daily and have blood vitamin A levels checked yearly by your doctor. Caution should be used when combining vitamin B3 (niacin) with a statin drug. Check with your doctor before starting this combination.

NUTRIENT DEPLETION/IMBALANCE

Statin drugs have been shown to deplete the body of coenzyme Q10 (CoQ10), which your body needs to create energy in cells, particularly heart cells. One study found that people taking atorvastatin (Lipitor) had blood CoQ10 levels reduced by 50 percent after 30 days. We recommend 100 to 200 mg daily of CoQ10 supplements to prevent deficiency for those using statin drugs.

Factors That Increase the Risk of Statin-Associated Myopathy

According to the *Journal of the American College of Cardiology*, people with the following conditions are at risk of muscle damage (myopathy) associated with taking statin drugs.

- Advanced age (especially more than 80 years) in patients (women more than men)
- Small body frame and frailty
- Multisystem disease (e.g., chronic renal insufficiency, especially due to diabetes)
- Taking multiple medications
- In a perioperative period—shortly before or after surgery
- Taking specific concomitant medications or consumption as listed below (check specific statin package insert for warnings)
  - Fibrates (especially gemfibrozil, but other fibrates too) for lowering cholesterol
  - Nicotinic acid (rarely)
  - Cyclosporine, an immune-suppressing drug
  - Azole antifungals such as fucanozole (Diflucan) or ketoconazole (Nizoral), commonly prescribed for fungal infections in various parts of the body
  - Macrolide antibiotics such as erythromycin and clarithromycin, commonly prescribed for respiratory tract and soft-tissue infections
  - Azithromycin (Zithromax)
  - Clarithromycin (Biaxin)
  - HIV protease inhibitors
  - Nefazodone (Serzone), an antidepressant
  - Verapamil (Calan, Calan SR, Covera-HS, Isoptin, Isoptin SR, Verelan, Verelan PM), generally prescribed for high blood pressure, angina (chest pain), irregular heart rhythm
  - Amiodarone, an antiarrhythmic medication

Myopathy risk in people who take statin drugs is also increased by drinking large quantities of grapefruit juice—usually more than one quart per day.

People who drink an excess of two drinks of alcohol per day are also predisposed to myopathy.

Bile Acid Sequestrants

Cholestyramine (Questran)

Colestipol (Colestid)

Colesevelam (Welchol)

HOW DO THEY WORK?

Bile acid sequestrants are pharmaceuticals used for lowering LDL cholesterol. They bind bile acids in the intestine for increased excretion through the stool. This causes the liver to convert more cholesterol into bile acids, which lowers the level of cholesterol in the blood.

WHAT ARE THE BENEFITS?

Low to high doses can lower LDL cholesterol by 10 to 30 percent and increase HDL cholesterol by 3 to 5 percent. They have no effect on triglycerides. Since they have mild cholesterol-lowering effects, they are often combined with statin drugs or niacin for a stronger therapeutic effect.

POTENTIAL SIDE EFFECTS

- Constipation
- Abdominal pain
- Bloating
- Vomiting
- Diarrhea
- Weight loss
- Excessive passage of gas (flatulence)

These drugs should not be used by pregnant or nursing women.

MAJOR CAUTIONS

Bile acid sequestrants decrease the absorption of fat-soluble vitamins. Long-term use may cause a deficiency of vitamins A, D, E, and K. Vitamins should be taken one hour before or four to six hours after the administration of a bile acid sequestrant.

KNOWN DRUG INTERACTIONS

This class of cholesterol-lowering drugs can bind to and decrease the absorption effectiveness of various medications including warfarin (Coumadin), thyroid hormones (Synthroid, Levoxyl), digoxin (Lanoxin), thiazide diuretics (Hydrodiuril, Oretic, Dyazide, Maxzide), and others.

FOOD OR SUPPLEMENT INTERACTIONS

Do not combine with cholesterol-lowering supplements.

NUTRIENT DEPLETION/IMBALANCE

In addition to depleting fat-soluble vitamins A, D, E, and K, this class of drugs can also cause a depletion of calcium, magnesium, folic acid, B12, zinc, iron, carotenoids, and omega-3 fatty acids. We recommend taking the following supplements:

- Vitamin A—take 5,000 IU daily.
- Vitamin D—take 1,000 IU daily.
- Vitamin E—take 200 IU of mixed vitamin E form.
- Calcium—take 500 to 1,200 mg daily.
- Magnesium—take 200 to 250 mg twice daily.

- Folic acid—take 400 mcg daily.
- B12—take 100 to 200 mcg daily.
- Carotenoids—take a mixed carotenoid formula daily or as part of a multivitamin.
- Omega-3 fatty acids—take 1,000 mg of combined EPA and DHA as found in fish oil.
- Iron—do not supplement unless testing by your doctor shows iron-deficiency anemia.

Fibric Acids

Gemfibrozil (Lopid)

Fenofibrate (Tricor)

Clofibrate (Atromid-S)

HOW DO THEY WORK?

The exact mechanism is unknown. They are thought to reduce the formation and increase the breakdown of cholesterol and triglycerides. They are mainly prescribed for people with very high triglycerides or for those who have low HDL cholesterol and high triglycerides.

WHAT ARE THE BENEFITS?

LDL cholesterol reduced 5 to 20 percent

HDL cholesterol increased 10 to 20 percent

Triglycerides decreased 20 to 50 percent

POTENTIAL SIDE EFFECTS

- Upset stomach, nausea, or vomiting
- Abdominal pain, constipation, diarrhea
- Increased risk of gallstones, inflamed liver, muscle inflammation (myositis)
- Vertigo
- Rash

These drugs should not be used by pregnant or nursing women.

MAJOR CAUTIONS

Gemfibrozil can interact with drugs that have blood-thinning effects (anticoagulants), causing bleeding.

Do not take clofibrate if you have liver disease, kidney disease, or biliary cirrhosis.

KNOWN DRUG INTERACTIONS

Fibric acids may increase the activity of diabetic medications. They also should not be combined with cholesterol-lowering statin drugs.

FOOD OR SUPPLEMENT INTERACTIONS

Alcohol should be avoided.

There is speculation that the nutritional supplement red yeast rice extract should not be combined with this drug.

NUTRIENT DEPLETION/IMBALANCE

Studies have shown that blood levels of coenzyme Q10 and vitamin E are reduced in men taking Gemfibrozil.

We recommend supplementing 100 to 200 mg of coenzyme Q10 and 200 IU of mixed vitamin E for those taking these medications.

Nicotinic Acid

Niaspan

Niacor

Slo-Niacin

HOW DO THESE DRUGS WORK?

Nicotinic acid is vitamin B3, also known as niacin. The exact mechanism is not well understood, but it may reduce the production of proteins that transport cholesterol and triglycerides in the blood.

WHAT ARE THE BENEFITS?

LDL cholesterol reduced by 5 to 25 percent

HDL cholesterol increased by 15 to 35 percent

Triglycerides decreased by 20 to 50 percent

POTENTIAL SIDE EFFECTS

- Stomach upset, gas, bloating, vomiting, diarrhea or nausea. (These side effects may be reduced by taking nicotinic acid with food.)
- Warmth and flushing of the neck, ears, and face along with itching, tingling, and headache.

Some doctors recommend taking aspirin or a nonsteroidal anti-inflammatory drug (NSAID) such as Motrin or Aleve before taking a dose of nicotinic acid to prevent this side effect, which generally lessens with time. We prefer that people who have this problem use over-the-counter flush-free niacin known as inositol hexaniacinate.

High doses of niacin should be avoided by pregnant or nursing women.

High doses of niacin rarely elevate blood homocysteine levels, a known risk factor for heart disease. Have your levels monitored by your doctor when taking niacin.

Niaspan may slow blood clotting and may need to be discontinued before surgery. Discuss this with your doctor.

MAJOR CAUTIONS

Niacin, especially the time-released or sustained-released versions, can irritate the liver and increase liver enzymes. There have been rare cases of liver failure or muscle injury. Blood tests for elevated liver enzymes should be performed before starting niacin therapy and every three to six months thereafter.

Do not use niacin if you have active liver disease or an active ulcer.

KNOWN DRUG INTERACTIONS

Niacin may increase blood glucose levels in diabetics. Therefore, diabetic medications may need to be adjusted when niacin is taken by diabetic patients.

The use of statin drugs may increase the risk of muscle damage when combined with niacin. Check with your doctor before combining these two medications.

Niaspan may lower blood pressure. Caution is advised if you are using blood pressure medications.

FOOD OR SUPPLEMENT INTERACTIONS

Drinking hot liquids or alcohol shortly before or after niacin is taken may increase the occurrence of flushing.

NUTRIENT DEPLETION/IMBALANCE

Long-term use of niacin is best accompanied by a blend of the other B vitamins commonly found in a multivitamin.

Selective Cholesterol Absorption Inhibitor

Ezetimibe (Zetia)

HOW DOES THIS DRUG WORK?

Ezetimibe (Zetia) is a new type of cholesterol-lowering drug. Zetia acts by blocking the absorption of dietary cholesterol through the intestines. It may be used alone or, for a stronger effect, be combined with a statin drug. For example, ezetimibe/simvastatin (Vytorin) is a combination of ezetimibe (Zetia) and simvastatin (Zocor).

WHAT ARE THE BENEFITS?

Zetia can lower LDL cholesterol up to 20 percent. It produces further reduction when combined with a statin drug. It has also been shown to reduce triglyceride levels and increase HDL cholesterol when combined with statin drugs.

POTENTIAL SIDE EFFECTS

- Diarrhea, abdominal pain
- Back pain, joint pain
- Sinusitis
- Rarely, hypersensitivity reactions, including angioedema (swelling of the skin and underlying tissues of the head and neck that can be life-threatening)
- Skin rash
- Pancreatitis and nausea

Ezetimibe (Zetia) should not be used by pregnant or nursing women.

MAJOR CAUTIONS

Muscle damage (myopathy or rhabdomyolysis) and hepatitis have rarely been associated with the use of ezetimibe.

KNOWN DRUG INTERACTIONS

Bile acid sequestrants such as gemfibrozil (Lopid), fenofibrate (Tricor), and clofibrate (Atromid-S) bind to ezetimibe and reduce its activity. Therefore, ezetimibe should be taken at least two hours after or one hour before taking these drugs.

Cyclosporin increases the levels of ezetimibe and may lead to greater side effects of ezetimibe.

FOOD OR SUPPLEMENT INTERACTIONS

None known with ezetimibe (Zetia). If combined with a statin drug, observe the cautions noted for statins (such as consumption of grapefruit juice) and have blood vitamin A levels checked yearly by your doctor. Caution should be used when combining vitamin B3 (niacin) with a statin drug. Check with your doctor before starting this combination.

NUTRIENT DEPLETION/IMBALANCE

None known with ezetimibe (Zetia). If combined with a statin drug, observe the cautions for statins—particularly the depletion of coenzyme Q10 (CoQ10). As noted, we recommend 100 to 200 mg daily of CoQ10 supplements to prevent deficiency for those using statin drugs.

Natural Alternatives to Cholesterol Drugs

Diet and Lifestyle Changes

Improved diet and increased exercise are both important in the natural treatment of high cholesterol. For some people, changes in diet and lifestyle will be sufficient to normalize their cholesterol levels. For others, these changes will help, but specific nutritional supplements will also be required.

1. Reduce saturated fat in the diet to less than 7 percent of daily calories. Saturated fat is found mainly in beef, veal, poultry (especially in dark meat, and when the skin is present). Saturated fat is also found in most dairy products except nonfat yogurt and cheese, and skim milk. Small amounts of saturated fat are found in coconut and palm oils, which should be used sparingly. Avoid products that contain trans fatty acids, which are found in deep-fried foods, bakery products, packaged snack foods, margarines (except margarines containing plant stanols or plant sterols), crackers, and vegetable shortening. If trans fats are present above 0.5 grams per serving, they will be listed on the label package. They are linked to cardiovascular disease, since they raise LDL cholesterol and triglycerides, and reduce HDL cholesterol. Cook with organic olive or canola oil.

2. Consume two servings a week of heart healthy omega-3 fatty acids found in fish such as anchovies, Atlantic herring, sardines, tilapia, and ocean or canned salmon. (For best seafood choices, see the nonprofit Web site www.oceansalive.org, which lists the safest fish to eat.)

3. Consume five to seven servings of fruits and vegetables daily. They contain fiber that helps lower cholesterol as well as antioxidants that prevent cholesterol oxidation.

4. Regularly consume foods such as beans, barley, oats, peas, apples, oranges, and pears, as they contain soluble fiber, which reduces the absorption of cholesterol from the intestines into the bloodstream. For example, a daily bowl of oatmeal can reduce total cholesterol by as much as 23 percent. It has also been shown to reduce the "bad" LDL cholesterol, while leaving beneficial HDL cholesterol alone. In addition, oats are a rich source of tocotrienols. These relatives of the vitamin E family prevent the oxidation of LDL cholesterol (which prevents LDL cholesterol from sticking to artery walls and causing plaque buildup) and reduce the production of cholesterol by the liver.

5. Consume nuts rich in monounsaturated fatty acids such as almonds and walnuts. For example, a study conducted at the Lipid Clinic in

Barcelona, Spain, showed that a walnut-rich diet reduced total cholesterol by as much as 7.4 percent and LDL cholesterol by as much as 10 percent. Other studies have found that walnuts significantly increase the elasticity of the arteries, which is a marker of healthier blood vessels. The Food and Drug Administration (FDA) allows walnuts to carry the health claim that "eating 1.5 ounces per day of walnuts as part of a diet low in saturated fat and cholesterol may reduce the risk of heart disease."

6. Consume ground flaxseeds (up to a quarter cup daily with 10 ounces of water), as they have been shown to reduce total and LDL cholesterol.

7. Consume 20 to 30 grams of soy protein daily (in food or protein powder form).

8. Reduce simple sugar in the diet (which has been shown to decrease the good HDL cholesterol). By cutting back on simple sugar, you also reduce the risk of elevated insulin levels, which lead to an increased production of cholesterol by the liver.

9. Exercise regularly. Thirty minutes of exercise, three to five times a week, has been shown to be effective for elevated cholesterol. Even walking has been shown to benefit cholesterol levels. Exercise decreases total and LDL cholesterol and increases the good HDL cholesterol.

10. Lose weight and body fat, and you'll also reduce cholesterol levels. You also improve insulin resistance, which is related to elevated cholesterol levels.

11. Stop smoking. Habitual smokers have lower levels of HDL cholesterol and increased risk of heart attacks.

12. Adopt stress-reduction techniques. Stress has been shown to elevate cholesterol in some individuals.

The medical community pays lip service to recommendations for diet and lifestyle changes as a first line of therapy for abnormal cholesterol levels. In our opinion, many patients instead are pressured to begin right away with drug therapy while diet and lifestyle changes are an afterthought. Patients are often told that, due to their "genetic" cholesterol problem, diet and lifestyle changes are not enough, that cholesterol-lowering medication is their sole recourse. While it is true that addressing diet and lifestyle may not be the whole answer for some individuals, there are several nontoxic nutritional supplements that often can help balance the cholesterol and lipid levels, bringing them into the normal range.

Work with a doctor willing to give targeted nutritional supplements, along with diet and lifestyle changes as described above, as a first line of therapy before resorting to drug therapy. (There are, of course, those people who have acute cardiovascular issues or special circumstances that require drug therapy.)

Testing Tip

When following a natural program for lowering cholesterol, we recommend that you get a baseline test to check your levels before you make lifestyle or dietary changes or start supplementation. After 8 to 12 weeks on the program, repeat the tests and compare results to your baseline levels to see how effectively you are responding.

Note that low hormone levels can cause elevation in cholesterol. This is particularly true for people who have low thyroid hormone and/or testosterone. Have these values tested by your doctor to see if they are contributing to elevated cholesterol levels.

Red Yeast Rice Extract

We have found red yeast rice extract to be a mainstay in the natural treatment of moderately elevated cholesterol and triglyceride levels. It has been shown in several studies to significantly lower total cholesterol, LDL cholesterol, and triglycerides. People who take red yeast rice extract may reduce cholesterol levels by 11 to 32 percent and triglyceride levels by 12 to 19 percent.

Red yeast rice is the fermented product of rice on which red yeast (*Monascus purpureus*) has been grown. A dietary staple in China and Japan, it is commonly used by Asian American communities in the United States as a natural food preservative for fish and meat.

Red yeast rice contains an ingredient called monacolin K, which inhibits the action of an enzyme in the liver (HMG-CoA reductase) involved in the synthesis of cholesterol. It is thought to have a similar effect to that of statin drugs such as lovastatin (Mevacor). Yet side effects such as elevated liver enzymes or muscle pain and weakness have not been found to be a problem.

The amount of monacolin K in red yeast rice is minute compared to what is found in lovastatin. Other ingredients in red yeast rice may also account for its powerful cholesterol-lowering properties, such as a family of eight other monacolins, sterols, and fatty acids.

A variety of human and animal studies have shown that red yeast rice is an effective supplement in lowering cholesterol levels. In a double-blind, randomized, placebo-controlled prospective study at the UCLA School of Medicine, researchers found that red yeast rice significantly reduced cholesterol levels. This 12-week study involved 83 healthy people (46 men and 37 women aged 34 to 78 years old) with high cholesterol levels, known as hyperlipidemia. The were treated with red yeast rice, 2,400 mg a day, or a placebo and instructed to consume a diet similar to the American Heart Association Step I diet. (This diet included 30 percent of energy from fat, less than 10 percent of calories from saturated fat, and less than 300 mg of daily cholesterol from food sources.) Blood lipid levels were measured before the start of the study and again at weeks 8, 9, 11, and 12. At weeks 8 and 12, total cholesterol, LDL cholesterol, and triglycerides were significantly reduced in the group supplementing red yeast rice extract compared to placebo.

There were no differences in HDL levels between the two groups.

The following chart is taken from that study, showing baseline values at the beginning of the research and cholesterol levels and trans-fat levels twelve weeks later.

	Baseline Values	After 12 Weeks
Total Chol	250	210
LDL Chol	173	135
TGs	133	112

There were no adverse side effects in the group taking red yeast rice extract and no significant differences in liver enzymes at the beginning and end of the 12-week study.

Beyond a cholesterol-lowering effect, red yeast rice extract has also been shown to reduce heart-related deaths. A study published in the *Journal of the American Geriatrics Society* examined the effect of red yeast rice extract on the risk of heart disease in Chinese people with a history of cardiovascular disease. The trial involved 1,445 Chinese people ages 65 to 75. About half of them were given 600 mg of xuezhikang two times per day and the other half were given a placebo two times per day for four years. The treatment group had a reduced rate of new coronary events including nonfatal heart attacks, sudden death from cardiac causes, and other heart-related deaths by almost 37 percent. Those taking red yeast rice extract were also 48 percent less likely to die from other causes such as cancer and stroke than were people in the placebo group.

DOSAGE

The concentration of red yeast rice extract used in the studies contained 10 to 13.5 milligrams of monacolins per day. The amount was 1,200 to 2,400 mg daily. We normally start patients at 1,200 mg twice daily and retest after two to three months. Some patients are able to maintain lower cholesterol levels at 1,200 mg daily. FDA regulations do not permit supplement companies to list the concentration of monacolins in their products. The only way to find out the concentration is to contact the manufacturer.

Tom, a 51-year-old engineer, was declined life insurance because a blood test showed that his cholesterol levels were too high. His medical doctor recommended that he take a statin drug to lower his cholesterol.

Being an advocate of natural therapies as a first line of treatment, Tom came to my clinic. When Dr. Stengler first saw Tom, Tom's tests showed a total cholesterol of 266. LDL cholesterol was 194, HDL cholesterol was 58, and the triglyceride level was 70. Interestingly, Tom maintained a good diet, limiting his intake of red meat and saturated fat. He also rode his bike regularly. It was obvious that Tom had "bad genetics" when it came to cholesterol.

Dr. Stengler put Tom on a regimen of 600 mg of red yeast rice extract, which he took twice daily along with 100 mg of coenzyme Q10. Four months later, Dr. Stengler retested his cholesterol levels. His total cholesterol had dropped to 167, LDL had plummeted to 94, and HDL cholesterol had increased to 62. His triglyceride level was reduced to 51. Tom was then able to get life insurance with his improved results. In addition to maintaining his usual diet and exercise schedule, Tom has continued using the same dosages of red yeast rice extract and coenzyme Q10. Two years later, his cholesterol levels remain healthy, and Tom has no side effects.

SAFETY

Red yeast may cause some mild side effects such as heartburn, dizziness, and gas. These symptoms may only be temporary. Those with an existing liver disorder should not use red yeast rice extract. Since its safety during pregnancy and breast-feeding is unknown, the extract should be avoided. As a precaution, we recommend those taking red yeast rice extract also supplement 50 mg to 100 mg of coenzyme Q10 to prevent any possible CoQ10 deficiency.

Plant Sterols

In September 2000, the FDA authorized the use of labeling for health claims about the role of plant sterol or plant stanol esters. It can now be said that foods or supplements containing these substances reduce the risk of coronary heart disease. Plant sterols and stanols are present in small quantities in many fruits, vegetables, nuts, seeds, cereals, legumes, vegetable oils, and other plant sources. Foods that may qualify for claims based on plant stanol ester content are spreads such as Benecol, salad dressings, and snack bars. Scientific studies show that 1.3 grams per day of plant sterol esters or 3.4 grams per day of plant stanol esters in the diet are needed to show a significant cholesterol-lowering effect.

Beta sitosterol is a type of plant sterol used in supplement form to lower cholesterol. Taking beta sitosterol supplements significantly reduces total and low-density lipoprotein (LDL) cholesterol levels. It does not have much effect on the good HDL cholesterol. Beta sitosterol works by inhibiting cholesterol absorption in the digestive tract by up to 50 percent. We recommend taking beta sitosterol in a plant sterol complex that contains other sterols such as campesterol, stigmasterol, and other sterols. Plant sterols can reduce LDL cholesterol by up to 14 percent.

DOSAGE

For a therapeutic effect, take 2 grams of plant sterols, or individual beta sitosterol, daily in divided doses with two meals a day. Doses of up to 3 grams can be used daily.

SAFETY

Plant sterols and stanols are Generally Recognized As Safe (GRAS) food-grade substances by the FDA. They have a safe history without any studies or reports showing harmful effects. Some research indicates that beta-carotene levels are slightly reduced with the use of these sterols and stanols. We recommend that if you take this type of supplement, you also eat foods rich in carotenoids such as carrots, tomatoes, and various types of melons. In addition, we recommend taking a multivitamin containing beta-carotene.

Garlic

Garlic has been used as a food and a supplement for many centuries. It is a tonic for the entire cardiovascular system. For achieving a modest reduction in cholesterol levels, the most well-studied form is aged garlic extract (AGE). While other forms of garlic have also been shown to reduce cholesterol, AGE has the most scientific credibility by far. Studies indicate that it inhibits the liver's ability to produce cholesterol, producing an effect that is similar to that of statin drugs. However it accomplishes this action without any known side effects. Researchers at Pennsylvania State University isolated an ingredient within AGE called S-allyl cysteine (SAC). They determined that SAC inhibited the formation of cholesterol by reducing the production of a liver enzyme called HMG-CoA.

When used for more than four weeks, garlic can lower total cholesterol levels between 4 and 12 percent. Studies on aged garlic extract have shown that it reduces total cholesterol between 7 and 31 percent, LDL cholesterol by 10 percent, and triglycerides by 10 percent. It has also been shown to reduce the oxidation of LDL cholesterol, an initiating factor in the development of plaque in the arteries.

Interestingly, investigators at the Research and Education Institute (REI) at Harbor-UCLA Medical Center have found in a human study that AGE supplementation reduces or inhibits plaque formation in the heart's arteries. In a year-long double-blind, randomized clinical trial, researchers administered 1,200 mg of AGE to a group of patients who had a history of bypass surgery and were currently taking statin therapies. A like number of patients in the control group received a placebo. Using electron beam tomography (special rapid X rays of heart arteries that give high-resolution images of moving objects such as the heart), researchers were able to evaluate artery health. After a year, the group taking AGE demonstrated a 67 percent slowing of calcified plaque in the coronary arteries. This group also had a reduction in homocysteine and LDL cholesterol, with a tendency toward increased HDL cholesterol.

DOSAGE

To reduce cholesterol and triglyceride levels, we recommend supplementing with AGE at a dose of 600 mg twice daily.

SAFETY

Garlic supplements are very safe. However, if you are on blood-thinning medications such as Coumadin, check with your doctor before using garlic supplements. Occasionally digestive upset occurs from garlic use. Also, garlic should not be used with the drugs chlorzoxazone and ticlopidine.

Niacin

See nicotinic acid in the drug therapy section of this chapter.

Fish Oil

Fish oil consistently lowers triglyceride levels, and high doses have been shown to lower total cholesterol and improve cholesterol ratios (the ratio of LDL to HDL and total cholesterol to HDL). In addition, it improves other cardiovascular risk markers such as VLDL (very-low-density lipoprotein, a type of cholesterol that increases cardiovascular risk when levels are high).

Several studies have shown that fish oil supplements can reduce triglyceride levels by a whopping 20 to 50 percent. The higher the dose of fish oil, the better the reduction.

In a preliminary trial, people who had been taking pravastatin (Pravachol) for high cholesterol were able to significantly lower their triglyceride levels and raise their levels of HDL "good" cholesterol by supplementing with either 900 mg or 1,800 mg of EPA (eicosapentaenoic acid, an omega-3 fatty acid found in fish oil) for three months in addition to pravastatin. Fish oil supplements have been shown to slow down or reduce atherosclerosis in human studies.

DOSAGE

For a therapeutic dosage to treat high triglycerides and cholesterol, we recommend taking fish oils providing eicosapentaenoic acid (EPA) 1,500 to 2,160 mg and docosahexaenoic acid (DHA) 1,200 to 1,440 mg. The amount of EPA and

DHA will be listed in supplement facts on the container. Also consider taking a garlic supplement combined with fish oil for an even better effect (see garlic section in this chapter).

SAFETY

Some people using fish oil have minor digestive problems such as burping or nausea. Fish oil has a blood-thinning effect, so check with your doctor if you are on blood-thinning medications such as Coumadin before starting fish oil supplementation.

Some people who take fish oil show an increase in LDL cholesterol, which may be offset by taking a garlic supplement.

Green Tea

Green tea, whether taken in liquid or supplement form, has been shown to lower LDL cholesterol, increase HDL cholesterol, and reduce triglycerides. It has also been shown to reduce the oxidation of LDL cholesterol. In addition, researchers have found that it inhibits abnormal blood clot formation.

Population studies indicate that higher consumption of green tea is associated with significantly lowered serum total cholesterol, triglycerides, LDL, and increased high-density lipoprotein (HDL) levels.

One Chinese study involving a total of 240 men and women 18 years or older on a low-fat diet with mild to moderate hypercholesterolemia were randomly assigned to receive a daily capsule containing theaflavin-enriched green tea extract (375 mg) or placebo for 12 weeks. LDL cholesterol was reduced by approximately 11 percent.

DOSAGE

Green tea as a beverage can be effective in reducing LDL oxidation and may reduce cholesterol. While very high dosages of up to ten cups daily may be required for some individuals to get a cholesterol-lowering effect, others can get a benefit from three cups daily. The capsule form containing 375 mg of theaflavin-enriched green tea extract is recommended for those who do not want to drink the tea.

SAFETY

Green tea is commonly consumed daily in Asian cultures and is not associated with significant adverse effects. An average serving of green tea contains 2 to 4 percent caffeine (10 to 80 mg of caffeine per cup). Since caffeine can act as a stimulant, it may cause or worsen anxiety, insomnia, tremors, heart palpitations, and restlessness in some people when consumed in high amounts. For sensitive individuals, decaffeinated green tea is available in beverage and supplement form.

Some people do experience digestive upset from green tea.

Green tea may reduce iron absorption. If you are taking iron supplements, wait for two hours before or after supplementation before you drink the tea.

References

Aberg, F, et al. 1998. Gemfibrozil-induced decrease in serum ubiquinone and alpha- and gamma-tocopherol levels in men with combined hyperlipidaemia. *European Journal of Clinical Investigations.* 28:235–42.

Adler, A, BJ Holub. 1997. Effect of garlic and fish-oil supplementation on serum lipid and lipoprotein concentrations in hypercholesterolemic men. *American Journal of Clinical Nutrition.* 65:445–50.

Budoff, M, et al. 2003. *Journal of the Federation of American Societies for Experimental Biology.* 17(5), LB360, 69.

Eritsland, J, et al. 1995. Long-term metabolic effects of n-3 polyunsaturated fatty acids in patients with coronary artery disease. *American Journal of Clinical Nutrition.* 61:831–6.

Heber, D, et al. 1999. Cholesterol-lowering effects of a proprietary Chinese red-yeast-rice dietary supplement. *American Journal of Clinical Nutrition.* February;69 (2):231–36.

Ide, N, BHS Lau. 1997. Garlic compounds inhibit low density lipoprotein (LDL) oxidation and protect endothelial cells from oxidized LDL-induced injury. *Journal of the Federation of American Societies for Experimental Biology.* 11(3): A122/#713.

———. 1997. Garlic compounds protect vascular endothelial cells from oxidized low-density lipoprotein-induced injury. *Journal of Pharmacy and Pharmacology.* 49:908–11

Ide, N, AB Nelson, and BHS Lau. 1997. Aged garlic extract and its constituents inhibit Cu+2-induced oxidative modification of low-density lipoprotein. *Planta Medica.* 63:263–4.

Imai, K, K Nakachi. 1995. Cross-sectional study of effects of drinking green tea on cardiovascular and liver diseases. *British Medical Journal.* 310:693–6.

Kawashima, Y, et al. 1989. Clinical study of kyoleopin for hyperlipemic patients. Treatment and new drug. *Shinryou-to-Shinyaku.* 26:377–388.

Lau, BHS, et al. 1987. Effect of an odor-modified garlic preparation on blood lipids. *Nutrition Research.* 7:139–149, 1987.

Law, M. 2000. Plant sterol and stanol margarines and health. *British Medical Journal.* 320:861–4.

Lovegrove, JA, et al. 2004. Moderate fish-oil supplementation reverses low-platelet, long-chain n-3 polyunsaturated fatty acid status and reduces plasma triacylglycerol concentrations in British Indo-Asians. *American Journal of Clinical Nutrition.* 79:974–82.

Morcos, NC. 1997. Modulation of lipid profile by fish oil and garlic combination. *Journal of the National Medical Association.* 89:673–8.

Mozaffarian, D, et al. 2006. Trans fatty acids and cardiovascular disease. *New England Journal of Medicine.* 354(15):1601–13.

Muggeo, M, et al. 1995. Serum retinol levels throughout 2 years of cholesterol-lowering therapy. *Metabolism.* 44:398–403.

Nakamura, N, et al. 1999. Joint effects of HMG-CoA reductase inhibitors and eicosapentaenoic acids on serum lipid profile and plasma fatty acid concentrations in patients with hyperlipidemia. *International Journal of Clinical and Laboratory Research.* 29:22–5.

Pasternak, RC, et al. 2002. ACC/AHA/NHLBI clinical advisory on the use and safety of statins. *Journal of the American College of Cardiology.* 40(3):567–72.

Pearlman, BL. 2002. The new cholesterol guidelines. Applying them in clinical practice. *Postgraduate Medicine.* 112(2):13–26.

Ros, E, et al. 2004. A walnut diet improves endothelial function in hypercholesterolemic subjects: A randomized crossover trial. *Circulation.* 109(13):1609–14.

Rundek, T, et al. 2004. Atorvastatin decreases the coenzyme Q10 level in the blood of patients at risk for cardiovascular disease and stroke. *Archives of Neurology.* 61:889–92.

Steiner, M., et al. 1996. A double-blind crossover study in moderately hypercholesteremic men that compared the effect of aged garlic extract and placebo administration on blood lipids. *American Journal of Clinical Nutrition.* 64: 866–870.

Von Schacky, C, et al. 1999. The effect of dietary omega-3 fatty acids on coronary atherosclerosis. A randomized, double-blind, placebo-controlled trial. *Annals of Internal Medicine.* 130:554–62.

Ye, P, et al. 2007. Effect of xuezhikang on cardiovascular events and mortality in elderly patients with a history of myocardial infarction: A subgroup analysis of elderly subjects from the China Coronary Secondary Prevention Study. *Journal of the American Geriatrics Society.* 55:1015–22.

Yeh, YY, et al. 1997. Garlic reduces cholesterol in hypocholesterolemic men maintaining habitual diets. In *Food Factors for Cancer Prevention.* H Ohigashi, et al, eds. (Tokyo: Springer-Verlag), 226–30.

11

Common Cold Drugs and Their Natural Alternatives

What Is the Common Cold?

The common cold is an acute infection of the upper respiratory tract caused by any of more than 200 viruses. Symptoms can vary but commonly include runny nose, fatigue, cough, sore throat, nasal congestion, sneezing, mild fever, mild headache, and watery eyes. Symptoms usually begin one to three days after exposure to the virus, which is transmitted by respiratory droplets (sneezing or coughing).

Several different over-the-counter medications are used by millions of people each year to reduce symptoms of a cold. In our experience, natural medicine not only helps cold sufferers to recover from a cold quicker but also can reduce people's susceptibility to becoming infected with a cold.

Common Cold Drugs

Analgesics

Aspirin (Bayer, Ecotrin, Bufferin)

Ibuprofen (Motrin, Advil)

Acetaminophen (Tylenol)

HOW DO THESE DRUGS WORK?

These are all nonsteroidal anti-inflammatory drugs, except acetaminophen, which reduce fever and have an analgesic effect that helps with mild to moderate pain. Pain, fever, and inflammation are promoted by the release of chemicals called prostaglandins. NSAIDs block the enzyme that makes prostaglandins (cyclooxygenase), resulting in lower levels of prostaglandins. As a result, inflammation, pain, and fever are reduced. The exact mechanism of acetaminophen is not known, but it increases the body's pain threshold and reduces fever through its action on the heat-regulating center of the brain.

WHAT ARE THE BENEFITS?

Reduced fever and minor aches that accompany a cold.

POTENTIAL SIDE EFFECTS

Most patients benefit from short-term use of NSAIDs and acetaminophen with a low risk of side effects. Serious side effects tend to be dose-related, and therefore one should use the lowest dose possible. The most common side effects of aspirin involve the digestive system (ulcerations, abdominal burning, pain, cramping, nausea, gastritis, and even serious gastrointestinal bleeding and liver toxicity) and ringing in the ears. Rash, kidney impairment, vertigo, and light-headedness can also occur. Aspirin should be avoided by patients with peptic ulcer disease or kidney disease. Aspirin can increase blood uric acid levels and should be avoided in patients with hyperuricemia (high blood uric acid levels) and gout. Talk with your doctor about discontinuing aspirin therapy before surgery due to its blood-thinning properties.

The most common side effects from ibuprofen are rash, ringing in the ears, headaches, dizziness, drowsiness, and digestive symptoms (abdominal pain, nausea, diarrhea, constipation and heartburn, ulceration of the stomach or intestines).

Side effects from acetaminophen are rare. Liver damage may occur with higher doses or when it is combined with alcohol or other drugs that affect liver function.

MAJOR CAUTIONS

Aspirin: Children and teenagers should avoid aspirin for flu or chicken pox symptoms because of the associated risk of Reye's syndrome, a serious disease of the liver and nervous system that can lead to coma. Talk with your doctor about discontinuing aspirin therapy before surgery due to its blood-thinning properties. Another possible complication of aspirin use is gastrointestinal bleeding. It can also cause kidney and liver toxicity.

Ibuprofen: Increased risk of ulceration of the stomach or intestinal bleeding. NSAIDs reduce the ability of blood to clot and therefore increase bleeding after an injury. NSAIDs reduce the flow of blood to the kidneys and impair function of the kidneys and should be avoided by those with kidney disease or congestive heart failure. Individuals with asthma are more likely to experience allergic reactions to ibuprofen and other NSAIDs. There is also an increased risk of water retention, blood clots, heart attacks, high blood pressure, and heart failure.

KNOWN DRUG INTERACTIONS

Aspirin should be avoided in patients taking blood-thinning medications such as warfarin (Coumadin), because of an increased risk of bleeding. Asthma patients can have worsening of breathing while taking aspirin. It can also increase the effect of diabetic medications resulting in abnormally low blood sugar levels.

Ibuprofen can interact negatively with lithium (Eskalith); high blood pressure medications; antibiotics such as aminoglycosides, for example, gentamicin (Garamycin); and blood-thinning medications such as warfarin (Coumadin).

Acetaminophen can have a reduced effect when combined with carbamazepine (Tegretol), isoniazid (INH, Nydrazid, Laniazid), rifampin (Rifamate, Rifadin, Rimactane), or cholestyramine (Questran). Acetaminophen should not be combined with alcohol or other drugs that have a high potential for liver damage. Large doses or prolonged use of acetaminophen should be avoided during warfarin (Coumadin) therapy.

FOOD OR SUPPLEMENT INTERACTIONS

Aspirin: The use of ginkgo biloba, vitamin E, fish oil, or coleus forskoli may increase the risk of bleeding while on aspirin therapy since they have blood-thinning effects. Alcohol should be avoided while using aspirin, as it has a blood-thinning effect and can erode the stomach lining.

The use of DGL (deglycyrrhizinated licorice) and zinc carnosine while using aspirin may prevent ulceration and bleeding of the lining of the digestive tract.

NUTRIENT DEPLETION/IMBALANCE

Folic acid, vitamin C, vitamin B12, and zinc can become deficient from aspirin use. We recommend the following supplements:

- Folic acid—take 400 mcg daily.
- Vitamin C—take 500 mg daily.
- B12—take 100 to 200 mcg daily.
- Zinc—take 15 mg daily.
- DGL—chew one 300-mg tablet twice daily before meals.
- Zinc carnosine—take 75 mg twice daily.

Topical Nasal Decongestants

Oxymetazoline (Afrin)

Phenylephrine (4-Way Fast Acting, Afrin Children's Pump Mist, Ah-chew

D, Little Colds, Little Noses Gentle Formula, Infants & Children, Neo-Synephrine 4-Hour, Rhinall, Vicks Sinex Ultra Fine Mist)

HOW DO THESE DRUGS WORK?

These topical nasal decongestants constrict blood vessels in your nose and sinuses, which improves drainage and decreased congestion.

WHAT ARE THE BENEFITS?

Decreased nasal congestion within a short period of time (a few minutes).

POTENTIAL SIDE EFFECTS

Burning, stinging, dryness, or irritation of the nose.

MAJOR CAUTIONS

Dizziness, fainting spells, difficulty breathing, irregular heartbeat, palpitations, chest pain, and swelling of the inside of the nose.

KNOWN DRUG INTERACTIONS

- Atropine
- Bromocriptine (Parlodel)
- Linezolid (Zyvox)
- Maprotiline (Ludiomil)
- Antidepressants
- Migraine medications
- High blood pressure medications
- Oxytocin
- Vasopressin

FOOD OR SUPPLEMENT INTERACTIONS

None known.

NUTRIENT DEPLETION/IMBALANCE

None known.

Oral Decongestants

Pseudoephedrine (Sudafed)

Phenylephrine (Sudafed PE)

Note: Phenylephrine and pseudoephedrine are both decongestants. Until recently, pseudoephedrine has been the more commonly used decongestant in many nonprescription cold and allergy medications. However, pseudoephedrine is also a key ingredient in making methamphetamine, a highly addictive illegal stimulant. Federal law now requires all nonprescription medications containing pseudo-ephedrine to be unavailable over the counter and kept behind the counter in the pharmacy. To purchase pseudoephedrine, one must show some form of government-issued identification and sign a logbook. Most products have been or are being reformulated with phenylephrine.

Pseudoephedrine and chlorpheniramine (Deconamine)

HOW DO THESE DRUGS WORK?

Pseudoephedrine and phenylephrine are nasal decongestants that relieve nasal or sinus congestion.

Deconamine is a combination of a decongestant (pseudoephedrine) and the antihistamine chlorpheniramine, which dries nasal and eye secretions.

WHAT ARE THE BENEFITS?

These medications can provide quick relief from a runny nose, sneezing, and nasal congestion.

POTENTIAL SIDE EFFECTS

Pseudoephedrine/phenylephrine: Overstimulation of the nervous system can result in difficulty sleeping, headache (mild), loss of appetite, nausea, stomach upset, restlessness, or nervousness.

Deconamine: In addition to the potential side effects listed above for pseu-doephedrine, the antihistamine in deconamine may cause drowsiness, rash, hives, perspiration, chills, dry mouth or throat, low blood counts, restlessness, ringing in the ears, stomach upset, and urinary frequency or difficulty.

Cold Medicine Ban

In October 2007 the U.S. Food and Drug Administration advisory panel had two days of hearings to consider banning the sale of over-the-counter cough and cold medicines for young children. The previous month, FDA safety experts published a 365-page report showing that decongestants and antihistamines have been linked with 123 pediatric deaths since 1969. Subsequently, leading drug makers announced a vol-untary withdrawal of oral cough and cold medicines marketed for use in infants. The FDA also announced that the makers of almost 200 unap-proved prescription medicines containing hydrocodone, a narcotic that is used to ease pain and cough, must cease making these products for chil-dren under age 6.

MAJOR CAUTIONS

Pseudoephedrine/phenylephrine:

- Bloody diarrhea and abdominal pain
- Chest pain
- Confusion
- Dizziness or fainting spells
- Hallucinations
- Numbness or tingling in the hands or feet
- Rapid or troubled breathing
- Seizures (convulsions)

Deconamine:

- Impaired ability to drive or operate machinery
- Worsening of glaucoma or asthma or chronic lung disease

KNOWN DRUG INTERACTIONS

Pseudoephedrine/phenylephrine:

- Ammonium chloride
- Amphetamine or other stimulant drugs
- Bicarbonate, citrate, or acetate products such as sodium bicarbonate, sodium acetate, sodium citrate, sodium lactate, and potassium citrate
- Bromocriptine
- Caffeine
- Furazolidone
- Linezolid
- Medicines for colds and breathing difficulties
- Diabetic medications
- Antidepressant MAO inhibitors, such as phenelzine (Nardil), tranylcypromine (Parnate), isocarboxazid (Marplan), and selegiline (Carbex, Eldepryl)
- Migraine medications
- Procarbazine
- Some medicines for chest pain, heart disease, high blood pressure, or heart rhythm problems
- Some medicines for weight loss, including some herbal products, ephedrine, or dextroamphetamine
- St. John's wort

- Theophylline
- Thyroid hormones

Deconamine should not be taken with MAO inhibitor antidepressant drugs. It should not be combined with other drugs containing pseudoephedrine such as Sudafed due to cardiovascular risks such as hypertension.

FOOD OR SUPPLEMENT INTERACTIONS

Avoid caffeine as found in chocolate, tea, and coffee. Tannin-rich foods that may interfere with the absorption of pseudoephedrine include green tea, black tea, uva ursi, black walnut, red raspberry, oak, and witch hazel.

NUTRIENT DEPLETION/IMBALANCE

None known.

Antihistamines

Diphenhydramine (Benadryl)

Brompheniramine (Dimetapp)

Chlorpheniramine (Chlor-Trimeton)

HOW DO THESE DRUGS WORK?

These medications have an antihistamine effect that has a drying effect on cells that secrete mucus and reduce sneezing.

WHAT ARE THE BENEFITS?

They dry mucus and reduce sneezing.

POTENTIAL SIDE EFFECTS

Drowsiness, dizziness, dry mouth, headache, loss of appetite, stomach upset, nausea, vomiting, diarrhea, or constipation

MAJOR CAUTIONS

- Agitation
- Nervousness
- Insomnia
- Blurred vision
- Fainting spells
- Irregular heartbeat, palpitations, or chest pain
- Muscle or facial twitches
- Pain or difficulty passing urine
- Seizures

KNOWN DRUG INTERACTIONS

- Alcohol
- Barbiturate medicines for inducing sleep or treating seizures (convulsions)
- Doxercalciferol
- Medicines for anxiety or sleeping problems, such as diazepam or temazepam
- Medicines for hay fever and other allergies
- Antidepressant medications
- Medicines for movement abnormalities as in Parkinson's disease, or for gastrointestinal problems

FOOD OR SUPPLEMENT INTERACTIONS

Do not combine with alcohol.

NUTRIENT DEPLETION/IMBALANCE

None known.

Mucus Thinner

Guaifenesin (Robitussin, Humibid, Humibid LA, Organidin NR, Fenesin)

HOW DO THESE DRUGS WORK?

Guaifenesin is a mucus thinner.

WHAT ARE THE BENEFITS?

As an expectorant, it is used to decrease mucus in the sinuses, lungs, and ears.

POTENTIAL SIDE EFFECTS

Side effects are not common. In doses higher than those typically used, nausea, vomiting, diarrhea, abdominal pain, or drowsiness may occur.

MAJOR CAUTIONS

At doses higher than normally recommended, one may experience nausea, vomiting, diarrhea, abdominal pain, or drowsiness.

KNOWN DRUG INTERACTIONS

None known.

FOOD OR SUPPLEMENT INTERACTIONS

None known.

NUTRIENT DEPLETION/IMBALANCE

None known.

Cough Suppressants

Dextromethorphan (component of over 100 cough and cold formulas including Benylin, Delsym, Pertussin, Robitussin)

HOW DO THESE DRUGS WORK?

Dextromethorphan acts on the brain to suppress the cough reflex.

WHAT ARE THE BENEFITS?

Reduced coughing.

POTENTIAL SIDE EFFECTS

- Dizziness
- Drowsiness
- Fatigue
- Nausea, vomiting
- Skin rash (not common)
- Stomachache

MAJOR CAUTIONS

- Confusion
- Restlessness or irritability
- Severe nausea, vomiting
- Slurred speech
- Seizures
- Shaky movements
- Slow or troubled breathing

KNOWN DRUG INTERACTIONS

- Alcohol
- Amiodarone
- Barbiturates
- Certain medicines for mental depression, anxiety, or other mental disturbances
- Furazolidone

Dextromethorphan Recreational Drug Use

Dextromethorphan is abused as a recreational drug, as it can give one a high sensation. It is considered safe in doses of 15 to 30 mg. Doses over 100 mg can cause side effects such as hallucinations.

- MAO inhibitors, such as phenelzine (Nardil), tranylcypromine (Parnate), isocarboxazid (Marplan), and selegiline (Carbex, Eldepryl)
- Linezolid
- Quinidine
- Sibutramine
- Sleeping pills or tranquilizers
- Terbinafine

FOOD OR SUPPLEMENT INTERACTIONS

None known.

NUTRIENT DEPLETION/IMBALANCE

None known.

Natural Alternatives to Common Cold Drugs

Diet and Lifestyle Changes

Drink plenty of water to remain hydrated and prevent dehydration. Herbal teas such as ginger and peppermint are great choices as well. Chicken soup and broths containing ginger, onions, and garlic help to drain the sinuses. Avoid simple sugars as found in soda pop, white bread and pastas, and candy, which can suppress immunity. Also limit dairy products, which may increase mucus. For nasal congestion use a humidifier. Lastly, make sure to get at least eight hours of sleep a night.

Reducing Cold Symptoms

Contrary to what the media and many doctors state, we find that natural therapies can on average shorten and decrease the symptoms of the common cold. In addition, since natural therapies often work by boosting immunity, we have observed that they help patients with colds to be less susceptible to complications of an upper respiratory tract infection such as bronchitis, sinusitis, and pneumonia.

Andrographis

This medicinal plant is native to India, and extracts made from it are available in the United States in health food stores. Several double-blind trials have shown that andrographis reduces the severity of symptoms in people with a cold. In a randomized, double-blind study, a group of 158 adults of both sexes with the common cold were given andrographis extract (1,200 mg a day) or placebo for five days. Patients filled out a symptom evaluation report at days zero, two, and four of the treatment. Researchers found great effectiveness in reducing the prevalence and intensity of the symptoms in uncomplicated common colds beginning at day two of treatment. No adverse effects were observed or reported. Other double-blind trials have shown benefit from andrographis when taken for the common cold. It has also been shown to be effective in preventing the common cold when taken continuously for two months.

DOSAGE

For treatment of the common cold, take 400 mg three times daily. For prevention of the common cold, take 200 mg daily.

SAFETY

Andrographis is generally well tolerated. Digestive upset may occur in some users. It should be used with caution by those who have ulcers or heartburn.

Echinacea

Studies of this popular immune-boosting herb for the treatment of upper respiratory tract infections have been mixed. A closer look at the data suggests that products that have standardization for key active constituents are most effective. For example, one randomized, double-blind clinical study involved 120 patients with initial symptoms of a cold. Participants took 20 drops of echinacea every two hours for the first day (and thereafter three times daily) or a placebo. After ten days, participants were questioned about the intensity of their illness, time to improvement, and time until cessation of treatment. The time taken to improve was significantly shorter in the echinacea group at four days, while those on placebo took an average of eight days to recover. No specific adverse events were reported.

A 2007 meta-analysis of 14 studies, published in *Lancet Infectious Disease*s, evaluated the effect of echinacea on the incidence and duration of the common cold. Researchers found after reviewing the data that echinacea decreased the odds of developing the common cold by 58 percent, and the duration of a cold by 1.4 days.

DOSAGE

Take 500 mg or 2 ml of the extract four times daily or as directed on the label.

Echinacea—Not Just for Colds

Echinacea has a long tradition among Native Americans of the Plains. They used this herb for infections, wounds, and even rattlesnake bites! In the late 1800s, settlers acquired medicinal knowledge from Native Americans. Today potent standardized versions are available. While media headlines state that echinacea is ineffective for the common cold, the truth is that studies using standardized doses of echinacea at therapeutic levels demonstrate convincingly that it is effective. Considering that conventional medicine has little to offer to treat the viruses that cause the common cold, this is good news.

SAFETY

Those with autoimmune diseases should consult with their doctor before supplementing echinacea. It should be avoided by those on immune-suppressant medications.

Vitamin C

This immune-enhancing vitamin has been the subject of controversy for several years regarding the prevention and treatment of the common cold. Vitamin C is important for proper white blood cell function as well as production of the antiviral chemical interferon. Studies have been mixed in showing its effectiveness of treating the common cold.

Australian and Finnish scientists analyzed data from 30 studies involving 11,350 participants to determine the effects of taking 200 mg or more daily of vitamin C on the prevention and treatment of colds. In the general population, vitamin C did not reduce the risk of catching a cold. However, people who were taking vitamin C when they contracted a cold experienced slight reductions in the duration and severity of their illness, compared to those taking a placebo. Among marathoners, skiers, and soldiers exposed to significant physical stress or frigid weather, participants who took vitamin C contracted 50 percent fewer colds.

A previous review of 21 controlled trials using 1 to 8 grams found that vitamin C reduced the duration of episodes and the severity of the symptoms of the common cold by an average of 23 percent.

DOSAGE

Take 1,000 mg two to four times daily.

SAFETY

Vitamin C may cause loose stool. Those with a history of kidney stones should check with their physician before supplementing vitamin C.

American Ginseng

At the University of Alberta, researchers conducted a randomized, double-blind, placebo-controlled study during the winter season. A total of 323 participants 18 to 65 years of age with a history of at least two colds in the previous year were recruited. The participants were instructed to take two capsules (400 mg) per day of either the North American ginseng extract or a placebo for a period of four months. The number of colds and cold symptoms was tracked. The total symptom score was 31.0 percent lower, and the total number of days that symptoms were reported was 34.5 percent less in the ginseng group than in the placebo group over the four-month intervention period. In addition, the ginseng extract was found to reduce the duration of a cold by 2.4 days.

Lomatium Dissectum

This herb has a rich history of use by Native Americans and naturopathic physicians for the treatment of upper respiratory tract infections and viral infections. Preliminary studies demonstrate that it has immune-boosting and antiviral properties. While we are unaware of formal studies, we have found it to be quite effective for reducing the severity and length of the common cold.

DOSAGE

Take 500 mg of the capsule form or 2 ml of the tincture four times daily.

SAFETY

Some users experience a body rash from lomatium, which clears up a few days after stopping it.

Zinc

Zinc lozenges have been shown to decrease the duration of the common cold in adults but not in children. Zinc supports normal immune function and interferes with viral replication. Positive studies have used zinc lozenges containing zinc gluconate, zinc gluconate-glycine, and most of all, zinc acetate.

DOSAGE

Take a lozenge containing 9 to 25 mg of zinc (acetate, gluconate, or gluconate-glycine) every two waking hours for up to seven days. Zinc lozenges work best when used at the first symptoms of a cold.

Relief from Cold Symptoms

Sore throat, runny nose, fatigue have you feeling down as the result of a cold? Natural therapies as described in this chapter can give you some quick relief. The key is taking the described medicines as recommended. We find that most people using natural remedies for the common cold generally take too low a dosage, whether it be echinacea or vitamin C. Higher doses of these natural supplements for short periods of time are quite safe for most people.

SAFETY

Zinc lozenges are very safe when used short term for the treatment of a cold. Digestive upset may occur in some users.

References

Caceres, DD, et al. 1997. Prevention of common colds with Andrographis Paniculata dried extract: A pilot, double-blind trial. *Phytomedicine.* 4:101–4.

———. 1999. Use of visual analogue scale measurements (VAS) to assess the effectiveness of standardized Andrographis paniculata extract SHA-10 in reducing the symptoms of common cold. A randomized, double-blind, placebo study. *Phytomedicine.* 6:217–23.

Douglas, RM, et al. 2007. Vitamin C for preventing and treating the common cold. *Cochrane Database of Systematic Reviews.* July;18(3):CD000980.

Hemilä, H. 1994. Does vitamin C alleviate the symptoms of the common cold?—a review of current evidence. *Scandinavian Journal of Infectious Diseases.* 26:1–6.

Hoheisel, O, et al. 1997. Echinagard treatment shortens the course of the common cold: A double blind, placebo-controlled clinical trial. *European Journal of Clinical Research.* 9:261–268.

Predy, GN, et al. 2005. Efficacy of an extract of North American ginseng containing poly-furanosyl-pyranosyl-saccharides for preventing upper respiratory tract infections: A randomized controlled trial. *Canadian Medical Association Journal.* 173:1043–8.

Shah, SA, et al. 2007. Evaluation of echinacea for the prevention and treatment of the common cold: A meta-analysis. *Lancet Infectious Diseases.* July;7(7):473–80.

12

Depression Drugs and Their Natural Alternatives

What Is Depression?

Depression is a condition that affects one's thoughts, feelings, moods, behavior, and physical health. It's a disorder that can interfere with daily life. Depression causes pain for those with the disorder and those who are close to them. There are two classic of symptoms of depression. One is a loss of interest in normal daily activities that one usually enjoys. The other is a depressed mood in which one feels sad and hopeless, and may have frequent episodes of crying. Additional symptoms that are usually present for two weeks or more include sleep problems, impaired concentration or memory, weight changes (weight gain or weight loss), restlessness or agitation, fatigue, low self-esteem, decreased interest in sex, and persistent thoughts of death or suicide. One may also experience anxiety along with depression. In addition, a variety of physical complaints may be caused by depression such as headache, backache, or digestive upset. It should be noted that the Food and Drug Administration requires a warning that antidepressant medications can sometimes cause or increase thoughts of suicide.

Depression is thought to affect approximately 10 percent of the U.S. population in any given year. At some point in their lives, 10 to 25 percent of women and 5 to 12 percent of men will become clinically depressed. It is twice as common in women and is the leading cause of disability for women. Men with depression are three times more likely to commit suicide than women.

Childhood and adolescent depression is common, too, and should be taken seriously. Childhood and teenage depression may show different symptoms such as pretending to be sick, refusing to go to school, or exhibiting behavior problems. Studies show that childhood depression tends to be a predictor of more severe illnesses in adulthood.

The main types of depression include:

Major depression

Dysthymia

Adjustment disorders

Bipolar disorder

Seasonal affective disorder (SAD)

Postpartum depression

Major Depression

This type lasts more than two weeks with symptoms that may include overwhelming feelings of sadness and grief, loss of interest or pleasure in activities that are normally pleasurable, and feelings of worthlessness or guilt. Physical ailments may accompany this type of depression such as insomnia, appetite change, fatigue, and difficulty concentrating.

Dysthymia

This is a less severe but more chronic form of depression. It is usually not disabling. One can have periods of feeling well. Those with dysthymia are at increased risk of major depression.

Adjustment Disorder

This is a when the response to a stressful event(s) or situation(s) causes signs and symptoms of depression or anxiety. This condition is considered chronic when it lasts for six months or longer.

Bipolar Disorder

This is characterized by recurring episodes of depression and mania (elation). It is also known as manic-depressive disorder.

Seasonal Affective Disorder (SAD)

This type of depression occurs as a result of reduced exposure to sunlight. It is therefore more common in the fall and winter months. Common symptoms include depression and fatigue.

Postpartum Depression

It is estimated that 10 to 15 percent of women experience postpartum depression after giving birth. Hormonal changes may be at the root of this condition.

Depression Drugs

Selective Serotonin Reuptake Inhibitors (SSRIs)

Citalopram (Celexa)

Escitalopram (Lexapro)

Fluoxetine tablets or capsules (Prozac)

Fluvoxamine (Luvox)

Paroxetine (Paxil, Paxil CR, Pexeva)

Sertraline (Zoloft)

HOW DO THESE DRUGS WORK?

These drugs block the reuptake of serotonin so that it remains active in the brain longer before being broken down and reabsorbed. The neurotransmitter serotonin gives one the sensation of well-being.

WHAT ARE THE BENEFITS?

Improvement in depression, generally with fewer side effects than with other categories of antidepressants. SSRIs have fewer side effects than the tricyclic antidepressants and monoamine oxidase (MAO) inhibitors, which we discuss below. Unlike MAO inhibitors, SSRIs do not interact with the amino acid tyramine found in certain foods. Also, SSRIs do not cause orthostatic hypotension and heart rhythm disturbances, as tricyclic antidepressants can. SSRIs are often the first-line pharmaceutical choice for depression.

POTENTIAL SIDE EFFECTS

- Nausea
- Diarrhea
- Agitation
- Insomnia
- Decreased sexual desire
- Delayed orgasm or inability to have an orgasm

MAJOR CAUTIONS

Tremors can be a side effect of SSRIs. Serotonergic syndrome, in which serotonin levels are too high, is a serious but rare condition associated with the use of SSRIs. Symptoms can include high fevers, seizures, and heart rhythm disturbances.

There is an association between bone loss and the use of SSRIs with older men and women. Suicidal thoughts or increased risk of suicide may occur from these medications.

KNOWN DRUG INTERACTIONS

- Astemizole (Hismanal)
- Cisapride (Propulsid)
- Pimozide (Orap)
- Terfenadine (Seldane)
- Thioridazine (Mellaril)
- MAO inhibitors such as phenelzine (Nardil), tranylcypromine (Parnate), isocarboxazid (Marplan), selegiline (Eldepryl)

FOOD OR SUPPLEMENT INTERACTIONS

Alcohol can increase the effect of drowsiness and dizziness associated with these medications, and should be avoided.

The following supplements increase levels of neurotransmitter such as serotonin. The combined effect with antidepressants may be too much, and they should be avoided.

- 5-HTP
- L-tryptophan
- St. John's wort

NUTRIENT DEPLETION/IMBALANCE

In one study, women taking 500 mcg of folic acid daily in addition to fluoxetine (Prozac) experienced significant improvement in their symptoms and had fewer side effects compared to women taking the drug only.

Fluoxetine (Prozac) has been shown to significantly lower melatonin levels. It has not been determined whether simultaneous supplementation is appropriate.

Ginkgo biloba extract has been shown to reduce sexual side effects in those taking SSRIs in both elderly men and women. Participants in the study used 200 to 240 mg of ginkgo biloba extract.

Selective Serotonin and Norepinephrine Reuptake Inhibitors (SNRIs)

Duloxetine (Cymbalta)

Venlafaxine (Effexor)

HOW DO THESE DRUGS WORK?

SNRIs work mainly by increasing the amounts of two neurotransmitters, serotonin and norepinephrine, in the brain. This improves alertness, energy, mood, and motivation.

WHAT ARE THE BENEFITS?

These drugs can be effective for severe and chronic cases of depression.

POTENTIAL SIDE EFFECTS

- Abdominal (stomach) pain or tenderness
- Itching
- Rash
- Dry mouth
- Constipation
- Dizziness
- Drowsiness
- Headache
- Increased sweating or flushing
- Loss of appetite, loss of weight
- Loss of sexual desire, erectile, or orgasm dysfunction
- Nausea
- Weakness or tiredness
- Weight gain or weight loss

MAJOR CAUTIONS

- Dark or brown urine
- Difficulty breathing
- Fainting spells
- Mania (overactive behavior), inability to sleep
- Restlessness, inability to sleep, or severe loss of sleep
- Suicidal thoughts
- Unexplained flulike symptoms
- Vomiting

- Yellowing of the skin or whites of the eyes
- Increased blood pressure
- Seizures

KNOWN DRUG INTERACTIONS

Do not take while on MAO inhibitors or Haldol for at least two weeks after their discontinuation. Caution should be used when taking this medication with the heart drug Lanoxin and the blood thinner Coumadin.

FOOD OR SUPPLEMENT INTERACTIONS

Do not combine with these medications, which can increase neurotransmitter levels:

- 5-hydroxytryptophan (5-HTP)
- L-tryptophan
- Sour date nut (*Ziziphus jujube*)
- St. John's wort

NUTRIENT DEPLETION/IMBALANCE

None known.

Tricyclic Antidepressants (TCAs)

This older group of antidepressants is used to treat depression and other mental conditions such as obsessive-compulsive disorder, panic attacks, post-traumatic stress disorder, attention deficit hyperactivity disorder, bed-wetting, and nerve pain.

Amitriptyline (Elavil, Endep, Vanatrip)

Amitriptyline injection (Elavil Injection, Vanatrip injection)

Amoxapine (Asendin)

Clomipramine (Anafranil)

Desipramine (Norpramin)

Doxepin (Adapin, Sinequan)

Imipramine (Tofranil)

Imipramine Pamoate (Tofranil PM)

Nortriptyline (Aventyl, Pamelor)

Nortriptyline Oral Solution (Aventyl Oral Solution)

Protriptyline (Vivactil)

HOW DO THESE DRUGS WORK?

TCAs work mainly by increasing the level of norepinephrine in the brain. They may also increase serotonin levels.

WHAT ARE THE BENEFITS?

They are used to treat moderate to severe depression.

POTENTIAL SIDE EFFECTS

- Blurred vision
- Constipation
- Dizziness
- Drowsiness
- Dry mouth
- Impaired sexual function
- Weight gain

MAJOR CAUTIONS

- Low blood pressure
- Glaucoma

KNOWN DRUG INTERACTIONS

These medications should not be combined with monoamine oxidase (MAO) inhibiting drugs as described in this chapter. Also, do not combine with epinephrine, and use caution when also taking cimetidine (Tagamet).

FOOD OR SUPPLEMENT INTERACTIONS

Do not combine with alcohol, as it can increase the side effects of drowsiness and dizziness associated with these medications.

NUTRIENT DEPLETION/IMBALANCE

The following nutrients may be depleted and should be supplemented while on these medications:

- Coenzyme Q10—take 100 to 200 mg daily
- Niacinamide
- Vitamin B1
- Vitamin B12
- Vitamin B2
- Vitamin B3
- Vitamin B5
- Vitamin B6

Take a B complex daily to guard against these potential B vitamin deficiencies.

Monoamine Oxidase Inhibitors (MAOIs)

Isocarboxazid (Marplan)

Phenelzine (Nardil)

Tranylcypromine (Parnate)

HOW DO THESE DRUGS WORK?

This group of antidepressants has been used since the 1950s. They increase the brain's level of neurotransmitters such as norepinephrine. They do this by inhibiting the enzyme monoamine oxidase that breaks down norepinephrine. Thus the amount of norepinephrine in the brain is increased.

WHAT ARE THE BENEFITS?

This class of drug can relieve depression as well as panic disorder and social phobias.

POTENTIAL SIDE EFFECTS

- Blurred vision or change in vision
- Constipation or diarrhea
- Difficulty sleeping
- Drowsiness or dizziness
- Dry mouth
- Increased appetite, weight increase
- Increased sensitivity to sunlight
- Muscle aches or pains, trembling
- Nausea or vomiting
- Sexual dysfunction
- Swelling of the feet or legs
- Tiredness or weakness

MAJOR CAUTIONS

MAOIs can impair the ability to break down tyramine, an amino acid found in aged cheese, wines, most nuts, chocolate, and some other foods. Like norepinephrine, tyramine can elevate blood pressure. MAOIs are not as commonly prescribed as other antidepressants. Other possible side effects:

- Agitation, excitability, restlessness, or nervousness
- Chest pain
- Confusion or changes in mental state
- Convulsions or seizures (uncommon)
- Difficulty breathing

- Difficulty passing urine
- Enlarged pupils, sensitivity of the eyes to light
- Fever, clammy skin, increased sweating
- Headache or increased blood pressure
- Light-headedness or fainting spells
- Muscle or neck stiffness or spasm
- Sexual dysfunction
- Slow, fast, or irregular heartbeat (palpitations)
- Sore throat and fever
- Yellowing of the skin or eyes

KNOWN DRUG INTERACTIONS

MAOIs can interact with over-the-counter cold and cough medications to cause dangerously high blood pressure.

FOOD OR SUPPLEMENT INTERACTIONS

- Aspartame
- Ephedra
- Scotch broom
- St. John's wort
- Tyramine-containing foods, which can elevate blood pressure when combined with these medications

NUTRIENT DEPLETION/IMBALANCE

Vitamin B6 may be depleted by these medications. Take 50 mg daily.

Atypical Antidepressants

The drugs in this class of antidepressants work in a variety of ways. They act like SSRIs and TCAs but have different mechanisms of action. Common examples include:

Bupropion (Wellbutrin)

Nefazodone (Serzone)

Trazodone (Desyrel)

Venlafaxine (Effexor)

HOW DO THESE DRUGS WORK?

Bupropion (Wellbutrin) works by inhibiting the reuptake of dopamine, serotonin, and norepinephrine and therefore increases the brain's levels of these neurotransmitters. This medication is unique in that its major effect is on dopamine.

Nefazodone (Serzone) works by inhibiting the reuptake of serotonin and norepinephrine and therefore increases the brain's levels of these neurotransmitters.

Trazodone's (Desyrel) mechanism is not exactly known but it likely inhibits the reuptake of serotonin and therefore increases the brain's level of this neurotransmitter.

Venlafaxine (Effexor) increases the brain's levels of serotonin and norepinephrine.

WHAT ARE THE BENEFITS?

These medications can relieve depression and offer treatment for people who do not respond to other pharmaceutical antidepressants.

POTENTIAL SIDE EFFECTS

Bupropion (Wellbutrin)

- Agitation
- Dry mouth
- Insomnia
- Headache
- Nausea
- Constipation
- Tremor
- Weight loss

Nefazodone (Serzone)

- Nausea
- Dizziness
- Insomnia
- Agitation
- Tiredness
- Dry mouth
- Constipation
- Light-headedness
- Blurred vision
- Confusion

Trazodone (Desyrel)

- Nausea
- Dizziness

- Insomnia
- Agitation
- Tiredness
- Dry mouth
- Constipation
- Light-headedness
- Headache
- Low blood pressure
- Blurred vision
- Confusion
- Impaired ejaculation, orgasm, and libido

Venlafaxine (Effexor)

- Nausea
- Headaches
- Anxiety
- Insomnia
- Drowsiness
- Loss of appetite
- Increased blood pressure

MAJOR CAUTIONS

Bupropion (Wellbutrin)

- Seizures
- Suicidal thinking and behavior
- Manic episodes or hallucinations

Nefazodone (Serzone)

- Rarely associated with priapism (prolonged penile erection) and blood clot formation within the penis
- Suicidal thinking and behavior

Trazodone (Desyrel)

- Priapism, a painful condition in which the penis or clitoris remains in an erect position for a prolonged period
- Suicidal thinking and behavior

Venlafaxine (Effexor)

- Suicidal thinking and behavior
- Confusion
- Seizures
- Mydriasis (prolonged dilation of the pupil of the eye)

KNOWN DRUG INTERACTIONS

Bupropion (Wellbutrin)

- Prochlorperazine (Compazine)
- Chlorpromazine (Thorazine) and other antipsychotic medications in the phenothiazine class
- During withdrawal from benzodiazepines, for example diazepam (Valium) or alprazolam (Xanax)
- Carbamazepine (Tegretol)
- Monoamine oxidase inhibitors
- Warfarin (Coumadin)

Nefazodone (Serzone)

- MAO inhibitor antidepressants, such as isocarboxazid (Marplan), phenelzine (Nardil), tranylcypromine (Parnate), and procarbazine (Matulane)
- Selegiline (Eldepryl)
- Fenfluramine (Pondimin), and dexfenfluramine (Redux)
- Terfenadine (Seldane)
- Triazolam (Halcion)
- Alprazolam (Xanax)
- Digoxin (Lanoxin)

Trazodone (Desyrel)

- MAO inhibitor antidepressants such as isocarboxazid (Marplan), phenelzine (Nardil), tranylcypromine (Parnate), and procarbazine (Matulane)
- Selegiline (Eldepryl)
- Digoxin (Lanoxin)
- Phenytoin (Dilantin)
- Carbamazepine (Tegretol)
- Ketoconazole (Nizoral)

- Ritonavir (Norvir)
- Indinavir (Crixivan)

Venlafaxine (Effexor)

- MAO inhibitor antidepressants such as isocarboxazid (Marplan), phenelzine (Nardil), tranylcypromine (Parnate), and procarbazine (Matulane)

FOOD OR SUPPLEMENT INTERACTIONS

Avoid the following:

- 5-hydroxytryptophan (5-HTP)
- L-tryptophan
- Sour date nut (*Ziziphus jujube*)
- St. John's wort

NUTRIENT DEPLETION/IMBALANCE

None known.

Natural Alternatives to Depression Drugs

Depression can be a life-threatening disorder and require medical supervision. Do not change your medication or treatment recommendations without the supervision of a medical professional.

Diet and Lifestyle Changes

One of the most important dietary considerations to prevent or improve depression is the balance of fats. The U.S. diet has an overabundance of saturated fats (as found in red meat and dairy products) and omega-6 fatty acids (polyunsaturated fatty acids) as found in vegetable cooking oils such as soy and corn oils. The brain is primarily composed of fatty acids and requires a constant dietary supply of omega-3 fatty acids. While omega-3 fatty acids are most recognized for their cardiovascular benefit, they are quite important for normal mood. Various studies, including a recent one in *Psychosomatic Medicine*, have demonstrated that a relative imbalance between omega-6 and omega-3 fatty acids is associated with symptoms of depression. Omega-3 fatty acids can be consumed through cold-water fish such as ocean salmon, sardines, and low-mercury-content tuna. Almonds, walnuts, pumpkin seeds, and flaxseeds are also healthy sources.

It is also important to reduce simple sugars in the diet, as they may worsen depression. Do eat regular meals so that blood sugar swings do not affect your mood. Avoid artificial sweeteners, which may aggravate depression in susceptible users.

Various studies have demonstrated that exercise is comparable in its benefit to that of depression drugs. Routine exercise (three hours a week) can profoundly reduce depression.

St. John's Wort

This herb has become very popular for the treatment of mild to moderate depression. Several studies have shown that extract of St. John's wort improves mood and decreases anxiety and insomnia related to mild to severe major depression. Even the American College of Physicians-American Society of Internal Medicine considers St. John's wort to be an option for short-term treatment of mild depression. Constituents in this herbal extract increase levels of the neurotransmitters serotonin, dopamine, and norepinephrine.

A variety of positive studies could be cited. A study published in the *British Medical Journal* reviewed 23 randomized clinical studies involving St. John's wort for depression. The researchers concluded that St. John's wort was equally as effective as pharmaceutical therapy for mild to moderate depression. Another double-blind, randomized, placebo-controlled study published in the *American Journal of Psychiatry* involved 186 patients given 300 mg of St. John's wort extract three times daily while 189 participants received a placebo for six weeks. Compared to placebo, St. John's wort was three times more effective in producing a significantly greater reduction in depression, and significantly more patients responded with treatment response or remission.

Another study published in *Pharmacopsychiatry* compared St. John's wort extract and paroxetine (Paxil) in patients suffering from moderate or severe depression. Both were similarly effective in preventing relapse in a continuation treatment after recovery from an episode of moderate to severe depression.

DOSAGE

Take 900 to 1,200 mg daily of a product standardized to 0.3 hypericin or 5 percent hyperforin.

SAFETY

Do not combine with the drug digitalis. It also should not be combined with pharmaceutical antidepressants or other medications that alter neurotransmitter levels. St.

Studies of St. John's Wort

One often cited study published in the *Journal of the American Medical Association* (*JAMA*) concluded that St. John's wort is not effective in treating major or severe cases of depression. It should be noted that St. John's wort has mainly been studied for the treatment of mild to moderate depression. Most practitioners do not use St. John's wort in treating severe depression. The placebo response in this study was very low, which brings into question the study design. In any event, one study on major depression cannot exclude the findings of over 25 positive studies.

John's wort may make the skin more sensitive to sunlight and therefore more susceptible to rashes and burns. We have not found this side effect to be common, but it is reported in the literature. It may also cause stomach upset, fatigue, itching, and sleep disturbance. It should be avoided by those with bipolar disease or those taking antiviral drugs to treat HIV. Other medications it should not be combined with include cyclosporine (Neoral, Sandimmune, SangCya), fexofenadine (Allegra), oral contraceptives, theophylline or aminophylline, omeprazole (Prilosec), or warfarin (Coumadin). St. John's wort should not be taken by those undergoing chemotherapy.

S-adenosylmethionine (SAMe)

This amino acid–like supplement has been shown in a variety of studies to be effective for the treatment of depression in several clinical trials. SAMe is a normal substance found in the body, including in the brain. It functions in the brain to make biochemical reactions possible for the formation of mood-elevating neurotransmitters such as serotonin and dopamine. Studies have shown SAMe to be comparable to tricyclic antidepressants for the treatment of depression. SAMe, a natural compound, is the most important methyl donor in the central nervous system. In several clinical trials, SAMe showed antidepressant activity. For example, a study published in the *American Journal of Clinical Nutrition* looked at the effect of SAMe for people diagnosed with major depressive episode. It involved two multicenter studies in which participants' depression was evaluated on the Hamilton Depression Rating. In the first study, 143 participants were given 1,600 mg daily of SAMe orally and 138 participants received 150 mg imipramine (Tofranil) orally per day for six weeks. In the second study, 147 participants received SAMe by injection and 148 received imipramine (Tofranil) for four weeks. In both studies, the positive results for both SAMe and imipramine (Tofranil) were about equal, but SAMe had significantly fewer side effects.

DOSAGE

For depression most studies used 1,600 mg daily. We have found that some patients get relief from depression at doses between 600 and 1,200 mg daily.

SAMe requires vitamins B12 and folic acid for proper metabolism. They can be taken as part of a high-potency multivitamin or B complex formulation.

SAFETY

SAMe is very safe. This has been confirmed even in studies using high doses intravenously. Users may rarely notice digestive upset such as loose stool, gas, or other digestive symptoms. It should not be taken with pharmaceutical antidepressants or Parkinson's medications unless a doctor instructs one to do so. It is recommended that it not be taken by those with bipolar disorder.

Dale, a 57-year-old carpenter, had suffered from moderate depression for several years. He had taken different pharmaceutical antidepressants but always discontinued them at some point due to side effects such as fatigue or dizziness. Wanting to try a safer, natural approach, he came to the clinic for a consultation. SAMe was recommended to him as a natural alternative, and within 10 days he noticed a nice uplift in his mood. Now ten months later, his depression continues to be alleviated and he still uses SAMe without side effects.

5-hydroxytryptophan (5-HTP)

5-hydroxytryptophan (5-HTP) has proven in our clinical experience to be effective for a high percentage of our patients with mild to moderate depression. The body manufactures 5-HTP from L-tryptophan, an amino acid found in food. The supplement 5-HTP is derived from the seeds of *Griffonia simplicifolia,* a West African plant. 5-HTP readily crosses the blood-brain barrier and increases synthesis of serotonin. 5-HTP has been shown to significantly improve symptoms of depression. One Japanese study of people with depression demonstrated that a daily dose of 150 to 300 mg of 5-HTP for three weeks was favorable in approximately 70 percent of participants.

DOSAGE

Take 150 to 300 mg daily in divided doses. 5-HTP should be taken on an empty stomach for best results.

SAFETY

5-HTP should not be combined with antidepressants or other serotonin-enhancing medications. It may cause digestive upset. 5-HTP should be avoided by those with Down's syndrome.

L-tryptophan is an amino acid that is a precursor to the formation of 5-HTP. L-tryptophan can also be used in the treatment of depression. We normally have patients supplement 5-HTP since it is closer in the biochemical pathway conversion to serotonin and is less expensive than L-tryptophan.

Fish Oil

The brain is composed of fats such as docosahexaenoic acid (DHA) that are required for normal function. As discussed above in the Diet and Lifestyle Changes section, omega-3 fatty acids are important for the prevention and treatment of depression. Since many people do not eat adequate amounts of omega-3 fatty acids, supplements of fish oil are desirable. Low blood levels of omega-3 fatty acids are associated with depression.

A study published in the *Archives of General Psychiatry* involved 70 patients with persistent depression despite ongoing treatment with an adequate dose of a standard antidepressant. Patients were randomized on a double-blind basis to placebo or fish oil at dosages of 1, 2, or 4 grams daily for 12 weeks in addition to unchanged medications. Researchers found that patients who took the lowest dose of fish oil at 1 gram daily showed significant improvements on all major measures of depression compared with those who took a placebo. More specifically, 69 percent of the patients who took the 1 gram dose had a 50 percent reduction in their symptoms, compared with only 25 percent of those who took a placebo.

Fish oil has also been shown in studies to be effective in the treatment of postpartum depression.

DOSAGE

Take 1 to 7 grams of combined EPA and DHA as found in fish oil.

SAFETY

Digestive upset such as burping, heartburn, or loose stool may occur from fish oil supplements. This may be improved by taking them with meals or using a hard-coated fish oil capsule. Fish oil has a blood-thinning effect, so check with your doctor before using it if you are on blood-thinning medications.

Vitamin B12 and Folic Acid

Deficiencies of these nutrients may cause symptoms of depression. Deficiencies of these nutrients are more common in vegetarians and seniors. A multivitamin may be sufficient to provide these nutrients and help depression. Researchers from the University of Sheffield assigned 225 older hospitalized patients (average age 75) to receive daily multivitamin and mineral supplements or a placebo along with the normal hospital diet. After six months, there was a significant increase in the number of patients with no symptoms of

---

Vitamin B12 Deficiency

Approximately 20 percent of seniors in the United States have a vitamin B12 deficiency. The ability to absorb this nutrient can diminish as people age. This certainly can predispose them to mood, fatigue, memory, and other problems. The solution is to take supplemental B12. The most effective method is either a B12 injection once monthly or the regular consumption of sublingual B12, which is absorbed in the veins underneath the tongue. Both techniques allow B12 to bypass the digestive tract for direct absorption into the bloodstream and cells.

depression in the supplement group (from 67 to 76 percent) compared to the placebo group and a decrease in patients with symptoms of mild (25 to 21 percent) or severe (8 to 3 percent) depression. Levels of folate and vitamin B12 increased significantly in those taking supplements and decreased in the placebo group.

References

Anghelescu, IG, et al. 2006. Comparison of Hypericum extract WS 5570 and paroxetine in ongoing treatment after recovery from an episode of moderate to severe depression: Results from a randomized multicenter study. *Pharmacopsychiatry.* November;39(6):213–9.

Blumenthal, JA, et al. 2007. Exercise and pharmacotherapy in the treatment of major depressive disorder. *Psychosomatic Medicine.* 69(7):587–96.

Childs, PA, et al. 1995. Effect of fluoxetine on melatonin in patients with seasonal affective disorder and matched controls. *British Journal of Psychiatry.* 166:196–8.

Cohen, AJ, B Bartlik. 1998. *Ginkgo biloba* for antidepressant-induced sexual dysfunction. *Journal of Sex and Marital Therapy.* 24:139–45.

Conklin, SM, et al. 2007. High omega-6 and low omega-3 fatty acids are associated with depressive symptoms and neuroticism. *Psychosomatic Medicine.* December;69(9): 932–4. Epub 2007 Nov. 8.

Coppen, A, J Bailey. 2000. Enhancement of the antidepressant action of fluoxetine by folic acid: A randomised, placebo-controlled trial. *Journal of Affective Disorders.* November;60(2):121–30.

Delle Chiaie, R, P Pancheri, and P Scapicchio. 2002. Efficacy and tolerability of oral and intramuscular S-adenosyl-L-methionine 1,4 butanedisulfonate (SAMe) in the treatment of major depression: Comparison with imipramine in two multicenter studies. *American Journal of Clinical Nutrition.* November;76(5):1172S–6S.

Gariballa, S, and S Forster. 2007. Effects of dietary supplements on depressive symptoms in older patients: A randomised double-blind placebo-controlled trial. *Clinical Nutrition.* 26(5):545–51.

Lecrubier, Y, et al. 2002. Efficacy of St. John's wort extract WS 5570 in major depression: A double-blind, placebo-controlled trial. *American Journal of Psychiatry.* August;159(8):1361–6.

Linde, K, et al. 1996. St. John's wort for depression—An overview and meta-analysis of randomized clinical trials. *British Medical Journal.* 313:253–58.

Maes, M, et al. 1999. Lowered omega-3 polyunsaturated fatty acids in serum phospholipids and cholesteryl esters of depressed patients. *Psychiatry Research.* 85:275–91.

Nakajima, T, Y Kudo, and Z Kaneko. 1978. Clinical evaluation of 5-hydroxy-L-tryptophan as an antidepressant drug. *Folia Psychiatrica et Neurologica Japonica.* 32:223–30.

Peet, M, DF Horrobin. 2002. A dose-ranging study of the effects of ethyl-eicosapen-taenoate in patients with ongoing depression despite apparently adequate treatment with standard drugs. *Archives of General Psychiatry.* October;59(10):913–9.

Shelton, RC, et al. 2001. Effectiveness of St. John's wort in major depression: A random-ized controlled trial. *Journal of the American Medical Association.* April 18;285(15): 1978–86.

Tiemeier, H, et al. 2003. P Plasma fatty acid composition and depression are associated in the elderly: The Rotterdam Study. *American Journal of Clinical Nutrition.* 78:40–6.

13

Diabetes Drugs and Their Natural Alternatives

What Is Diabetes?

Diabetes is a chronic disease that continues to increase in frequency for both children and adults in the United States. With diabetes, blood glucose levels are abnormally elevated. This is due to a deficiency of the glucose-transporting hormone insulin, or to the inability of the body's cells to properly utilize insulin. According to the American Diabetes Association, a whopping 7 percent (21 million) of the U.S. population has diabetes. One-third of people who have diabetes are unaware they have it and require testing to identify the disease. Pre-diabetes, the stage before type 2 diabetes, is very common, affecting up to 40 percent of the U.S. population. It is more commonly being identified and treated with diet, lifestyle changes, exercise, nutritional supplements, and pharmaceuticals.

Glucose is required for cell energy production. When glucose does not get into the cells, a host of health problems can occur. Following are signs and symptoms of diabetes:

- Increased thirst and frequent urination
- Extreme hunger
- Weight loss
- Fatigue
- Blurred vision
- Slow-healing sores or frequent infections

Types of Diabetes

Type 1 diabetes results from a deficiency of the hormone insulin. It is estimated that 5 to 10 percent of Americans who are diagnosed with diabetes have type 1 diabetes.

Type 2 diabetes results from insulin resistance, in which the cells do not readily accept insulin. In severe cases, insulin deficiency may occur as well.

Gestational diabetes occurs during pregnancy and affects about 4 percent of all pregnant women.

Pre-diabetes is a condition that occurs when a person's blood glucose levels are higher than normal but not at a level found with type 2 diabetes. This is estimated to affect up to 40 percent of the U.S. population.

Diabetes is diagnosed by blood tests. See the following tables:

FASTING PLASMA GLUCOSE TEST

Plasma Glucose Result (mg/dL)	Diagnosis
99 and below	Normal
100 to 125	Pre-diabetes (impaired fasting glucose)
126 and above	Diabetes

Another test is the oral glucose tolerance test (OGTT). After fasting, a person's glucose level is tested and then one drinks a glucose-rich beverage. Blood glucose levels are evaluated after two hours.

ORAL GLUCOSE TOLERANCE TEST

2-Hour Plasma Glucose Result (mg/dL)	Diagnosis
139 and below	Normal
140 to 199	Pre-diabetes (impaired glucose tolerance)
200 and above	Diabetes

It is important to screen for diabetes regularly and to monitor those with diabetes closely. Poor glucose control with diabetes can lead to complications such as:

- High blood sugar (hyperglycemia)
- Diabetic ketoacidosis (increased ketones in the urine)
- Low blood sugar (hypoglycemia)
- Heart and blood vessel disease
- Nerve damage (neuropathy)

- Kidney damage (nephropathy)
- Eye damage
- Foot damage
- Skin and mouth conditions
- Osteoporosis
- Increased risk of Alzheimer's disease

Diabetes Drugs

Alpha-glucosidase inhibitors

Acarbose (Precose)

Miglitol (Glyset)

HOW DO THESE DRUGS WORK?

These medications slow down the action of digestive enzymes that digest carbohydrates. This prevents the carbohydrates from being metabolized into sugar, which keeps blood sugar levels more normal after eating.

WHAT ARE THE BENEFITS?

Reduced blood sugar levels that are not controlled by diet and exercise.

POTENTIAL SIDE EFFECTS

- Abdominal pain
- Diarrhea
- Flatulence

Other possible but rare side effects are an increase in liver enzymes and a decrease in red blood cells.

MAJOR CAUTIONS

- Paralytic ileus (paralysis of a portion of the small intestine)
- Elevated liver enzymes
- Decreased hematocrit (red blood cells)

KNOWN DRUG INTERACTIONS

- Acetaminophen
- Charcoal
- Cholestyramine
- Colestipol

- Digoxin
- Neomycin
- Other diabetic medications (causing too-low glucose levels)
- Pancreatic enzymes, amylase, or other digestive enzyme supplements
- Ranitidine (Zantac) and propranolol (Inderal)
- Warfarin

FOOD OR SUPPLEMENT INTERACTIONS

Carbohydrate-blocking supplements such as phaseolamin, starch blockers, wheat amylase inhibitors, and white kidney bean extract.

NUTRIENT DEPLETION/IMBALANCE

- Calcium—take 500 mg daily.
- Vitamin B6—take 50 to 100 mg daily.

Glucose-lowering supplements such as chromium, vanadium, cinnamon extract, fenugreek, *Gymnema sylvestre*, bitter melon extract, ginseng, and others may enhance the effect of a diabetic medication. Check with your doctor before combining together.

Biguanides

Metformin (Glucophage)

Metformin Extended-Release (Fortamet, Glucophage XR, Glumetza)

HOW DO THESE DRUGS WORK?

The exact mechanism of this class of diabetic drugs is not known. They reduce insulin resistance in muscle cells and decrease the release of glucose from the liver. In addition, they reduce the absorption of glucose in the small intestine. Biguanides may also enhance insulin sensitivity inside the cell and stimulate the removal of glucose.

WHAT ARE THE BENEFITS?

Since biguanides do not stimulate insulin secretion, they do not cause low blood sugar (hypoglycemia). They can also benefit obese patients who require weight loss. They can also help women with polycystic ovary syndrome (PCOS) to induce ovulation.

POTENTIAL SIDE EFFECTS

One out of three users will experience one or more of the following symptoms:

- Nausea
- Vomiting

- Gas
- Bloating
- Diarrhea
- Loss of appetite

MAJOR CAUTIONS

Lactic acidosis is a rare but serious side effect that occurs in one out of every 30,000 patients. It is fatal in 50 percent of cases. Symptoms include weakness, trouble breathing, abnormal heartbeats, unusual muscle pain, stomach discomfort, light-headedness, and feeling cold.

KNOWN DRUG INTERACTIONS

- Alcohol
- Cephalexin (Keflex, Keftab)
- Cimetidine (Tagamet)
- Digoxin (Lanoxin)
- Dofetilide (Tikosyn)
- Entecavir
- Morphine (Kadian, Avinza)
- Nifedipine (Adalat, Procardia)
- Procainamide (Pronestyl, Procan-SR, Procanbid)
- Propantheline (Pro-Banthine)
- Quinidine (Quinaglute, Quinidex, Quinora)
- Quinine (Quinerva, Quinite, QM-260)
- Ranitidine (Zantac)
- Trimethoprim (Trimpex, Proloprim, Primsol)
- Trospium (Sanctura)
- Vancomycin (Vancocin)
- Diuretics

FOOD OR SUPPLEMENT INTERACTIONS

- Alcohol
- Dehydroepiandrosterone (DHEA)
- Guar gum
- Ginkgo biloba (may be combined under doctor's supervision)

Glucose-lowering supplements such as chromium, vanadium, cinnamon extract, fenugreek, *Gymnema sylvestre*, bitter melon extract, ginseng, and others may enhance the effect of a diabetic medication. Check with your doctor before combining together.

NUTRIENT DEPLETION/IMBALANCE

- Vitamin B12—take 100 mcg daily.
- Folic acid—take 400 mcg daily.
- Calcium—take 500 mg daily.

Dipeptidyl Peptidase-4 Inhibitor

Sitagliptin (Januvia)

HOW DOES THIS DRUG WORK?

This medication increases insulin after you eat to lower your blood sugar. It also reduces the amount of sugar made by your liver after you eat.

WHAT ARE THE BENEFITS?

Reduction in glucose levels. It is often combined with other type 2 diabetic drugs. It is not combined with insulin.

POTENTIAL SIDE EFFECTS

- Upper respiratory tract infection
- Headache
- Nausea
- Diarrhea

MAJOR CAUTIONS

- Abdominal pain

KNOWN DRUG INTERACTIONS

- Alcohol
- Digoxin (Lanoxin)
- Exenatide (Byetta)
- Insulin
- Nateglinide (Starlix)
- Repaglinide (Prandin)

FOOD OR SUPPLEMENT INTERACTIONS

- Alcohol
- Glucose-lowering supplements such as chromium, vanadium, cinnamon extract, fenugreek, *Gymnema sylvestre*, bitter melon extract, ginseng, and others may enhance the effect of a diabetic medication. Check with your doctor before combining together.

NUTRIENT DEPLETION/IMBALANCE

None known.

Insulin

Insulin is a hormone that can be replaced for those with type 1 diabetes, in whom pancreatic output is deficient. It may also be used in cases of type 2 diabetes in which glucose levels cannot be controlled with oral medications.

Mixed (Humalog Mix 75/25)

Humulin 50/50

Humulin 70/30

Iletin II Mixed

NovoLog Mix, Novolin 70/30

Insulin Aspart injection (NovoLog)

Insulin lispro protamine injection (Humalog Mix 50/50)

Insulin inhalation powder (Exubera)

Insulin detemir injection (Levemir)

Insulin injection (Humulin, Iletin II, Novolin, Velosulin)

Insulin glulisine injection (Apidra)

Insulin, regular (Humulin R, Novolin R, Regular Iletin II)

Insulin aspart; Insulin aspart protamine injection (NovoLog 70/30, NovoLog Mix 70/30)

Insulin lispro (Humalog)

Insulin glargine injection (Lantus)

HOW DO THESE DRUGS WORK?

Insulin transports glucose into the cells to be used as fuel for the production of energy. The drug is injected under the skin, normally in the abdomen.

WHAT ARE THE BENEFITS?

Lowers glucose for those diabetics who cannot produce enough insulin or for those with type 2 diabetes with very high glucose levels.

POTENTIAL SIDE EFFECTS

- Hypoglycemia (low blood sugar)
- Skin reactions (redness, swelling, itching, or rash at the site of injection)
- Worsening of diabetic retinopathy
- Changes in the distribution of body fat
- Sodium retention
- General body swelling

MAJOR CAUTIONS

- Allergic reactions
- Blurred vision
- Loss of consciousness with hypoglycemia

KNOWN DRUG INTERACTIONS

The following drugs can increase the effect of insulin:

- Alcohol
- MAO inhibitors such as phenelzine (Nardil)
- Beta-blockers such as propranolol (Inderal)
- Salicylates such as aspirin (Bayer) or salsalate (Disalcid)
- Anabolic steroids such as methyltestosterone (Android)
- Tetracycline antibiotics such as doxycycline (Vibramycin) and guanethidine (Ismelin)
- Oral hypoglycemic drugs such as glyburide (Diabeta)
- Sulfa antibiotics such as sulfadiazine
- ACE inhibitors such as captopril (Capoten)

Drugs that may reduce the effectiveness of insulin include:

- Diltiazem (Cardizem)
- Niacin
- Corticosteroids such as prednisone
- Estrogens
- Oral contraceptives
- Thyroid hormones such as levothyroxine (Synthroid)
- Isoniazid
- Epinephrine
- Thiazide diuretics such as hydrochlorothiazide and furosemide (Lasix)

FOOD OR SUPPLEMENT INTERACTIONS

- Alcohol
- Niacin
- Chromium (may reduce the amount of insulin required)
- Tobacco (smoking)
- Glucose-lowering supplements such as chromium, vanadium, cinnamon extract, fenugreek, *Gymnema sylvestre*, bitter melon extract, ginseng, and others may enhance the effect of a diabetic medication. Check with your doctor before combining together.

NUTRIENT DEPLETION/IMBALANCE

- Dehydroepiandrosterone (DHEA)

Meglitinides

Nateglinide (Starlix)

Repaglinide (Prandin)

HOW DO THESE DRUGS WORK?

These diabetic medications stimulate the pancreas to produce more insulin.

WHAT ARE THE BENEFITS?

Reduction in glucose levels with a faster onset and a shorter duration of action than the sulfonylurea class of diabetic medications.

POTENTIAL SIDE EFFECTS

- Runny nose
- Cough
- Flu-like symptoms
- Dizziness
- Joint pain

MAJOR CAUTIONS

- Hypoglycemia

KNOWN DRUG INTERACTIONS

- Nonsteroidal anti-inflammatory agents (NSAIDs) such as ibuprofen and aspirin
- MAO inhibitors such as phenelzine (Nadril)
- Beta-blocking drugs such as propranolol (Inderal)
- Thiazide diuretics such as hydrochlorothiazide
- Steroids such as prednisone
- Thyroid hormone such as levothyroxine
- Epinephrine
- Albuterol (Ventolin)

FOOD OR SUPPLEMENT INTERACTIONS

Glucose-lowering supplements such as chromium, vanadium, cinnamon extract, fenugreek, *Gymnema sylvestre*, bitter melon extract, ginseng, and others may enhance the effect of a diabetic medication. Check with your doctor before combining together.

NUTRIENT DEPLETION/IMBALANCE

None known.

Sulfonylureas

Glipizide (Glucotrol)

Tolazamide (Tolinase)

Glimepiride (Amaryl)

Tolbutamide (Orinase)

Glyburide (Diabeta, Glynase, Micronase)

Glipizide Extended-Release (Glucotrol XL)

Acetohexamide (Dymelor)

Chlorpropamide (Diabinese)

HOW DO THESE DRUGS WORK?

This group of medications stimulates the pancreatic output of insulin to lower glucose levels.

WHAT ARE THE BENEFITS?

Reduced glucose levels for people with type 2 diabetes.

POTENTIAL SIDE EFFECTS

- Headache
- Dizziness
- Diarrhea
- Gas
- Skin rashes

MAJOR CAUTIONS

- Hepatitis
- Jaundice
- Low blood sodium
- Hypoglycemia

KNOWN DRUG INTERACTIONS

- Alcohol
- Cholestyramine
- Fluconazole (Diflucan)
- Nonsteroidal anti-inflammatory drugs such as ibuprofen
- Sulfa drugs

- Warfarin (Coumadin)
- Miconazole
- Beta-blockers such as propranolol
- Thiazide diuretics
- Corticosteroids
- Thyroid medicines
- Estrogens
- Niacin
- Phenytoin (Dilantin)
- Calcium channel blocking drugs such as diltiazem

FOOD OR SUPPLEMENT INTERACTIONS

- Niacin.
- Magnesium.
- Glucose-lowering supplements such as chromium, vanadium, cinnamon extract, fenugreek, *Gymnema sylvestre*, bitter melon extract, ginseng, and others may enhance the effect of a diabetic medication. Check with your doctor before combining together.

NUTRIENT DEPLETION/IMBALANCE

None known.

Sulfonylurea/Biguanide Combination

Glyburide and Metformin (Glucovance)

Glipizide and Metformin (Metaglip)

HOW DO THESE DRUGS WORK?

These drugs combine two diabetic medication categories: biguanides and sulfonylureas. They work to stimulate insulin secretion and improve the cells' sensitivity to insulin.

WHAT ARE THE BENEFITS?

More aggressive diabetic treatment and better compliance by combining the two medications.

POTENTIAL SIDE EFFECTS

See the list of side effects under biguanide and sulfonylurea medication classes in this chapter.

MAJOR CAUTIONS

See the list of major cautions under biguanide and sulfonylurea medication classes in this chapter.

KNOWN DRUG INTERACTIONS

See drug interactions under biguanide and sulfonylurea medication classes in this chapter.

FOOD OR SUPPLEMENT INTERACTIONS

See food or supplement interactions under biguanides and sulfonylurea medication classes in this chapter.

NUTRIENT DEPLETION/IMBALANCE

See nutrient depletion/imbalance under biguanide and sulfonylurea medication classes in this chapter.

Thiazolidinediones

Rosiglitazone maleate (Avandia)

Pioglitazone hydrochloride (Actos)

Rosiglitazone maleate and glimepiride (Avandaryl)

Rosiglitazone maleate and metformin hydrochloride (Avandamet)

Pioglitazone hydrochloride and glimepiride (Duetact)

HOW DO THESE DRUGS WORK?

This class of diabetic medications improves the cells' response to glucose and insulin for lowered blood glucose levels.

Rosiglitazone Maleate

On June 14, 2007, an article in the *New England Journal of Medicine* reviewed 42 trials that had been completed with rosiglitazone maleate (Avandia). Researchers tracked heart attacks and death from cardiovascular causes. The average age of death in these trials was 56 years. The researchers concluded that rosiglitazone maleate (Avandia) "was associated with a significant increase in the risk of myocardial infarction (heart attack) and with an increase in the risk of death from cardiovascular causes that has borderline significance."

WHAT ARE THE BENEFITS?

Improved insulin sensitivity and reduced blood glucose levels.

POTENTIAL SIDE EFFECTS

- Upper respiratory tract infection
- Headache
- Back pain
- Hyperglycemia (high blood glucose levels)
- Fatigue
- Sinusitis
- Diarrhea
- Hypoglycemia (low blood sugar levels)
- Edema (fluid retention)
- Anemia
- Weight gain
- Elevated total and LDL cholesterol
- Sore throat
- Muscle pain
- Tooth pain

MAJOR CAUTIONS

- Increased risk of heart failure
- Anemia
- Liver toxicity
- Increased fracture risk in women

KNOWN DRUG INTERACTIONS

- Rifampin (Rifadin, Rimactane)
- Gemfibrozil (Lopid)

FOOD OR SUPPLEMENT INTERACTIONS

Glucose-lowering supplements such as chromium, vanadium, cinnamon extract, fenugreek, *Gymnema sylvestre*, bitter melon extract, ginseng, and others may enhance the effect of a diabetic medication. Check with your doctor before combining together.

NUTRIENT DEPLETION/IMBALANCE

None known.

Rosiglitazone and Bone Fractures

A study published in the *Journal of the American Medical Association* found that the rosiglitazone class of diabetic medications (Avandia, Avandaryl, Avandamet) were more likely to cause bone fractures. The study compared women taking the diabetic medications metformin or glyburide as compared to rosiglitazone. Most of the fractures seen in the women taking rosiglitazone affected bones in the upper arm, hand, or foot. The study was conducted on 4,351 patients recently diagnosed with type 2 diabetes that lasted between four and six years.

Thiazolidinedione/Biguanide Combination

Rosiglitazone (Avandia) and metformin (Avandamet)

HOW DO THESE DRUGS WORK?

This is a combination of the diabetic classes thiazolidinedione and biguanide. Rosiglitazone (Avandia) improves the cells' response to glucose and insulin for lowered blood glucose levels. Metformin (Avandamet) reduces insulin resistance in muscle cells and decreases the release of glucose from the liver. In addition, it reduces the absorption of glucose in the small intestine. Metformin (Avandamet) may also enhance insulin sensitivity inside the cell and stimulate the removal of glucose.

WHAT ARE THE BENEFITS?

This is a more aggressive prescription for lowering blood glucose for those with type 2 diabetes.

POTENTIAL SIDE EFFECTS

See the list of side effects under thiazolidinedione and biguanide medication classes in this chapter.

MAJOR CAUTIONS

See major cautions under thiazolidinedione and biguanide medication classes in this chapter.

KNOWN DRUG INTERACTIONS

See known drug interactions under thiazolidinedione and biguanide medication classes in this chapter.

FOOD OR SUPPLEMENT INTERACTIONS

See food or supplement interactions under thiazolidinedione and biguanide medication classes in this chapter.

NUTRIENT DEPLETION/IMBALANCE

See nutrient depletion/imbalance under thiazolidinedione and biguanide medication classes in this chapter.

Natural Alternatives to Diabetes Drugs

Our experience is that natural therapies such as diet changes, exercise, and specific nutritional supplements are very helpful in helping to better manage type

1 and type 2 diabetes. When followed closely, they can effectively reverse pre-diabetes. It is important to consult with your doctor before starting a nutritional protocol for diabetes, as it's quite possible your medication dosages will need to be lowered over time. Proper monitoring is very important.

Diet and Lifestyle Changes

Without question, proper diet and exercise are critical components in controlling diabetes. Make sure to eat three meals a day at regular times, keeping portions moderate. Never skip breakfast, which leads to blood glucose fluctuations in the morning. Keep your snacks small, choosing nuts, seeds, protein drinks, vegetables, or fruit. Focus on having at least two servings of fruits and three or more servings of vegetables per day. Many diabetics notice better glucose control by including small portions of protein at every meal. Examples include nuts such as almonds, walnuts, and cashews, and fish, chicken, turkey, or other lean meat. Foods shown to reduce glucose levels include vinegar (use in salad dressings), grapefruit, peanuts and peanut butter, chile, and cinnamon.

It is particularly important to limit refined carbohydrates such as found in white flours, candy, fruit juice, soda pop, and so on. Natural sweeteners such as Luo Han Guo, stevia, and xylitol are excellent substitutes for baking or beverage sweeteners and do not adversely affect blood glucose levels. They are commonly available in health food stores.

A regular exercise program must be followed for those with diabetes. It reduces insulin and glucose levels, and shrinks fat cells, making glucose control more effective. It also protects against cardiovascular disease and osteoporosis, which people with diabetes are more susceptible to. Talk with your physician about an exercise plan that lasts 30 minutes or more daily.

Chromium

Several studies demonstrate chromium's effectiveness in the treatment of type 2 diabetes. Following are two of the more recent studies.

A study published in *Diabetes Care* involved 37 people with type 2 diabetes. Participants were randomized to receive a sulfonylurea diabetic drug plus placebo or sulfonylurea plus 1,000 micrograms of chromium for six months. Those receiving the medication plus chromium had significantly improved insulin sensitivity and glucose control. Those receiving the medication plus placebo had a significant increase in body weight, percent body fat, and total abdominal fat. Another study looked at the effect of chromium supplementation on elderly people with diabetes, with an average age 73 years. The participants supplemented with 200 micrograms twice daily for three weeks while a control group took nothing. Significant differences in the fasting blood level of glucose compared to the baseline (190 mg/dL versus 150 mg/dL) were found at the end of the study.

Lipoic Acid

This antioxidant is a valuable nutrient for people with diabetes. A 12-week clinical study in patients with type 2 diabetes on medication found that 1,200 mg daily of a time-released lipoic acid resulted in a significant reduction of plasma fructosamine. This is a marker of short-term glucose balance, with a lower level indicating better glucose control. The study also found a trend toward reduced C-peptide, an indication of increased insulin sensitivity.

Lipoic acid is also quite effective for diabetic retinopathy. Taking 600 mg to 1,200 mg a day orally and intravenously has been shown to reduce symptoms of peripheral neuropathy such as burning, pain, numbness, and prickling of the feet and legs.

DOSAGE

Take 600 to 1,200 mg daily in divided doses.

SAFETY

This supplement is quite safe. It may cause minor digestive upset in some individuals.

Ginseng

Both American ginseng (*Panax quinquefolius*) and Asian ginseng (*Panax ginseng*) have been shown to be beneficial for type 2 diabetes. In a double-blind, placebo-controlled study, 36 type 2 diabetic patients were treated for eight weeks with Asian ginseng (100 or 200 mg) or placebo. A dose of 200 mg daily was shown to decrease fasting blood glucose levels and hemoglobin A1c (HbA1c) in patients with type 2 diabetes. Several studies have also shown American ginseng to be effective for type 2 diabetes when taken 40 minutes before a meal.

DOSAGE

- Asian ginseng (4 to 7 percent ginsenosides)—take 200 mg daily.
- American ginseng—take 3,000 mg within two hours of a meal.

Asian vs. American Ginseng

Asian and American ginseng have similar active constituents known as ginsenosides. However, the ratio of these ginsenosides differs in the two species. Asian ginseng contains a higher percent of Rb1 ginsenosides, which are stimulating. Both herbs have direct blood glucose–lowering benefits. Also, both support functioning of the adrenal gland, an organ that is involved in energy production as well as glucose control.

SAFETY

Asian ginseng may increase blood pressure in some individuals.

PGX

A special type of fiber developed by researchers from the University of Toronto has been shown to be helpful in lowering glucose and cholesterol levels for those with metabolic syndrome and type 2 diabetes.

DOSAGE

Take 2.5 to 5 grams daily with meals.

SAFETY

Digestive upset such as gas, bloating, or constipation may occur, which can be reduced by taking water with PGX or reducing the dosage.

Pycnogenol

Pycnogenol, a standardized extract from the bark of the French maritime pine, has been shown in preliminary studies to modestly decrease blood glucose and hemoglobin A1c levels in people with type 2 diabetes. Positive studies have used 50 to 200 mg daily. Also, a study published in *Angiology* looked at the effect of pycnogenol in people who had diabetes and poor circulation (microangiopathy) as measured in their feet. Patients received pycnogenol at a dose of 50 mg three times daily for four weeks. There was good improvement in the microcirculation of the feet, a common site of diabetic ulcers.

DOSAGE

Take 150 to 200 mg daily.

SAFETY

Caution when using with blood-thinning medications, as pycnogenol has a mild blood-thinning effect.

Peter had recently been diagnosed with type 2 diabetes and was using the medication metformin (Glucophage). An aggressive holistic protocol including dietary changes, daily exercise, and a variety of nutritional supplements resulted in him being able to reduce his metformin dosage by 50 percent. In addition, his daily blood sugar values were mostly normal, whereas before they had spiked much higher on medication alone. He continues to do well and has lost 20 pounds since starting our holistic program.

PETER'S STORY

References

Cesarone, MR, et al. 2006. Improvement of diabetic microangiopathy with Pycnogenol: A prospective, controlled study. *Angiology.* 57:431–6.

Evans, JL, ID Goldfine. 2000. a-Lipoic acid: A multi-functional antioxidant that improves insulin sensitivity in patients with type 2 diabetes. *Diabetes Technologies and Therapeutics* 2:401–13.

Hampton, T. 2007. Diabetes drugs tied to fractures in women. *Journal of the American Medical Association.* April 18;297(15):1645.

Jacob, S, et al. 1999. Oral administration of RAC-alpha-lipoic acid modulates insulin sensitivity in patients with type 2 diabetes mellitus: A placebo-controlled pilot trial. *Free Radical Biology and Medicine.* 27:309–314.

Liu, X, HJ Zhou, P Rohdewald. 2004. French maritime pine bark extract pycnogenol dose-dependently lowers glucose in type 2 diabetic patients (letter). *Diabetes Care.* 27:839.

Liu, X, et al. 2004. Antidiabetic effect of Pycnogenol French maritime pine bark extract in patients with diabetes type II. *Life Sciences.* 75:2505–13.

Martin, J, et al. 2006. Chromium picolinate supplementation attenuates body weight gain and increases insulin sensitivity in subjects with type 2 diabetes. *Diabetes Care.* 29:1826–32.

Nissen, SE, K Wolski. 2007. Effect of rosiglitazone on the risk of myocardial infarction and death from cardiovascular causes. *New England Journal of Medicine.* June 14;356(24):2457–71.

Rabinovitz, H, et al. 2004. Effect of chromium supplementation on blood glucose and lipid levels in type 2 diabetes mellitus elderly patients. *International Journal for Vitamin and Nutrition Research.* 74:178–82.

Ruhnau, KJ, et al. 1999. Effects of 3-week oral treatment with the antioxidant thioctic acid (alpha-lipoic acid) in symptomatic diabetic polyneuropathy. *Diabetic Medicine.* 16:1040–3.

Sotaniemi, EA, E Haapakoski, A Rautio. 1995. Ginseng therapy in non-insulin dependent diabetic patients. *Diabetes Care.* 18:1373–5.

Vuksan, V, et al. 2000. American ginseng (Panax quinquefolius L) reduces postprandial glycemia in nondiabetic subjects and subjects with type 2 diabetes mellitus. *Archives of Internal Medicine.* April 10;160(7):1009–13.

———. 2000. Beneficial effects of viscous dietary fiber from Konjac-mannan in subjects with the insulin resistance syndrome: Results of a controlled metabolic trial. *Diabetes Care.* January;23(1):9–14.

———. 1999. Konjac-mannan (glucomannan) improves glycemia and other associated risk factors for coronary heart disease in type 2 diabetes. A randomized controlled metabolic trial. *Diabetes Care.* June;22(6):913–9.

Ziegler, D, et al. 2004. Treatment of symptomatic diabetic polyneuropathy with the antioxidant alpha-lipoic acid: A meta-analysis. *Diabetic Medicine.* 21:114–21.

14

Eczema Drugs and Their Natural Alternatives

What Is Eczema?

Eczema is a general term used to describe a range of persistent, usually chronic, inflammatory skin conditions (dermatitis). The most common form of eczema is atopic dermatitis, which is characterized by dry, red, extremely itchy patches on the skin. Symptoms usually come and go, brought on by various triggers (see page 198); in people with eczema, these triggers cause an overexaggerated immune response.

Eczema has various causes. It is known, however, that there is a hereditary predisposition; that is, you are more likely to have eczema if your parents or other family members have ever had eczema, hay fever, asthma, or food allergies. Research has shown that dysbiosis, an imbalance of the flora in the digestive tract, can be the root of abnormal immune response. This has been shown most clearly in young children.

Eczema manifests differently in every person; and in each person it may even affect different parts of the body and vary in intensity over the course of his or her life. Generally, eczema is known for its intense itch. Symptoms depend on the type and severity of the eczema and usually include the following:

- Dry, itchy skin commonly occurring on the face, behind the ears, inside the elbows, and behind the knees
- Red, inflamed skin that itches or burns

- Scaly, crusted skin or thick, callused skin resulting from excessive scratching
- Blisters that itch, burn, or ooze

Eczema is extremely common in infancy, affecting 10 to 20 percent of all infants diagnosed. In fact, nearly 60 percent of people with eczema had their first symptom before they turned 1 year old! Fortunately, most children with eczema are symptom-free by the time they reach adolescence; but for others, eczema continues into adulthood. Currently, the National Institutes of Health estimates that some form of eczema affects 15 million people in the United States.

Common eczema triggers may include, but are not limited to:

- Irritants—bathing with nonmoisturizing soaps, irritating chemicals or fabrics
- Allergens—dust mites, pet dander, pollen, molds, juices, foods
- Infections—bacterial, viral, fungal
- Environmental factors—extremes in temperature, perspiration, stress
- Nutritional—nutrient deficiencies or imbalances such as essential fatty acids, zinc
- Poor digestion and detoxification

    Imbalances in the gut ecology (low levels of good bacteria and abnormally high levels of harmful bacteria and fungus)

    Constipation

With conventional treatment, there is no cure for eczema, so the goal of treatment is symptom management. Moisturizing creams and tar products are commonly used to treat very mild eczema and prevent flare-up. For more severe cases, the primary classes of drugs used to help control eczema include: antihistamines, topical corticosteroids, calcineurin inhibitors, and oral corticosteroids. We find natural therapies superior to pharmaceutical therapy for the long-term treatment of eczema.

Eczema Drugs

Antihistamines

Loratadine (Claritin, Alavert)

Fexofenadine (Allegra)

Hydroxyzine (Atarax)

Diphenhydramine (Benadryl)

HOW DO THESE DRUGS WORK?

For most eczema sufferers, itching is the most aggravating symptom. Antihistamines reduce itching by protecting tissues from the effects of histamine—a pro-inflammatory substance released during an allergic reaction.

POTENTIAL SIDE EFFECTS

Antihistamines frequently cause dry mouth and nose, and sleepiness. Other common side effects include dizziness, headache, loss of appetite, upset stomach, vision changes, and irritability.

MAJOR CAUTIONS

Major cautions primarily involve function of the brain or nervous system. Symptoms may include hallucinations, slurred speech, severe dizziness or fainting, tremors, tachycardia, shortness of breath, disorientation, severe sleepiness, inability to urinate, and very dilated pupils.

MEDICAL PRECAUTIONS

People with the following conditions or disorders should discuss their risks with their physician:

- Glaucoma (narrow angle)
- Stomach ulcers
- Difficulty urinating (e.g., from enlarged prostate)
- Heart disease
- High blood pressure
- Seizures
- Lung problems
- Overactive thyroid
- Pregnancy
- Breast-feeding

KNOWN DRUG INTERACTIONS

Combining antihistamines with tranquilizers or sedatives will cause increased drowsiness. It is important to talk to your doctor if you take medications for depression, seizures, or pain. Antihistamines should not be combined with other medications for colds, hay fever, or allergies.

FOOD OR SUPPLEMENT INTERACTIONS

Limit alcohol intake to avoid excessive drowsiness. Consumption of fruit juices—including grapefruit, orange, and apple—may decrease absorption of fexofenadine (Allegra). Simultaneous use of St. John's wort and fexofenadine may cause increased blood levels of the drug.

NUTRIENT DEPLETION/IMBALANCE

None known.

Topical Corticosteroids

Hydrocortisone (Alphaderm)

Betamethasone dipropionate (Diprosone, Diprolene)

Betamethasone valerate (Valisone)

Clobetasol (Temovate, Cormax)

HOW DO THESE DRUGS WORK?

Topical corticosteroids (also called steroids) are absorbed into the skin cells where applied. They then stop these skin cells from producing various inflammation-causing chemicals that are normally released when they react to allergens or irritation. By preventing these inflammatory chemicals from being released in the skin, corticosteroids reduce inflammation and relieve associated symptoms. Topical steroids can be divided into four different strengths: mild, moderate, potent, and very potent; they are the mainstay of treatment for eczema.

POTENTIAL SIDE EFFECTS

Burning, stinging, redness, and itching commonly occur when these drugs are first applied, but usually subside within a few days. Thereafter, the most common side effect with prolonged use is thinning, fragile skin. Other adverse effects include striae, purplish skin blotches (purpura), acne, dermatitis around the mouth, rosacea-like rash, increased hair growth, hypopigmentation (whitening), skin infection, allergic contact dermatitis to corticosteroids, skin tolerance to corticosteroid effect, and glaucoma and cataracts when used around the eyes.

MAJOR CAUTIONS

High-strength steroids used over large areas may be significantly absorbed into the body. Systemic absorption of topical corticosteroids has produced hypothalamic-pituitary-adrenal (HPA) axis imbalance, resulting in Cushing's syndrome symptoms, high blood sugar, and glucose in the urine (glucosuria) in some patients.

MEDICAL PRECAUTIONS

People with the following conditions or disorders should discuss their risks with their physician:

- Glaucoma
- Infection or sores on the area to be treated

- Pregnancy
- Breast-feeding

KNOWN DRUG INTERACTIONS

Oral corticosteroids and other skin medications should not be used concomitantly with topical corticosteroids.

FOOD OR SUPPLEMENT INTERACTIONS

Animal research suggests that applying aloe gel along with a topical corticosteroid may enhance anti-inflammatory activity in the skin. Orally, licorice (*Glycyrrhiza glabra*) has immune-stimulating effects, which can decrease the response to corticosteroids; however, when glycyrrhetinic acid (a chemical found in licorice) is applied to the skin, it may increase the activity of hydrocortisone.

NUTRIENT DEPLETION/IMBALANCE

Nutrient depletions/imbalances are primarily a concern with systemic absorption of the corticosteroid. See the section on Oral Corticosteroids.

Topical Immunomodulators/Topical Calcineurin Inhibitors

Pimecrolimus (Elidel, Douglan)

Tacrolimus (Protopic)

HOW DO THESE DRUGS WORK?

Topical calcineurin inhibitors are a newer class of steroid-free drugs that work by suppressing the immune system in the affected area and subsequently the inflammatory process. Because they are a type of immunosuppressant (reducing T-cell and mast cell activity), they decrease the effects of your body's immune system, which can relieve itching and improve the rash associated with eczema.

WHAT ARE THE BENEFITS?

Effective topical relief of eczema without the use of systemic medications.

POTENTIAL SIDE EFFECTS

The most common side effects are reactions at the site of application, including burning, itching, and redness. Other side effects that may occur include sore throat, stuffy nose, headache, cough, respiratory tract and viral infections, and skin infection. Severe flushing and photosensitive reactivity are also observed.

MAJOR CAUTIONS

In 2006, the U.S. Food and Drug Administration issued a public health advisory regarding the potential risk of lymph node or skin cancer from these drugs. In addition, concomitant exposure to sunlight or ultraviolet light may increase the risk of serious side effects.

MEDICAL PRECAUTIONS

People with the following conditions or disorders should discuss their risks with their physician:

- History of skin infections
- Immune system problems
- Netherton's syndrome
- Pregnancy
- Breast-feeding
- Children under 2 years of age

KNOWN DRUG INTERACTIONS

Drug interactions with these medications have not been well studied. Nonetheless, the combination with any other topical medication could potentially cause adverse interactions. Furthermore, it is advised that using pimecrolimus with drugs that utilize the same liver enzymes for elimination from the body—such as ketoconazole, itraconazole, erythromycin, and fluconazole—could elevate levels of pimecrolimus and increase its toxicity.

Elidel and Protopic Warning

The FDA has issued its strongest black box warning on the packaging of Elidel and Protopic. The warning advises doctors to prescribe short-term use of Elidel and Protopic only after other available eczema treatments have failed in adults and children over the age of 2.

FOOD OR SUPPLEMENT INTERACTIONS

None known.

NUTRIENT DEPLETION/IMBALANCE

None known.

Oral Corticosteroids

Cortisone (Cortone)

Dexamethasone (Decadron)

Hydrocortisone (Cortef)

Methylprednisolone (Medrol)

Prednisolone (Prelone)

Prednisone (Deltasone)

HOW DO THESE DRUGS WORK?

Corticosteroids mimic the effects of cortisone and hydrocortisone—hormones your body produces naturally in your adrenal glands. By mimicking these hormones, they block the production of immune system substances that trigger allergic and inflammatory actions, such as prostaglandins. It should be noted that oral corticosteroids are generally not prescribed unless topical treatments have not worked and the eczema is severe; yet they do have their place in treatment.

WHAT ARE THE BENEFITS?

These medications give quick relief of moderate to severe eczema.

POTENTIAL SIDE EFFECTS

Dizziness, nausea, indigestion, increased appetite, weight gain, weakness, or sleep disturbances are common side effects that usually disappear as your body adjusts to the medication. More serious adverse effects that require attention include peptic ulceration, vomiting of blood, black or tarry stools, puffing of the face, swelling of the ankles or feet, unusual weight gain, prolonged sore throat or fever, muscle weakness, breathing difficulties, mood changes, vision changes, cataracts, and glaucoma.

MAJOR CAUTIONS

Common side effects with long-term therapy include suppression of the HPA and growth retardation, Cushing's syndrome (bloating), muscle wasting, skin thinning, hyper-pigmentation, easy bruising, fluid retention, suppressed immune function and predisposition to infection, poor wound healing, glucose intolerance, and osteoporosis.

MEDICAL PRECAUTIONS

People with the following conditions or disorders should discuss their risks with their physician:

- Liver or kidney disease
- Diabetes
- Heart problems
- Intestinal problems
- Ulcers
- High blood pressure
- Underactive thyroid
- Myasthenia gravis
- Herpes eye infection
- Tuberculosis

- Seizures
- Blood clots
- Osteoporosis (brittle bones)
- Eye problems
- Allergies
- Pregnancy
- Breast-feeding

KNOWN DRUG INTERACTIONS

Aspirin, arthritis medication, blood thinners, diuretics, rifampin, phenobarbital, estrogen (e.g., birth control pills), phenytoin, ketoconazole, and drugs for diabetes may all have undesirable interactions with oral corticosteroids. It is crucial to tell your physician about all over-the-counter or prescription medications you are taking.

FOOD OR SUPPLEMENT INTERACTIONS

Avoid ephedra and magnesium supplements because they may decrease the absorption or activity of corticosteroids. Herbs that cause mineral losses such as diuretic herbs, laxative herbs, buckthorn, and alder buckthorn may compound mineral losses associated with corticosteroid use. Licorice may prolong drug activity, resulting in increased side effects; other research suggests that glycyrrhizin (an active constituent of licorice) decreases the immune-suppressing activity of corticosteroids.

In regard to food, using salt may enhance the sodium and water retention associated with corticosteroids, alcohol can increase stomach irritation, and grapefruit juice may increase blood levels of corticosteroids by delaying absorption.

NUTRIENT DEPLETION/IMBALANCE

Nutrients depleted by corticosteroids include calcium, vitamin D, potassium, magnesium, vitamin B6, and chromium. There may also be increased urinary loss of vitamin K, vitamin C, selenium, and zinc. Furthermore, suppressed production of melatonin has been recorded with corticosteroid treatment. We recommend the following supplements:

- Calcium—500 mg for children, 500 to 1,200 mg daily for adults
- Vitamin D—400 IU for children, 1,000 IU for adults
- Magnesium—200 to 250 mg for children, 250 to 500 mg for adults
- Vitamin B6—as part of children's multivitamin, 50 mg for adults
- Chromium—as part of multivitamin for children, 200 mcg for adults
- Vitamin K—as part of multivitamin for children, 500 mcg for adults

- Vitamin C—200 mg for children, 500 mg for adults
- °Selenium—as part of multivitamin for children and adults
- Zinc—as part of multivitamin for children, 15 mg for adults

Natural Alternatives to Eczema Drugs

Diet and Lifestyle Changes

Foods rich in skin-healthy essential fatty acids are very important. This includes ground flaxseeds, cold-water fish such as sardines and wild salmon, pumpkin seeds, almonds, and walnuts. Healthy oils such as from flaxseed and hemp seed are great additions to salads and supply inflammation-fighting omega-3 fatty acids. The diet should be rich in detoxifying fruits, vegetables, and lean poultry. Avoid frequent consumption of saturated fat found in red meat and dairy products. Foods that commonly aggravate eczema include citrus fruits, cow's milk, soy, chocolate, alcohol, gluten-containing foods (wheat, rye, barley), and sometimes spicy foods. Work with a holistic doctor to have your food sensitivities tested. In addition, high levels of stress can worsen the inflammatory response, so regular exercise and other stress-reducing techniques are important. Lastly, be aware of chemicals (soaps and detergents) that may be causing a reaction with your skin and triggering eczema.

Fish Oil

Fish oil is a rich source of inflammation-fighting omega-3 fatty acids. More specifically, eicosapentaenoic acid, one type of omega-3 fatty acid, is a powerful inhibitor of inflammatory chemicals in the body.

A double-blind trial researched the effect of fish oil (1.8 grams of EPA) given to a group of eczema sufferers. After 12 weeks, those supplementing fish oil experienced significant improvement.

DOSAGE

Adults should take fish oil containing 1.8 grams to 2.4 grams of EPA (eicosapentaenoic acid) per day. Children should use half this amount or the amount recommended by their doctor.

SAFETY

If you are on blood-thinning medications, check with your doctor before supplementing fish oil.

Gamma Linoleic Acid (GLA)

GLA is found in supplements such as evening primrose oil, black currant oil, and borage oil. GLA is converted to compounds that have anti-inflammatory and antiproliferative properties. A metabolite of GLA known as dihomogam-malinolenic acid appears to modulate or balance an overactive immune system. While studies are mixed in regards to its effectiveness, we find it is very helpful for about 15 percent of patients who have eczema.

DOSAGE

Adults should take 1,000 mg of GLA daily. Children should use half this amount or the amount recommended by their doctor.

SAFETY

A small percent of users may experience digestive upset. If you are on blood-thinning medications, consult with your doctor first before using.

Probiotics

Friendly bacteria known as probiotics are a normal and essential part of the body's immune, digestive, and detoxification systems. In the digestive tract, these friendly bacteria play an important role in reducing the absorption of allergens and maintaining a balanced immune system. One trial looked at the effect of giving 20 billion lactobacilli twice per day to breast-feeding mothers whose

Healthy Bacteria

Over 100 trillion bacteria are found in the human digestive tract. The introduction of the healthy bacteria occurs during the birth process from the birth canal and first breaths of air. Adults can get a steady supply of these friendly organisms from foods such as yogurt, sauerkraut, cottage cheese, kefir, and miso. In addition, certain foods contain fiber that promotes the growth of these healthy bacteria. Such growth promoters are known as "prebiotics." Examples include bananas, garlic, onions, soybeans, Jerusalem artichoke, and chicory. Supplements that contain these good bacteria are known as "probiotics." Research continues to demonstrate that friendly flora normalizes immune activity, synthesizes nutrients such as B vitamins, and supports detoxification, all of which can help skin conditions such as eczema.

infants had eczema. Researchers found significant improvement of the infants' eczema after one month. A different double-blind trial found that a probiotic preparation containing 1 billion organisms of *Lactobacillus fermentum* taken twice a day reduced the severity of eczema in a group of young children with moderate or severe eczema.

Homeopathy

We have found certain homeopathic remedies to be quite helpful for the treatment of eczema. The most common is homeopathic Sulfur. It is used for eczema characterized by red, dry, itchy skin that is made worse from bathing and warm environments. People benefiting from this remedy often have itching so bad, they want to scratch their skin until it bleeds.

There are a variety of different homeopathic remedies that can be helpful for eczema. It is best to consult with a practitioner trained in homeopathy for an individual recommendation.

DOSAGE

Take two pellets of a 30C potency twice daily for up to two weeks to see if there are any positive results. If you notice improvement, stop using unless symptoms return.

SAFETY

Homeopathic Sulfur is very safe for adults and children. Some people notice an initial worsening of their symptoms followed by marked improvement of their eczema. If you do not notice improvement within two weeks of starting this homeopathic remedy, discontinue its use.

Calendula

Calendula flowers have been traditionally recommended by herbalists for a variety of skin conditions such as eczema. Medicinal use of calendula reduces inflammation, prevents infection, and is well tolerated. Flavonoids, which are plant pigments, are thought to give calendula its anti-inflammatory properties.

DOSAGE

Calendula is applied topically as a gel or cream to the areas of eczema. Apply one to three times daily for reduced itching and skin healing.

SAFETY

Calendula is well tolerated. As with any topical application, there is always the potential for an allergic reaction.

Todd, a 10-year-old, had suffered for several years with eczema. When we saw him at the clinic, he had severe eczema over many parts of his body, including his face, neck, arms, and legs. Over the years he had been on topical and oral steroids. Topical creams were of little benefit. At times he suffered skin infections due to the scratching of his skin. A natural protocol was begun that involved the elimination of food sensitivities such as gluten and cow's milk, as well as supplementation with fish oil, homeopathic Sulfur, and probiotics. Over the next two months, his skin dramatically improved, and one year later his eczema was 90 percent improved. Now two years later, he continues to do well on natural treatment only.

References

Bjørneboe, A, et al. 1987. Effect of dietary supplementation with eicosapentaenoic acid in the treatment of atopic dermatitis. *British Journal of Dermatology.* 117:463–9.

———. 1989. Effect of n-3 fatty acid supplement to patients with atopic dermatitis. *Journal of Internal Medicine Supplement.* 225:233–6.

Majamaa, H, E Isolauri. 1997. Probiotics: A novel approach in the management of food allergy. *Journal of Allergy and Clinical Immunology.* 99:179–85.

Weston, S, et al. 2005. Effects of probiotics on atopic dermatitis: A randomised controlled trial. *Archives of Disease in Childhood.* 90:892–7.

15

Erectile Dysfunction (Impotence) Drugs and Their Natural Alternatives

What Is ED?

Erectile dysfunction (ED), also known as impotence, is the inability of a man to maintain a firm erection long enough to have sex. Although this condition is more common in older men, it can occur at any age. Contrary to what you may have read, its causes are more often physical than psychological. This condition affects approximately 18 million American men.

A variety of different diseases may cause ED. The most common is vascular disease, which refers to the blood vessels. This includes atherosclerosis (hardening of the arteries), hypertension, and high cholesterol. These diseases account for 70 percent of physically related causes of ED, since they restrict blood flow to the penis. Diabetes, kidney disease, and neurological disease (such as multiple sclerosis or Parkinson's disease) are also common causes. Others include prostate enlargement, prostate cancer treatments (radiation, surgery), spinal cord injuries, hormonal imbalances, and drug use.

ED Drugs

Alkaloids

Yohimbine (Actibine, Aphrodyne, Dayto Himbin, Yocon, Yohimex, Yomax)

HOW DO THESE DRUGS WORK?

Yohimbine is type of chemical known as an alkaloid. It naturally occurs in the bark of the evergreen forest tree. This chemical increases penile blood flow.

WHAT ARE THE BENEFITS?

Research seems to indicate that yohimbine works better for those men who have erectile dysfunction from stress or anxiety.

POTENTIAL SIDE EFFECTS

- Dizziness
- Flushing
- Headache
- Irritability
- Nausea
- Nervousness
- Restlessness
- Sweating
- Tremor

MAJOR CAUTIONS

- Anxiety or agitation
- Shortness of breath
- Chest pain
- Heart palpitations
- High blood pressure
- Increased heart rate
- Skin rash, itching
- Vomiting

KNOWN DRUG INTERACTIONS

- High blood pressure medications
- Antidepressant medications

FOOD OR SUPPLEMENT INTERACTIONS

Avoid consuming tyramine-containing foods such as aged cheeses, red wine, beer, hard liquor, salami, or pepperoni, as the combination with yohimbine may result in headaches, increased blood pressure, or irregular heartbeat.

- Yohimbe supplements
- St. John's wort

NUTRIENT DEPLETION/IMBALANCE

None known.

Phosphodiesterase Enzyme Inhibitors

Vardenafil (Levitra)

Sildenafil tablets (Viagra)

Tadalafil (Cialis)

HOW DO THESE DRUGS WORK?

This class of drugs enhances the effect of a chemical known as nitric oxide. This results in increased penile blood flow and longer time of blood engorgement of the penile tissues.

WHAT ARE THE BENEFITS?

Quick onset of action leading to an erection. Vardenafil (Levitra) and sildenafil tablets (Viagra) can be taken 30 to 60 minutes before sexual relations. Tadalafil (Cialis) can be used 24 hours prior to sexual relations.

POTENTIAL SIDE EFFECTS

- Flushing of the face
- Headaches
- Stomach pain
- Nasal congestion
- Nausea
- Diarrhea
- Inability to differentiate between the colors green and blue
- Abnormal ejaculation

MAJOR CAUTIONS

- Low blood pressure
- Erections lasting more than four hours
- Chest pain or palpitations
- Shortness of breath
- Dizziness
- Eyelid swelling

FOOD OR SUPPLEMENT INTERACTIONS

- Grapefruit juice

> ## ED Drugs and Hearing Loss
>
> In November 2007, in response to a request from the FDA, the makers of vardenafil (Levitra), sildenafil tablets (Viagra), and tadalafil (Cialis) agreed to revise labeling due to reports of users experiencing a sudden decrease or loss of hearing. This was accompanied in some cases by tinnitus and dizziness.

NUTRIENT DEPLETION/IMBALANCE

None known.

Prostaglandin E Analogs

Alprostadil pellets (Muse)

Alprostadil injection (Caverject, Edex Kit)

HOW DO THESE DRUGS WORK?

The drug Alprostadil is used to relax smooth muscles of the penis, increase penile blood flow, and prevent platelet aggregation. These biochemical reactions help a man achieve and maintain an erection. There are two different methods of administration. Alprostadil pellets (Muse) involve inserting a suppository into the urethra. Alprostadil injection (Caverject, Edex Kit) is injected into the penis.

WHAT ARE THE BENEFITS?

An erection within five minutes after application that usually lasts 30 to 60 minutes.

POTENTIAL SIDE EFFECTS

- Pain in the penis or testicle
- Penile bleeding
- Dizziness
- Heart palpitations
- Flu-like symptoms
- Headache

MAJOR CAUTIONS

- Fainting
- Painful erection for hours
- Caution for those with heart disease

KNOWN DRUG INTERACTIONS

- Anticoagulant medications such as heparin or warfarin

FOOD OR SUPPLEMENT INTERACTIONS

None known.

NUTRIENT DEPLETION/IMBALANCE

None known.

Testosterone

Testosterone gel (AndroGel)

Testosterone transdermal (Androderm, Testoderm, Testoderm TTS)

HOW DO THESE DRUGS WORK?

Testosterone is a hormone that plays a role in libido and erection.

WHAT ARE THE BENEFITS?

Men with low testosterone may notice a benefit in erections when prescribed testosterone replacement.

POTENTIAL SIDE EFFECTS

- Digestive upset such as nausea and vomiting
- Headache
- Hair loss
- Acne
- Frequent erections

MAJOR CAUTIONS

- Swelling
- Trouble breathing
- Urination problems
- Mood changes such as depression or irritability
- Dizziness
- Breast pain or enlargement
- Weight gain
- Change in size or shape of the testicles
- Men with prostate cancer should not use testosterone therapy

KNOWN DRUG INTERACTIONS

- Fluconazole (diflucan)
- Cyclosporine (Gengraf, Neoral)
- Medicines for prostate enlargement or prostate cancer
- Warfarin (Coumadin)

FOOD OR SUPPLEMENT INTERACTIONS

None known.

NUTRIENT DEPLETION/IMBALANCE

None known.

We recommend that men who use testosterone also supplement with indole 3 carbinole, a phytonutrient that helps the liver metabolize estrogen, which may build up as a result of testosterone use.

MEDICATIONS THAT CAN CAUSE ERECTILE DYSFUNCTION

Antidepressant and other psychiatric medications:

- Amitriptyline (Elavil)
- Buspirone (Buspar)
- Chlordiazepoxide (Librium)
- Chlorpromazine (Thorazine)
- Clorazepate (Tranxene)
- Desipramine (Norpramin)
- Diazepam (Valium)
- Doxepin (Sinequan)
- Fluoxetine (Prozac)
- Fluphenazine (Prolixin)
- Imipramine (Tofranil)
- Lorazepam (Ativan)
- Meprobamate (Equanil)
- Mesoridazine (Serentil)
- Nortriptyline (Pamelor)
- Oxazepam (Serax)
- Phenelzine (Nardil)
- Phenytoin (Dilantin)
- Thioridazine (Mellaril)
- Thiothixene (Navane)
- Tranylcypromine (Parnate)
- Trifluoperazine (Stelazine)

Antihistamine medications:

- Dimenhydrinate (Dramamine)
- Diphenhydramine (Benadryl)
- Hydroxyzine (Vistaril)
- Meclizine (Antivert)
- Promethazine (Phenergan)

Antihypertensive and diuretic medications:

- Atenolol (Tenormin)
- Bethanidine

- Chlorothiazide (Diuril)
- Chlorthalidone (Hygroton)
- Clonidine (Catapres)
- Enalapril (Vasotec)
- Guanabenz (Wytensin)
- Guanethidine (Ismelin)
- Guanfacine (Tenex)
- Haloperidol (Haldol)
- Hydralazine (Apresoline)
- Hydrochlorothiazide (Esidrix)
- Labetalol (Normodyne)
- Methyldopa (Aldomet)
- Metoprolol (Lopressor)
- Minoxidil (Loniten)
- Phenoxybenzamine (Dibenzyline)
- Phentolamine (Regitine)
- Prazosin (Minipress)
- Propranolol (Inderal)
- Reserpine (Serpasil)
- Spironolactone (Aldactone)
- Triamterene (Maxzide)
- Verapamil (Calan)

Among the antihypertensive medications, thiazides are the most common cause of ED, followed by beta-blockers. Alpha-blockers are, in general, less likely to cause this problem.

Parkinson's disease medications:
- Benztropine (Cogentin)
- Biperiden (Akineton)
- Bromocriptine (Parlodel)
- Levodopa (Sinemet)
- Procyclidine (Kemadrin)
- Trihexyphenidyl (Artane)

Chemotherapy medications:
- Antiandrogens (Casodex, Flutamide, Nilutamide)
- Busulfan (Myleran)

- Cyclophosphamide (Cytoxan)
- Ketoconazole
- LHRH agonists (Lupron, Zoladex)

Other medications:
- Aminocaproic acid (Amicar)
- Atropine
- Clofibrate (Atromid-S)
- Cyclobenzaprine (Flexeril)
- Cyproterone
- Digoxin (Lanoxin)
- Disopyramide (Norpace)
- Estrogen
- Finasteride (Propecia, Proscar)
- Furazolidone (Furoxone)
- H2-blockers (Tagamet, Zantac, Pepcid)
- Indomethacin (Indocin)
- Lipid-lowering agents
- Licorice
- Metoclopramide (Reglan)
- NSAIDs (ibuprofen, etc.)
- Orphenadrine (Norflex)
- Prochlorperazine (Compazine)

Opiate analgesics (painkillers):
- Morphine
- Methadone
- Fentanyl (Innovar)
- Meperidine (Demerol)
- Codeine
- Oxycodone (Oxycontin, Percodan)
- Hydromorphone (Dilaudid)

Recreational drugs:
- Alcohol
- Amphetamines
- Barbiturates

- Cocaine
- Marijuana
- Heroin
- Nicotine

The information provided above is from the National Institutes of Health, www.nlm.nih.gov/medlineplus/ency/article/004024.htm.

Natural Alternatives to Erectile Dysfunction Drugs

Diet and Lifestyle Changes

Some men with erectile dysfunction have poor circulation due to arteriosclerosis. See chapter 10 on cholesterol drugs and their natural alternatives. One study found 8 ounces of pomegranate juice daily to be helpful in about half of men with mild to moderate erectile dysfunction. Although overall statistical significance was not achieved in this pilot study, the authors felt that a larger study for a longer period of time may achieve statistical significance.

Regular exercise, stress-reduction techniques, and quitting smoking are important lifestyle aspects of the holistic treatment of erectile dysfunction.

Korean Red (Asian) Ginseng

This herb has been used in historic medical traditions to treat erectile dysfunction. In a double-blind, placebo-controlled, crossover study of 45 men with clinically diagnosed erectile dysfunction, 60 percent of the participants reported that Korean red (Asian) ginseng improved erection. The dose used was 900 mg three times daily.

DOSAGE

Take 900 mg three times daily of a nonstandardized preparation, or follow the label directions for more concentrated, standardized versions.

SAFETY

Side effects may include insomnia; headache; and, rarely, increased blood pressure.

Ginkgo Biloba

The extract of this herb has been shown to have a vasodilation effect. Studies have shown it to be effective for ED. This includes for men on antidepressant medications.

DOSAGE

Take 120 mg twice daily of a 24 percent flavoglycoside extract.

SAFETY

Do not combine ginkgo biloba with blood-thinning medication such as Coumadin, since ginkgo has blood-thinning effects.

Arginine

This amino acid increases nitric oxide levels, which dilates the arteries and improves blood flow.

A prospective, randomized, double-blind, placebo-controlled study looked at the effect of six weeks of 5 grams a day orally of L-arginine on 50 men with erectile dysfunction (ED). Nine of 29 (31 percent) of men taking L-arginine and 2 of 17 controls reported a significant subjective improvement in sexual function. It should be noted that all nine men treated with L-arginine and who had improvement had had an initially low urinary nitric oxide, and this level had doubled by the end of the study. Taking the supplement pycnogenol at a dose of 40 mg three times daily may improve the effectiveness of a lower dose of L-arginine of 1.7 grams daily.

L-arginine Safety

There has been concern about the safety of L-arginine due to a study done at Johns Hopkins University Medical Center. Researchers gave L-arginine supplements (up to 3,000 mg three times daily) to 55 study participants, while 59 people got placebos. The study was cut short because, after six months, there had been six deaths among participants taking L-arginine—and no deaths in the placebo group. In response, researchers recommended that this supplement not be used following a heart attack.

It should be noted that the six deaths may have been due to chance. Two died from a heart attack or its complications, two succumbed to blood infections unrelated to L-arginine, and two died from unknown causes. We agree that people who have had a heart attack should not take L-arginine, at least until further studies are done. But for people with no history of heart attack, we believe that 3,000 mg of L-arginine, taken two to three times daily, is safe and effective in treating hypertension and congestive heart failure, as well as improving blood flow in people with diabetes and in treating erectile dysfunction. Also note that those prone to herpes skin breakouts should use L-arginine with caution as it may worsen this condition.

DOSAGE

Take 5 grams daily or 1.7 grams along with 120 mg of pycnogenol daily.

SAFETY

Men with a history of heart disease should check with their doctor first before using L-arginine.

Carnitine

The combination of two forms of carnitine has been shown to be effective for elderly men with ED associated with low testosterone. The randomized, double-blind study involved 120 men who were given either testosterone undecanoate 160 mg per day, propionyl-L-carnitine 2 g per day plus acetyl-L-carnitine 2 g per day, or placebo. The study lasted six months. Those receiving the carnitine combination had more significant improvement in the treatment of erectile dysfunction. In addition, the testosterone group had increased prostate size while the carnitine group did not.

DOSAGE

Take 2 grams daily of propionyl-L-carnitine along with 2 grams per day of acetyl-L-carnitine.

SAFETY

The carnitines are quite safe.

Jose, a 63-year-old carpenter, came to the clinic seeking a natural approach to ED. For most of his life he had relied on herbs and other natural approaches to help with health problems. His request was for an effective, economical, natural approach so that he would be able to resume relations with his wife. His testosterone level was checked, and was shown to be slightly below an average value. Jose was prescribed Korean Red (Asian) ginseng along with regular consumption of pomegranate juice. After three weeks he noticed an improvement in his libido and ED. After six weeks of treatment he found this natural approach to be extremely effective for his ED.

JOSE'S STORY

References

Cavallini, G, et al. 2004. Carnitine versus androgen administration in the treatment of sexual dysfunction, depressed mood, and fatigue associated with male aging. *Urology*. 63:641–6.

Chen, J, et al. 1999. Effect of oral administration of high-dose nitric oxide donor L-arginine in men with organic erectile dysfunction: Results of a double-blind, randomized, placebo-controlled study. *British Journal of Urology.* Int;83:269–73.

Cohen, AJ, B Bartlik. 1998. Ginkgo biloba for antidepressant-induced sexual dysfunction. *Journal of Sex and Marital Therapy.* 24:139–43.

Forest, CP, H Padma-Nathan, HR Liker. 2007. Efficacy and safety of pomegranate juice on improvement of erectile dysfunction in male patients with mild to moderate erectile dysfunction: A randomized, placebo-controlled, double-blind, crossover study. *International Journal of Impotence Research.* 19: 564–67; doi:10.1038/sj.ijir.3901570; published online June 14, 2007.

Hong, B, et al. 2002. A double-blind crossover study evaluating the efficacy of Korean red ginseng in patients with erectile dysfunction: A preliminary report. *Journal of Urology.* 168:2070–3.

Sohn, M, and R Sikora. 1991. Ginkgo biloba extract in the therapy of erectile dysfunction. *Journal of Sex Education and Therapy.* 17:53–61.

Stanislavov, R, V Nikolova. 2003. Treatment of erectile dysfunction with pycnogenol and L-arginine. *Journal of Sex and Marital Therapy.* 29:207–13.

16

Glaucoma Drugs and Their Natural Alternatives

What Is Glaucoma?

Glaucoma actually refers to a group of diseases in which fluid pressure inside the eye rises. This can lead to damage of the eye's optic nerve and result in vision loss and blindness. Glaucoma is characterized by a subtle loss of side vision, known as peripheral vision. Untreated, it can progress to a loss of central vision and blindness. It is usually associated with elevated pressure in the eye, known as intraocular pressure (IOP). It can also occur with normal IOP. This is thought to be due to poor blood flow to the optic nerve.

Eye tone and shape are regulated by IOP. A normal range is between 8 and 22 mm (millimeters) of mercury. High pressure increases damage to the delicate nerve fibers of the optic nerve. The front of the eye is filled with a clear fluid called the aqueous humor. It nourishes the structures in the front of the eye. When the aqueous humor cannot drain through the tiny channels of the eye properly, pressure builds up.

It is estimated that over 3 million Americans have glaucoma, but only half of those know they have it. In addition, 9 to 12 percent of all cases of blindness in the United States are due to glaucoma. According to the World Health Organization, glaucoma is the second leading cause of blindness in the world.

There are many different types of glaucoma. In general, they can be classified as either open-angle glaucomas (generally chronic) or closed-angle glaucomas (usually sudden or acute). Glaucoma usually affects both eyes but can progress more rapidly in one eye. The most common form is chronic open-angle glaucoma. It is associated with aging and progresses with no or few symptoms until it becomes advanced. Without treatment, loss of peripheral vision can lead to a decrease in central vision and ultimately the loss of central vision.

Risk Factors

- Age. Those older than 60 are at increased risk. African Americans have an increased risk after age 40.
- Race. African Americans, Mexican Americans, Japanese Americans, and Asian Americans are at increased risk of various types of glaucoma.
- Family history of glaucoma.
- Certain medical conditions. Diabetes, high blood pressure, heart disease, and hypothyroidism increase one's risk.
- Physical injuries. Eye trauma such as being hit in the eye, eye disorders such as detached retina, and eye surgery are all risk factors for glaucoma.
- Nearsightedness.
- Prolonged corticosteroid use. Using corticosteroids for long periods of time increases risk.
- Structural abnormalities of the eye.

Regular eye exams are important to diagnose glaucoma so it can be treated early to prevent serious vision loss. Those with glaucoma need to be monitored regularly.

Glaucoma Drugs

Eye Drops

Beta-blockers

Timolol ophthalmic (Betimol, Timoptic, Timoptic-XE)

Levobunolol Ophthalmic (AKBeta, Betagan)

Carteolol Ophthalmic (Ocupress)

Betaxolol Ophthalmic (Betoptic, Betoptic S)

Metipranolol Ophthalmic (OptiPranolol)

HOW DO THESE DRUGS WORK?

They decrease the rate of flow of aqueous humor into the eyeball.

WHAT ARE THE BENEFITS?

Decreased intraocular pressure.

POTENTIAL SIDE EFFECTS

- Burning, stinging, or itching of the eyes or eyelids
- Vision changes
- Light sensitivity

MAJOR CAUTIONS

- Confusion, hallucinations
- Difficulty breathing, wheezing
- Difficulty sleeping, nightmares
- Dizziness or fainting spells
- Irregular heartbeat, palpitations, chest pain
- Skin rash, itching, peeling skin
- Slow heart rate (less than 50 beats per minute)
- Swelling of the legs or ankles
- Caution for those with asthma, emphysema, bradycardia (slow heart rate), low blood pressure, fatigue, and impotence

KNOWN DRUG INTERACTIONS

- Atropine (Atropisol, Isopto Atropine)
- Clonidine (Catapres)
- Ergotamine
- High blood pressure medications
- Cough and cold medications
- Diabetic medications
- Antidepressant and other psychiatric medications
- Heart arrhythmia medications
- Monoamine oxidase (MAO) inhibitors (Azilect, Eldepryl, Emsam, Marplan, Nardil, Parnate, Zelapar)
- Theophylline (Theo-Dur, Respbid, Slo-Bid, Theo-24, Theolair, Uniphyl, Slo-Phyllin)

FOOD OR SUPPLEMENT INTERACTIONS

None known.

NUTRIENT DEPLETION/IMBALANCE

One study found that 90 mg of coenzyme Q10 supplementation reduced timolol-induced cardiovascular side effects without interfering with treatment of glaucoma.

Prostaglandin Analogs

Bimatoprost (Lumigan)

Latanoprost (Xalatan)

Travoprost (Travatan)

HOW DO THESE DRUGS WORK?
These drugs increase the rate at which the aqueous fluid flows out of the eye.

WHAT ARE THE BENEFITS?
Decreased intraocular pressure.

POTENTIAL SIDE EFFECTS
- Burning, stinging, or itching of the eyes or eyelids
- Changes in eye, eyelash, or eyelid color
- Dry eyes
- Increased flow of tears
- Light sensitivity

MAJOR CAUTIONS
- Vision changes
- Inflamed or infected eyes or eyelids

KNOWN DRUG INTERACTIONS
None known.

FOOD OR SUPPLEMENT INTERACTIONS
None known.

NUTRIENT DEPLETION/IMBALANCE
None known.

Carbonic Anhydrase Inhibitors

Methazolamide (GlaucTabs, Neptazane)

Brinzolamide (Azopt)

Dorzolamide ophthalmic (Trusopt)

Acetazolamide (AK-Zol, Diamox)

Acetazolamide Sustained-Release (Diamox Sequels)

Acetazolamide Injection (Diamox Injection)

HOW DO THESE DRUGS WORK?

This group of drugs decreases the rate at which the aqueous humor flows into the eye. They are available in topical eye drops or oral tablets or capsules.

WHAT ARE THE BENEFITS?

Decreased intraocular pressure.

POTENTIAL SIDE EFFECTS

Topical Dorzolamide Ophthalmic (Trusopt):

- Burning, stinging, or discomfort immediately after using the solution
- Dry eyes
- Increased flow of tears
- Sensitivity of the eyes to light

Oral capsules or tablets:

- Nausea
- Loss of appetite
- Constipation
- Frequent urination
- Drowsiness
- Weakness
- Headache

MAJOR CAUTIONS

Topical Dorzolamide Ophthalmic (Trusopt):

- Blurred vision
- Fever
- Inflamed or infected eyes or eyelids
- Muscle and joint aches
- Redness, blistering, peeling, or loosening of the skin, including inside the mouth
- Skin rash
- Fatigue or weakness

Oral capsules or tablets:

- Fever
- Sore throat
- Unusual bleeding or bruising
- Skin rash

- Painful urination
- Tingling or tremors of the hands or feet

KNOWN DRUG INTERACTIONS

Oral capsules or tablets:

- Amphotericin B
- Aspirin
- Barbiturate medicines
- Carbamazepine (Tegretol)
- Ciprofloxacin (Cipro)
- Digoxin (Lanoxin)
- Dextroamphetamine or amphetamine
- Mecamylamine (Inversine)
- Methenamine (Hiprex, Mandelamine, Urex)
- Mexiletine (Mexitil)
- Phenytoin (Dilantin)
- Pseudoephedrine
- Quinidine (Quinaglute, Quinidex, Quinora)
- Quinine (Quinerva, Quinite, QM-260)
- Prednisone or cortisone
- Diuretics

NUTRIENT DEPLETION/IMBALANCE

None known.

Carbonic Anhydrase Inhibitor and Beta-Blocker Combination Ophthalmic

There is currently one combination topical eye medication on the market. It combines two medications that are effective at lowering IOP (intraocular pressure). The advantage of a combination medication is that it is more convenient than using two separate topical eye medications.

Dorzolamide and timolol ophthalmic (Cosopt).

HOW DO THESE DRUGS WORK?

This class of drugs includes a combination of dorzolamide and timolol ophthalmic (Cosopt) to lower intraocular eye pressure.

WHAT ARE THE BENEFITS?

A more aggressive approach for decreasing intraocular pressure.

POTENTIAL SIDE EFFECTS

See side effects earlier in this chapter for dorzolamide ophthalmic (Trusopt) and timolol ophthalmic (Betimol, Timoptic, Timoptic-XE).

MAJOR CAUTIONS

See major cautions earlier in this chapter for dorzolamide ophthalmic (Trusopt) and timolol ophthalmic (Betimol, Timoptic, Timoptic-XE).

KNOWN DRUG INTERACTIONS

See drug interactions earlier in this chapter for dorzolamide ophthalmic (Trusopt) and timolol ophthalmic (Betimol, Timoptic, Timoptic-XE).

FOOD OR SUPPLEMENT INTERACTIONS

See food or supplement interactions earlier in this chapter for dorzolamide ophthalmic (Trusopt) and timolol ophthalmic (Betimol, Timoptic, Timoptic-XE).

NUTRIENT DEPLETION/IMBALANCE

See nutrition depletion/imbalance earlier in this chapter for dorzolamide ophthalmic (Trusopt) and timolol ophthalmic (Betimol, Timoptic, Timoptic-XE).

Sympathomimetics

Apraclonidine (Iopidine)

Brimonidine opthalmic solution (Alphagan)

Dipivefrin ophthalmic (Propine)

HOW DO THESE DRUGS WORK?

These eye drops decrease the formation of aqueous humor in the eye, along with increasing the flow of aqueous humor out of the eye.

WHAT ARE THE BENEFITS?

Decreased intraocular pressure.

POTENTIAL SIDE EFFECTS

- Blurred vision
- Burning, stinging, itching of the eyes immediately after use
- Change in taste
- Drowsiness
- Dry eyes

- Dry nose or dry mouth
- Headache
- Nausea, diarrhea, upset stomach
- Light sensitivity of the eys

MAJOR CAUTIONS
- Allergic reaction (rash, itching, hives)
- Conjunctivitis (pink eye)
- Inflamed, swollen, painful, or infected eyes or eyelids

KNOWN DRUG INTERACTIONS
- Monoamine oxidase (MAO) inhibitors such as Parnate (tranylcypromine), Marplan (isocarboxazid), or Nardil (phenelzine)
- Barbiturate medicines
- Beta-blockers
- Cyclosporine
- Digoxin (Lanoxin)
- Medicines for colds
- High blood pressure medications
- Depression medications
- Medicines for anxiety or sleeping problems
- Muscle relaxants
- Some antipsychotic medications
- Some pain medications

FOOD OR SUPPLEMENT INTERACTIONS
- Alcohol

NUTRIENT DEPLETION/IMBALANCE
None known.

Parasympathomimetics (also known as Miotics)

Pilocarpine ophthalmic (Isopto Carpine, Pilocar, Pilopine HS)

HOW DO THESE DRUGS WORK?
These drugs increase the aqueous outflow from the eye.

WHAT ARE THE BENEFITS?
Decreased intraocular pressure.

POTENTIAL SIDE EFFECTS

- Blurred vision
- Runny nose
- Chills
- Dizziness
- Eye irritation, burning, or itching
- Flushing
- Headache
- Increased sweating
- Nausea, vomiting
- Sensitivity
- Stomach upset
- Trembling
- Urgent need to urinate
- Weakness

MAJOR CAUTIONS

- Difficulty breathing
- Irregular heartbeat

KNOWN DRUG INTERACTIONS

- Atropine
- Acetazolamide
- Epinephrine
- Timolol

FOOD OR SUPPLEMENT INTERACTIONS

None known.

NUTRIENT DEPLETION/IMBALANCE

None known.

Natural Alternatives to Glaucoma Drugs

Mild cases of glaucoma may respond well to the following natural alternatives. These recommendations can also be used in addition to pharmaceutical treatments. In all cases, proper monitoring by an eye specialist is required.

Diet and Lifestyle Changes

Caffeine may increase intraocular pressure, so avoid coffee, chocolate, and caffeinated teas and sodas. Fish may decrease intraocular pressure. Consume cold-water fish such as sardines and wild salmon three times weekly. If this is difficult to do, supplement with fish oil that contains 1,000 mg of combined EPA and DHA.

Vitamin C

Vitamin C has been shown to reduce intraocular pressure in those with glaucoma.

DOSAGE

Take 1,000 mg two to four times daily.

SAFETY

Reduce the dosage if you experience loose stool.

Magnesium

This mineral dilates blood vessels and may improve blood flow. One trial found that magnesium had a mild benefit on improving vision in people with glaucoma. The dose used in the study was 245 mg of magnesium per day.

DOSAGE

Take 200 mg twice daily.

SAFETY

Too much magnesium may cause loose stool. Reduce the dosage if this occurs.

Ginkgo Biloba

Ginkgo biloba is a well-known vasodilator that improves circulation. In addition, it has potent antioxidant properties. A study in *Ophthalmology* looked at the effect of ginkgo extract in patients with a type of glaucoma known as normal tension glaucoma (NTG). This prospective, randomized, placebo-controlled, double-masked crossover trial involved 27 patients with bilateral visual field damage resulting from NTG. Participants received 40 mg of ginkgo biloba extract three times daily for four weeks, followed by a wash-out period of eight weeks, then four weeks of placebo treatment (identical capsules filled with 40 mg fructose). Gingko biloba extract treatment resulted in a significant improvement in visual field ratings. The authors concluded, "Ginkgo biloba extract administration appears to improve preexisting visual field damage in some patients with NTG."

Ginkgo biloba has been used by Chinese herbalists and physicians for over 3,500 years. It has several health benefits due to its special type of flavonoids (plant pigments). Ginkgo acts as a vasodilator and improves circulation, particularly to the brain and extremities. It is likely that this circulatory benefit would help those with glaucoma.

Lipoic Acid

Patients with stages I and II open-angle glaucoma (OAG) were involved in a study using lipoic acid. Of a total of 45 participants, 26 participants were given lipoic acid in a daily dose of 75 mg for two months and 19 were given 150 mg daily for one month. The study also included a control group of 31 patients with OAG. Approximately 47.5 percent of the eyes examined had improvement in those receiving 150 mg of lipoic acid.

Bonnie, a 64-year-old retiree, had recently been diagnosed with a mild case of open-angle glaucoma. Her desire was to try a nondrug approach and we agreed, provided she follow up with repeat testing from her ophthalmologist. A two-month multifactorial approach with supplements of vitamin C, magnesium, and ginkgo biloba resulted in her eye pressure dropping to the lower range. She continues to take these supplements, and repeat testing proves her eye pressure remains in the normal range.

BONNIE'S STORY

References

Filina, AA, et al. 1995. Lipoic acid as a means of metabolic therapy of open-angle glaucoma. *Vestnik oftalmologii.* 111(4):6–8.

Gaspar, AZ, P Gasser, J Flammer. 1995. The influence of magnesium on visual field and peripheral vasospasm in glaucoma. *Ophthalmologica.* 209:11–13.

Quaranta, L, et al. 2003. Effect of Ginkgo biloba extract on preexisting visual field damage in normal tension glaucoma. *Ophthalmology.* 110:359–62.

Ringsdorf, WM, Jr, E Cheraskin. 1981. Ascorbic acid and glaucoma: A review. *Journal of Holistic Medicine.* 3:167–72.

Takahashi, N, et al. 1989. Effect of coenzyme Q10 on hemodynamic response to ocular timolol. *Journal of Cardiovascular Pharmacology.* 14:462–8.

17

Headache Drugs and Their Natural Alternatives

What Are Headaches?

Headaches are all too common with Americans. According to the National Headache Foundation, over 45 million Americans suffer from chronic, recurring headaches. About 20 percent of children and adolescents also have significant headaches.

There are several types of headaches. This chapter focuses on primary headaches, which are headaches not caused by other diseases. They include tension, migraine, and cluster headaches. Secondary headaches are associated with other diseases. An example would be a headache caused by high blood pressure. There are various causes for each type of headache.

Tension headaches are by far the most common type. Most adults, as many as 90 percent, have or will experience this type of headache. They are caused by tension in the muscles of the head, neck, shoulder, and face, and are characterized by a generalized mild to moderate pain over the head. Many people describe the feeling as having a tight band around their head or pain in the back of their neck at the base of the skull. Stress is a primary cause, but other triggers may include:

- Depression and anxiety
- Lack of sleep or changes in sleep routine
- Skipping meals
- Poor posture

- Working in awkward positions or holding one position for a long time
- Lack of physical activity
- Occasionally, hormonal changes related to menstruation, pregnancy, menopause, or hormone use
- Medications used for other conditions, such as depression or high blood pressure
- Overuse of headache medication
- Temporomandibular disorder (pain and tenderness in the jaw joints)
- Grinding teeth

Researchers now believe that tension headaches may result from imbalances in certain brain chemicals such as serotonin. This is similar to migraine headaches. Therefore root causes beyond just tight muscles and poor stress-coping mechanisms may need to be addressed.

Cluster headaches are much rarer, affecting 0.1 percent of the population. Approximately 85 percent of cluster headache sufferers are men. They can affect people at any age, but they occur most commonly between ages 20 and 40. These are one-sided headaches that are intense for a number of days or weeks or even months, and then disappear and reoccur later. As the name implies, they occur in a cyclical, or cluster, pattern. Some 10 to 15 percent of cluster headaches occur daily for more than a year with no remission, or with pain-free periods lasting less than one month. Cluster attacks typically occur with clocklike regularity during a 24-hour day. Since the cycle of cluster headaches often follows the seasons of the year, researchers suspect dysfunction within a part of the brain called the hypothalamus. This is the location of the body's biological clock, which controls various hormonal and neurotransmitter rhythms of the body. Among the many functions of the hypothalamus is control of the sleep-wake cycle and other internal rhythms.

Abnormalities of the hypothalamus may explain the timing and cyclical nature of cluster headache. Studies have detected increased activity in the hypothalamus during the course of a cluster headache. This activity isn't seen in people with other headaches such as migraines.

Studies also indicate that cluster headache sufferers have abnormal levels of certain hormones, including melatonin and testosterone, during cluster periods. These hormonal changes are believed to be due to a problem with the hypothalamus. Other studies show activity in the hypothalamus during cluster attacks, but what causes these abnormalities in the first place remains unknown.

Migraine headaches are the second most common type of primary headache. An estimated 30 million people in the United States will experience migraine headaches, and they affect children as well as adults. Before puberty, boys and girls are affected equally by migraine headaches, but after puberty, more women than men are affected. Most migraine sufferers are between the ages of 15 and 55. Migraine pain is severe and occurs on one side of the head.

Headaches often last from 4 to 72 hours. They usually have a pulsating or throbbing pain and are made worse from exertion. The may be accompanied by nausea or vomiting and/or oversensitivity to light and sound. About 20 percent of migraine sufferers experience an aura, which may be perceived as flashing lights, blind spots, and wavy lines or dots in the field of vision. It should be noted that some people suffer from "mixed" headache disorders, in which tension headaches trigger migraine headaches. There are several causes of migraine headaches that may include:

- Changes in altitude, weather, or time zone.
- Dehydration.
- Fatigue.
- Sleep problems.
- Glaring lights or eyestrain.
- Head trauma, such as a car accident.
- Hormonal imbalances.
- Medications such as birth control pills or those used for erectile dysfunction. Migraine medications when overused may cause migraines as well.
- Perfumes or other powerful odors.
- Stress.
- Nutritional deficiencies.

Tension Headache Drugs

The following drugs are used for the treatment of acute tension headaches. Some of these medications are also used for migraine headaches. Analysis of migraine drugs is found later in this chapter.

Analgesics

There are two major classes of over-the-counter analgesics. These include acetaminophen (Tylenol) and nonsteroidal anti-inflammatory drugs (NSAIDs). The two types of NSAIDs are aspirin and nonaspirin. Examples of nonaspirin NSAIDs are ibuprofen (Advil, Nuprin, Motrin IB, and Medipren) and naproxen (Aleve). Some NSAIDs are available by prescription only, as they contain higher dosages.

Common NSAIDs include:

Aspirin

Salsalate (Amigesic)

Diflunisal (Dolobid)

Ibuprofen (Motrin, Advil)

Ketoprofen (Orudis)

Nabumetone (Relafen)

Piroxicam (Feldene)

Naproxen (Aleve, Naprosyn)

Diclofenac (Voltaren)

Indomethacin (Indocin)

Sulindac (Clinoril)

Tolmetin (Tolectin)

Etodolac (Lodine)

Ketorolac (Toradol)

Oxaprozin (Daypro)

Celecoxib (Celebrex)

HOW DO THESE DRUGS WORK?

The exact mechanism of how acetaminophen works is unknown. It seems to raise the body's threshold of tolerance to pain. Unlike the NSAIDs, it does not reduce inflammation.

NSAIDs work by blocking enzymes that are involved in the production of chemicals in the body known as prostaglandins. Certain prostaglandins promote pain and inflammation. By reducing the activity of cyclooxygenase (COX) enzymes, these medicines reduce pain and inflammation.

WHAT ARE THE BENEFITS?

Quick pain relief with medications that are easily accessible over the counter.

POTENTIAL SIDE EFFECTS

Acetaminophen can cause elevated liver enzymes or liver damage. This is typically at higher doses or when combined with alcohol, recreational drugs, or other pharmaceuticals.

For NSAIDs the most common side effects are nausea, vomiting, diarrhea, constipation, decreased appetite, rash, dizziness, headache, and drowsiness. They can also cause fluid retention and swelling of tissue.

MAJOR CAUTIONS

Acetaminophen can cause liver damage. This risk is increased with higher dosages and when combined with alcohol. Avoid its use for those with acute or chronic liver disease.

With NSAIDs there is a small risk of kidney failure, liver failure, ulcers, and prolonged bleeding after an injury or surgery. People allergic to NSAIDs may develop shortness of breath. People with asthma have a higher risk of experiencing a serious allergic reaction to NSAIDs. Those with a serious allergy to one NSAID are likely to experience a similar reaction to a different NSAID. The use of aspirin in children and teenagers with a viral infection or recent viral infection (especially chicken pox, common cold, or the flu) has been associated with the development of Reye's syndrome. This is a reaction in which one can suffer increased pressure within the brain and, often, massive accumulations of fat in the liver and other organs. Therefore, aspirin and nonaspirin salicylates (e.g., salsalate) should not be used in children and teenagers with suspected or confirmed chicken pox, common cold, or the flu.

KNOWN DRUG INTERACTIONS

Acetaminophen: The drugs cholestyramine (Questran), carbamazepine (Tegretol), isoniazid (INH, Nydrazid, Laniazid), and rifampin (Rifamate, Rifadin, Rimactane) can reduce the levels of acetaminophen and may decrease its effectiveness. Higher-than-recommended doses of acetaminophen may result in severe liver damage. The potential for liver damage from acetaminophen is increased when it is combined with alcohol or other drugs (recreational or pharmaceutical). Acetaminophen can increase the blood-thinning effect of warfarin (Coumadin).

NSAIDs: These can reduce blood flow to the kidneys and reduce the action of diuretics and decrease the elimination of lithium (Eskalith) and methotrexate (Rheumatrex). NSAIDs also decrease the ability of the blood to clot and therefore increase bleeding time. Bleeding complications are even more of a risk when NSAIDs are combined with other medications that have a blood-thinning effect. NSAIDs can also increase blood pressure. In February 2007 the American Heart Association issued new guidelines discouraging the use of regular nonsteroidal anti-inflammatory drugs (NSAIDs) in patients with known heart disease or those thought to be at high risk of getting heart disease.

FOOD OR SUPPLEMENT INTERACTIONS

Ibuprofen can cause salt and water retention. Therefore people should watch and minimize their sodium intake while using ibuprofen.

Hibiscus tea should not be consumed when taking acetaminophen, as it may decrease the levels of the drug.

Deglycyrrhizinated licorice (DGL) may help protect against ulceration of the digestive tract while using these medications, especially aspirin.

NUTRIENT DEPLETION/IMBALANCE

Milk thistle, vitamin C, and N-acetylcysteine may help prevent liver damage from acetaminophen. It should be noted that hospitals use oral and intravenous N-acetylcysteine to treat overdoses of acetaminophen. NSAIDs have been shown to deplete vitamin C and folic acid. Use these supplements under the guidance of a doctor.

- Milk thistle—take 250 to 300 mg twice daily.
- Vitamin C—take 500 mg daily.
- N-acetylcysteine—take 500 mg daily.
- Folic acid—take 400 micrograms daily.

Migraine Headache Drugs

Acetaminophen and NSAIDs described in the previous tension headache section can be used for migraine headaches. However, stronger treatment provided by specific migraine medications usually is needed for the relief of acute migraine headaches. The two categories include triptans and ergot preparations. Both classes of drugs counteract the dilation of the temporal arteries.

Triptans

Sumatriptan (Imitrex)

Zolmitriptan (Zomig)

Rizatriptan (Maxalt)

Naratriptan (Amerge)

Almotriptan (Axert)

Frovatriptan (Frovalan)

HOW DO THESE DRUGS WORK?

This class of drugs works by attaching to serotonin receptors on the blood vessels and nerves to reduce inflammation and constrict the blood vessels. Depending on the drug, they are available in injection, oral tablet, and nasal spray. Triptans are best used early in a migraine attack, preferably before the onset of pain.

WHAT ARE THE BENEFITS?

When used early, triptans can abort more than 80 percent of migraine headaches within two hours.

POTENTIAL SIDE EFFECTS

Common side effects include facial flushing, tingling of the skin, and a sense of tightness around the chest and throat. Less common side effects include drowsiness, fatigue, and dizziness.

MAJOR CAUTIONS

This class of migraine drugs carries the serious risk of heart attack and stroke. This is more of a concern in those who have atherosclerosis, in which arterial plaque occludes blood flow to the heart and brain. Triptans constrict the cerebral and heart arteries, and in those with existing arterial narrowing such as in atherosclerosis, the decreased blood flow can be a problem. These medications should be avoided by anyone with a history of heart attack, stroke, angina, transient ischemic attacks (TIAs), intermittent claudication, and with strong risk factors for cardiovascular disease. Also, triptans should not be used by pregnant women and young children.

KNOWN DRUG INTERACTIONS

Triptans should not be combined with pharmaceutical antidepressants including selective serotonin reuptake inhibitors (SSRIs) such as fluoxetine (Prozac), paroxetine (Paxil), sertraline (Zoloft), citalopram (Celexa), and fluvoxamine (Luvox); and monoamine oxidase (MAO) inhibitors such as phenelzine (Nardil) and tranylcypromine (Parnate). This can lead to serotonin levels that are too high, which may cause confusion, fever, tremor, high blood pressure, diarrhea, and sweating.

Propranolol (Inderal) can raise rizatriptan blood levels. Cimetidine (Tagamet) can increase zolmitriptan blood levels.

FOOD OR SUPPLEMENT INTERACTIONS

Avoid the use of the serotonin supportive supplements 5-hydroxytryptophan (5-HTP) and L-tryptophan. Also avoid the use of ginkgo biloba, as it affects blood circulation to the head. Avoid alcohol use with Imitrex.

NUTRIENT DEPLETION/IMBALANCE

- Vitamin B2 (riboflavin)—take 25 to 50 mg daily or as part of B complex.
- Coenzyme Q10—take 100 to 200 mg daily.

Natural Alternatives to Headache Drugs

Diet and Lifestyle Changes

Even mild levels of dehydration may trigger headaches. Make sure to drink adequate quality water throughout the day.

Food sensitivities may trigger migraine headaches (and possibly tension headaches). Although one could be sensitive to any food that is triggering headaches, the following foods are most commonly involved. If you frequently consume these foods, try omitting one or more at a time to see if your headaches improve. Holistic doctors can test you for food sensitivities as well.

- Alcohol, especially red wine and beer
- Artificial sweeteners

- Caffeine
- Chocolate
- Dairy products, especially aged cheese
- Pickled foods
- Shellfish
- Wheat
- MSG (monosodium glutamate), a flavoring often used in Asian cooking, packaged meats and vegetables, soups and snack foods
- Nitrites, a type of preservative commonly found in bacon, sausage and hot dogs, plus smoked or cured deli meats, fish, and poultry

Migraine and tension headaches can also be triggered by hypoglycemia, or low blood sugar. Make sure to limit your consumption of refined carbohydrates and to eat regular meals and snacks throughout the day.

Regular exercise is helpful for many people in preventing headaches related to stress and muscle tightness.

Environmental allergies may trigger tension and migraine headaches. Work with a holistic doctor to identify and treat these types of reactions.

Massage, chiropractic, acupuncture, craniosacral therapy, and other types of bodywork can be helpful therapies for all three types of headaches.

Magnesium

A deficiency of this mineral can lead to abnormal blood vessel constriction that occurs before a headache. It also is required for healthy neurotransmitter balance. People with migraine headaches tend to have lower blood magnesium levels. In a double-blind trial of 81 people with migraines, 600 mg of magnesium per day was significantly more effective than placebo at reducing the frequency of migraines. We also find that magnesium supplements are effective for those with tension headaches, as magnesium works to relax tight muscles and calms the nervous system.

DOSAGE

Take 200 mg two to three times daily. It can also be taken in combination with calcium.

SAFETY

The most common side effect with too much magnesium is digestive upset, particularly diarrhea. This symptom improves when the dosage is lowered.

Riboflavin (Vitamin B2)

This water-soluble B vitamin is involved in the metabolism of amino acids and fats, along with vitamin B6 (pyridoxine) and folic acid, to produce energy in cells. Its mechanism in preventing migraine headaches is unknown. A Belgian study published in *Cephalalgia: An International Journal of Headache*, involved 49 migraine patients who took 400 mg of riboflavin as a single oral daily dose for at least three months. Treatment resulted in an overall improvement of 68 percent. In a follow-up trial with the same group, 55 migraine patients took either a placebo or 400 mg of riboflavin daily. Frequency of migraine episodes and the number of days with headache decreased by at least half in 59 percent of patients in the riboflavin group, compared with 15 percent of patients in the placebo group. There is also some evidence that combining riboflavin with beta-blockers (cardiovascular drugs sometimes given to reduce the frequency and severity of migraines) may boost the drugs' effectiveness without increasing their adverse side effects.

DOSAGE

Take 400 mg daily.

SAFETY

No toxic effects have been reported.

Coenzyme Q10

A study done at Thomas Jefferson University followed 31 migraine patients who were given 150 mg of CoQ10 daily. After three months of treatment, participants reported that the average number of attacks per month fell from 4.85 to 2.81, and that the number of days the migraines lasted also was significantly reduced. In another study from the same institution, double-blind and placebo controlled, 42 patients took either placebo or CoQ10 at 100 mg three times a day for three months. Migraine frequency diminished by half in 47 percent of the patients taking CoQ10, compared with 14 percent of placebo users. CoQ10 users also reported less nausea.

DOSAGE

Take 150 mg daily.

SAFETY

Coenzyme Q10 is very safe and well tolerated.

Butterbur

This botanical contains anti-inflammatory compounds known as sesquiterpenoids. *Petasites hybridus* root (butterbur) has been shown to prevent migraine headaches. A study published in *Neurology* included people ages 18 to 65 who had had at least two to six migraine attacks over the preceding three months.

> ### Energy-Deficient Brain Cells and Migraines
>
> A more recent theory as to why migraines occur in some people is a lack of energy production within brain cells. It is thought that poor energy production causes the release of pain signals that promote brain inflammation and neurotransmitter and circulation changes that initiate migraines. Nutrients such as coenzyme Q10, magnesium, and vitamin B2 help with cellular energy production.

Participants who took butterbur standardized to contain 75 mg twice daily for four months had their migraine attack frequency decrease an average of 48 percent as compared to 26 percent for the placebo group.

There is also evidence that butterbur extract can decrease the frequency of migraine headaches in children ages 6 to 17 years. The multicenter, prospective, open-label study involved 108 children and adolescents between the ages of 6 and 17. Participants suffered from migraines diagnosed for at least one year. Patients were treated with 50 to 150 mg of the butterbur root extract, depending on age, for a period of four months. Treatment progression was recorded in migraine journals especially designed for children and adolescents, and 77 percent of all patients reported a reduction in the frequency of migraine attacks of at least 50 percent. Overall attacks were reduced by 63 percent. Some 91 percent of patients felt substantially or at least slightly improved after four months of treatment. About 90 percent of each, doctors and patients, reported well-being or even improved well-being. Undesired effects (7.4 percent) included mostly burping. No serious adverse events occurred and no adverse event caused a premature stopping of the study.

DOSAGE

Adults take 75 mg twice daily. Give children 50 to 75 mg twice daily.

SAFETY

Butterbur appears to be well tolerated.

5-hydroxytryptophan

This amino acid is converted in the body into serotonin, which plays a role in pain control and inflammation involved with migraine and tension headaches. Several studies demonstrate that 5-HTP can be of mild benefit in the prevention of these headaches.

MICHELLE'S STORY

Michelle, a 45-year-old teacher, had suffered with migraines for more than five years. She would normally experience two or more migraines a month. Pharmaceutical medications would often stop the migraines if taken early enough in the course of a migraine. She tried a variety of different natural therapies including chiropractic, acupuncture, and a strict diet, without much success. The triad of magnesium, vitamin B2, and coenzyme Q10 reduced her migraine frequency by approximately 90 percent and without any side effects.

DOSAGE

Take 400 to 600 mg daily in divided doses on an empty stomach.

SAFETY

This supplement should not be combined with any pharmaceuticals that affect serotonin levels such as antidepressants and anti-anxiety medications. It should not be taken simultaneously with migraine medications. Digestive upset is an occasional side effect.

Feverfew

There are several studies that demonstrate that botanical feverfew can reduce the frequency of migraine headaches, including symptoms of pain, nausea, vomiting, and sensitivity to light and noise. It is commonly used by the public as a natural, over-the-counter migraine prevention remedy. A recent study found that the combination of feverfew and white willow bark extract was quite effective in preventing migraine headaches. Published in *Clinical Drug Investigations*, this prospective, open-label study involved 12 patients diagnosed with migraine without aura. For 12 weeks, participants were given 300 mg of white willow extract and 300 mg of feverfew. Attack frequency was reduced by 61.7 percent at 12 weeks in 9 of 10 patients, with 70 percent of patients having a reduction of at least 50 percent. Attack intensity was reduced by 62.6 percent at 12 weeks in 10 of 10 patients, with 70 percent of patients having a reduction of at least 50 percent. Attack duration decreased by 76.2 percent at 12 weeks in 10 of 10 patients. The treatment was well tolerated.

DOSAGE

Use a product containing 250 to 500 micrograms of parthenolides daily.

SAFETY

Feverfew appears to be very safe in studies that have been conducted.

Melatonin

This hormone has effects on blood flow and pain signals. It also is thought to lower core body temperature. Those with cluster headaches tend to have higher body heat. Also, patients with migraine headaches tend to have lower melatonin production. Sleep problems may be a trigger of migraine headaches in some individuals. Taking 10 mg every evening has been shown to reduce the frequency of episodic (not chronic) cluster headaches. Lower dosages do not seem to be beneficial. Melatonin at a dose of 3 mg each evening has been shown to benefit those with episodic migraine headaches and reduce their duration and intensity.

DOSAGE

For episodic cluster headache prevention, take 10 mg each evening before bedtime on an empty stomach.

For episodic migraine headache prevention, take up to 3 mg each evening before bedtime on an empty stomach.

SAFETY

Melatonin is quite safe and available over the counter. It should not be used by pregnant or nursing women unless under the supervision of a doctor. It should not be used by children unless directed to do so by a doctor.

References

Leone, M, et al. 1996. Melatonin versus placebo in the prophylaxis of cluster headache: A double-blind pilot study with parallel groups. *Cephalalgia.* 16:494–6.

Lipton, RB, et al. 2004. Petasites hybridus root (butterbur) is an effective preventive treatment for migraine. *Neurology.* 63(12):2240–4.

Peres, MFP, et al. 2004. Melatonin, 3 mg, is effective for migraine prevention. *Neurology.* 63:757.

Pothmann, R, U Danesch. 2005. Migraine prevention in children and adolescents: Results of an open study with a special butterbur root extract. *Headache.* March;45(3):196–203.

Rozen, TD, et al. 2002. Open label trial of coenzyme Q10 as a migraine preventive. *International Journal of Headache.* March; 22(2): 137–41.

Sandor, PS, et al. 2005. Efficacy of coenzyme Q10 in migraine prophylaxis: A randomized controlled trial. *Neurology.* 64:713–5.

Schoenen, J, Jacquy J, Lenaerts M. 1998. Effectiveness of high-dose riboflavin in migraine prophylaxis. A randomized controlled trial. *Neurology.* 50:466–70.

Schoenen, J, M Lenaerts, E Bastings. 1994. High-dose riboflavin as a prophylactic treatment of migraine: Results of an open pilot study. *Cephalalgia.* 14:328–9.

Shrivastava, R, JC Pechadre, GW John. 2006. Tanacetum parthenium and Salix alba (Mig-RL) combination in migraine prophylaxis: A prospective, open-label study. *Clinical Drug Investigations.* 26(5):287–96.

Weaver, K. 1990. Magnesium and migraine. *Headache.* 30:168 [letter].

18

Herpes Drugs and Their Natural Alternatives

What Is Herpes?

"Herpes" is the shortened name given to herpes simplex virus (HSV)—a common, contagious viral infection that causes sores or blemishes on the face or in the genital area. Herpes simplex infection on the face is the most common, usually caused by HSV-1. Its symptoms are commonly known as "cold sores" or "fever blisters," which typically appear on the lips. Genital herpes is characterized by recurrent clusters of blisters and lesions in the genital area, usually caused by HSV-2. Under a microscope, HSV-1 and HSV-2 are virtually identical, and both types infect the body's mucosal surfaces and then "hide out" in the nervous system when symptoms resolve. The main difference between the two infections is the primary site of infection: in the genital area or on the face. It was once widely believed that HSV-1 could not cause herpes in the genital area, and that HSV-2 could not cause herpes on the face, but the fact of the matter is that either infection can be transmitted to either mucosal surface.

While generally not dangerous, herpes is very contagious and can cause stress and emotional trauma. Very rarely, herpes can cause severe or fatal disease if the infection travels to the eyes or brain (herpes encephalitis). The danger of such severe effects is highest in newborns exposed to genital herpes during passage through the birth canal, or in people with poor immune function, for example, someone with HIV.

How Do You Get Herpes?

Any direct skin-to-skin contact (kissing, touching, intercourse) or transfer of bodily fluids can transmit herpes (HSV-1 or HSV-2). A person is most contagious when early warning signs (called prodrome: tingling, redness, etc.), active sores, and healing lesions are present. However, herpes can be spread even in the absence of symptoms, because a person who has herpes could potentially always be "shedding" active virus.

Oral herpes is estimated to affect 50 to 80 percent of the adult U.S. population. And genital herpes affects one in five American adolescents and adults, but only one-third of those infected are aware that they have the virus because their symptoms are mild, and some may have no symptoms at all. Research indicates that more than 500,000 Americans are diagnosed with genital herpes every year; and unfortunately, the group seeing the largest increase is young teens.

An important aspect of herpes infection is that it's chronic, meaning the infection is lifelong. Although the immune system attacks the herpes virus and can resolve symptoms, it cannot rid the body of herpes completely. This is because the virus "hides," inactive (or dormant), in nerve cells, evading the immune system. When conditions are right, the virus is "triggered" and becomes active again, causing symptoms. Triggers, as well as signs and symptoms, vary widely from person to person.

If signs and symptoms occur during the first outbreak, they can be quite pronounced. Symptoms of herpes usually develop within 2 to 20 days after contact with the virus and may last several weeks. Generally, typical initial and recurrent symptoms include:

Tingling, itching sensation

Red, sensitive skin

Flu-like symptoms (swollen glands, headache, muscle ache, fever)

Appearance of one or more painful blisters or bumps

Blisters that open and then heal as new skin forms

Herpes cannot be cured. Infected people can suffer several outbreaks every year. Outbreaks can be reduced by using effective treatments, minimizing stress, avoiding triggers (e.g., excessive sun exposure, physical trauma, allergens, nutritional deficiencies), and supporting a strong immune function. Conventional treatment primarily involves oral and/or topical antiviral therapy that is used during an outbreak (episodically) or daily (suppressive therapy). These medications may reduce the occurrence of blisters, shorten their duration, and reduce associated pain.

Synthetic Nucleoside Analogs

Acyclovir (Zovirax oral, intravenous, and topical)

Penciclovir (Denavir topical cream)

Famciclovir (Famvir)

Valacyclovir (Valtrex)

HOW DO THESE DRUGS WORK?

Nucleoside analogs are the first line of treatment for herpes. They specifically target herpes-infected cells, where they prevent the formation and spread of new virus by stopping new viral DNA from forming. It's important to note here that these medicines only work on active, replicating virus—not on dormant virus hidden in nerve cells.

WHAT ARE THE BENEFITS?

These medications help lessen the severity of a primary outbreak and can reduce healing time. They also decrease the number of days of painful symptoms, and in some cases, how long a person can spread the virus. In addition, oral suppressive (or daily) therapy can reduce the number of outbreaks by 70 to 80 percent. Although oral antiviral medication is generally prescribed for genital herpes, it is not uncommon for doctors to prescribe these medications to patients who have severe cases of facial herpes.

POTENTIAL SIDE EFFECTS

Oral medications: Upset stomach, loss of appetite, nausea, vomiting, diarrhea, headache, dizziness, fatigue or weakness, and painful periods are common side effects that may resolve as your body adjusts to the medication. More serious side effects may include mental/mood changes, difficulty sleeping, confusion, speech problems, shaky movement, vision changes, numbness or tingling of the hands or feet, back pain, joint pain, sore throat, skin rash, or hair loss.

Topical medications: Common side effects include burning, stinging, redness, and mild numbness where applied.

MAJOR CAUTIONS

With oral medications, changes in urine, easy bruising or bleeding, seizures, loss of consciousness, and signs of other infection (fever, sore throat, chills, etc.) can indicate serious problems. In rare cases Valtrex may cause a blood disorder or a severe kidney problem, especially in people with HIV or in transplant recipients. Allergy to these oral or topical drugs is unlikely, but symptoms such as rash, itching, swelling, dizziness, or trouble breathing are indicative of a severe allergic reaction.

MEDICAL PRECAUTIONS

People with the following conditions or disorders should discuss their risks with their physician:

Topical Drugs

- Allergy to valacyclovir, penciclovir, or polyethylene glycol

Oral Drugs

- Immune dysfunction
- Human immunodeficiency virus infection (HIV)
- Acquired immunodeficiency syndrome (AIDS)
- Kidney or liver disease
- Blood disorders
- Galactose intolerance or glucose-galactose malabsorption (inherited conditions in which the body is not able to tolerate lactose)
- Old age
- Pregnancy
- Breast-feeding

KNOWN DRUG INTERACTIONS

Various oral nucleoside analogs may interact with some or all of the following medications: amphotericin B (Fungizone); aminoglycoside antibiotics such as amikacin (Amikin), gentamicin (Garamycin), kanamycin (Kantrex), neomycin (Nes-RX, Neo-Fradin), paramomycin (Humatin), streptomycin, and tobramycin (Tobi, Nebcin); aspirin and other nonsteroidal anti-inflammatory medications such as ibuprofen (Advil, Motrin), and naproxen (Aleve, Naprosyn); cyclosporine (Neoral, Sandimmune); medications to treat HIV or AIDS such as zidovudine (Retrovir, AZT); pentamidine (NebuPent); cimetidine (Tagamet), and probenecid (Benemid); sulfonamides such as sulfamethoxazole and trimethoprim (Bactrim); tacrolimus (Prograf); vancomycin; and digoxin (Lanoxin). Many other medications may also interact.

FOOD OR SUPPLEMENT INTERACTIONS

With oral medications, alcohol should be avoided because of the dizziness associated with these medications. St. John's wort should be avoided due to known interactions between this herb and certain antiviral medications. Herbs with antiviral properties, including cat's claw, cloves, cardamom seed, mountain laurel, oak bark, sage leaf, and scarlet pimpernel may increase the effects of antiviral drugs. In vitro and animal studies suggest that the following supplements may help Zovirax work better: citrus root bark, flavonoids, *Geum japonicum*, *Rhus javanica*, *Syzygium aromaticum*, *Terminalia chebula*, and *Tripterygium wilfordii*.

NUTRIENT DEPLETION/IMBALANCE

None known.

Topical Fusion Inhibitor

Docosanol (Abreva): This over-the-counter topical drug is used specifically for the treatment of herpes lesions on the lips. Where applied, it prevents the herpes virus from entering healthy cells. Abreva is the only FDA-approved over-the-counter cream clinically proven to help speed the healing process. In clinical trials, Abreva reduced cold sore healing time to a median of 4.1 days versus 4.8 days with placebo. It also shortened the duration of pain, burning, itching, and tingling symptoms. There are not any side effects, precautions, or interactions associated with the use of Abreva.

Topical Analgesics and Anesthetics

These topical drugs may provide some relief from pain and discomfort. Such treatments include Blistex lip ointment, Campho-phenique, Herpecin-L, Viractin, and Zilactin. In some cases, such over-the-counter treatments may actually delay the healing time of lesions because they can irritate the area with repeated applications.

Vaccines

Herpes vaccines are being investigated and may be available in three to five years. GlaxoSmithKline Biologicals began a Phase 3 trial, called the "HERPEVAC Trial for Women," in November 2002. In addition, over 56 countries utilize isoniplex (Isoprinosine)—a vaccine approved for use in HSV infections due to its antiviral action and its ability to stimulate the body's immune response. Isoniplex is currently under investigational trials in primary and recurrent HSV cases in the United States. Unfortunately, those who already have the virus will be unlikely to gain any benefit, as vaccines will only prevent the infection in new patients.

Natural Alternatives to Herpes Drugs

Many people with oral herpes (HSV-1) find that natural therapies are quite effective in greatly reducing the frequency and severity of outbreaks. Many of our patients have found that natural therapy works so well that cold sore outbreaks are uncommon. One of the authors of this book has not had a cold sore outbreak for over 15 years with the type of program outlined in this chapter. Most people afflicted with genital herpes (HSV-2) use pharmaceutical antiviral medication to suppress outbreaks and shorten their course and severity of symptoms. Since these drug therapies do not affect the dormant HSV-2 virus, it could be helpful to use natural therapies that improve the immune system's ability to keep the virus suppressed. Also, natural therapies may be used simultaneously with pharmaceutical treatment for a quicker recovery. There are individuals who respond so well to natural therapy that they do not require drug therapy for genital herpes outbreaks. In any event, anyone infected with HSV-2 should be under the care of a physician.

Diet and Lifestyle Changes

One common dietary approach recommended by practitioners of natural medicine is for patients to limit foods containing the amino acid L-arginine. Test tube studies demonstrate that the herpes virus is promoted by L-arginine and suppressed by L-lysine. Foods that are high in the amino acid L-arginine include nuts, wheat, chocolate, and peas. Increase your intake of foods rich in L-lysine, which include legumes, turkey, fish, chicken, red meat, and most vegetables. While no human studies have ever shown this dietary approach to be helpful, we have seen it benefit many patients with herpes.

Simple sugars such as white flours, fruit juices, candy, and soda pop should be minimized, as they suppress immune function.

L-lysine

This amino acid has been shown in several studies to reduce the recurrence and severity of both types of herpes outbreaks, and to shorten their healing time. In one small double-blind trial, 3,000 mg per day of lysine in divided doses led to a decrease in severity of symptoms and a reduction in healing time of both oral and genital herpes.

DOSAGE

For acute outbreaks take 1,000 mg three times daily between meals. For prevention take 500 to 1,000 mg twice daily between meals.

SAFETY

There are no known safety problems with L-lysine.

Lemon Balm

The topical application of lemon balm is helpful in the treatment of oral and genital herpes. This plant appears to have antiviral effects. A double-blind,

LYNN'S STORY

Lynn, a 38-year-old receptionist, had been experiencing multiple breakouts of cold sores on the corner of her mouth for a year. On the advice of a friend, she began supplementation of L-lysine and found that the frequency of her outbreaks decreased by 90 percent. When she did have an outbreak, she increased the dosage and found that it greatly reduced the severity and duration of the breakout.

placebo-controlled, randomized trial published in the journal *Phytomedicine* demonstrated that topical lemon balm was effective for the treatment of cold sores. The study involved 66 patients with a history of recurrent cold sores (at least four episodes per year); 34 of them received treatment and 32 were given placebo. The cream had to be smeared on the affected area four times daily over five days. Using the cream was found to shorten the healing period and prevent the infection from spreading, while having a rapid effect on the typical symptoms of herpes such as itching, tingling, burning, stabbing, swelling, tautness, and redness.

DOSAGE

Apply lemon balm cream to the affected area four times daily until the lesions have healed.

SAFETY

Topical application of lemon balm cream has been shown to be very safe. There is always the possibility of a sensitivity reaction to any topical treatment.

Propolis

This is the resinous substance that is collected by bees from the buds and bark of trees. It contains antimicrobial and anti-inflammatory flavonoids.

Topical use of propolis has been shown to be effective for genital herpes. A randomized, single-blind, masked investigator, controlled multicenter study involving 90 men and women with recurrent genital herpes (HSV-2 type) compared propolis ointment against acyclovir ointment and placebo on their healing ability and capacity to remedy symptoms. Thirty individuals were randomized to each group. On day ten of treatment, the participants were

---

The Buzz about Bee Propolis

Bee propolis is quite an interesting medicinal substance. Also referred to as "bee glue," it is the product of bees gathering a resinous substance from the buds and barks of certain trees, particularly conifer and poplar trees. It is then mixed with saliva secretions from worker bees, as well as wax flakes, and spread on the beehive walls. Besides forming a physical barrier, propolis protects the colony against infectious agents such as viruses, fungi, and bacteria. Propolis also plays an important role as a coating for the area of the hive where the queen bee lays her eggs. Due to its ability to fight infections, Russian scientists have nicknamed it "Russian penicillin."

examined; 24 out of 30 individuals in the propolis group, 14 out of 30 in the acyclovir group, and 12 out of 30 in the placebo group had healed. The healing process and reduction in symptoms appeared to be faster in the propolis group.

DOSAGE

Apply propolis cream or spray to the affected area four times daily until the lesions have healed.

SAFETY

Topical application of propolis has been shown to be very safe. There is always the possibility of a sensitivity reaction to any topical treatment.

Zinc

The mineral zinc is known to have immune-boosting properties. The topical application of zinc sulfate ointment has been shown to reduce the severity and duration of symptoms in both oral and genital herpes.

DOSAGE

Apply zinc sulfate ointment to the affected area four times daily until the lesions have healed.

SAFETY

Topical application of zinc has been shown to be very safe. There is always the possibility of a sensitivity reaction to any topical treatment.

Aloe Vera

This commonly used medicinal plant can be used topically for oral and genital herpes. A double-blind trial using a 0.5 percent *aloe vera* cream found that applying the cream three times a day shortened the healing time of genital herpes outbreaks.

DOSAGE

Apply aloe vera gel to the affected area four times daily until the lesions have healed.

SAFETY

Topical application of aloe has been shown to be very safe. There is always the possibility of a sensitivity reaction to any topical treatment.

Homeopathic Herpes Nosode

This type of treatment involves taking the homeopathic form of the herpes virus. It stimulates a response by the immune system to mount an attack against the herpes virus. While there are no formal studies we are aware of, the authors have found it helpful in preventing reoccurring oral and genital herpes outbreaks. Work with a practitioner trained in homeopathy for this type of treatment.

References

Eby, GA, WW Halcomb. 1985. Use of topical zinc to prevent recurrent herpes simplex infection: Review of literature and suggested protocols. *Medical Hypotheses.* 17:157–65.

Griffith, RS, et al. 1987. Success of L-lysine therapy in frequently recurrent herpes simplex infection. *Dermatologica.* 175:183–90.

Kneist, W, B Hempel, S Borelli. 1995. [Clinical, double-blind trial of topical zinc sulfate for herpes labialis recidivans (article in German)]. *Arzneimittelforschung.* 45:624–6.

Koytchev, R, RG Alken, S Dundarov. 1999. Balm mint extract (Lo-701) for topical treatment of recurring herpes labialis. *Phytomedicine.* October;6(4):225–30.

Syed, TA, M Afzal, et al. 1997. Management of genital herpes in men with 0.5 percent *Aloe vera* extract in a hydrophylic cream: A placebo-controlled, double-blind study. *Journal of Dermatological Treatment.* 8:99–102.

Vynograd, N, I Vynograd, Z Sosnowski. 2000. A comparative multi-centre study of the efficacy of propolis, acyclovir and placebo in the treatment of genital herpes (HSV). *Phytomedicine.* 7:1–6.

Hypothyroid Drugs and Their Natural Alternatives

What Is Hypothyroidism?

Prescription medications for hypothyroidism are very common in the United States. According to the American Association of Clinical Endocrinologists, studies have shown that as many as 10 percent of women and 3 percent of men have hypothyroidism.

The thyroid gland is located at the base of the neck below the Adam's apple. It secretes thyroid hormones that have pronounced effects on the cells of your body. The two main thyroid hormones include T3 (liothyronine) and T4 (L-thyroxine). Another thyroid hormone, known as thyroid-stimulating hormone (TSH), regulates the secretion of T3 and T4. This hormone is secreted by the pituitary gland when the pituitary receives messages from the brain (hypothalamus) that blood levels of thyroid hormones are getting low. When the hypothalamus senses low blood levels of thyroid hormones, it signals the pituitary gland to release more TSH; and this in turn signals the thyroid gland to release more of T4 and T3 hormone.

Thyroid hormones control the metabolic activity in every cell. This is important for temperature control, weight regulation, heart rate, and energy production. Thyroid activity even influences one's mood and neurotransmitter balance, and affects the balance of other hormones in the body. Hypothyroidism occurs when the thyroid gland is underactive, leading to a shortage of thyroid hormones. The most common cause is a disease known as Hashimoto's thyroiditis. This is an autoimmune condition in which the body's immune

> ## Subclinical Hypothyroidism
>
> It is our experience that many cases of hypothyroidism are undiagnosed. A common scenario is when a patient has several hypothyroid symptoms but no abnormal blood test results. Doctors usually refuse to treat patients for hypothyroidism when they have no abnormalities in their tests. Many of these patients have what we term subclinical hypothyroidism. That is to say, they exhibit symptoms of low thyroid but their blood tests have not revealed a deficiency. Many of these patients' symptoms improve tremendously from thyroid support with natural therapy (including nutritional supplements) or from carefully monitored thyroid hormone replacement.

system produces antibodies to the thyroid gland. The attack on the thyroid gland leads to the suppression of thyroid hormone production and secretion. Other reasons for hypothyroidism may include iodine deficiency and other nutritional deficiencies, stress, pregnancy, medications such as lithium or estrogen therapy, and an underfunctioning pituitary gland.

Hypothyroidism is most common in middle-aged and older women. It can occur in any age group, though, including infants and teenagers. Untreated hypothyroidism can be life-threatening.

Common symptoms of hypothyroidism include fatigue, weight gain, dry skin, hair loss, constipation, intolerance to cold, and poor memory. Since thyroid hormones affect all cells of the body, there are many other signs and symptoms including:

- Anxiety
- Arthritis
- Brittle nails
- Cold hands and feet
- Eyebrow loss (especially the outer third)
- High cholesterol
- Heart palpitations
- Infertility
- Headaches
- Depression
- Low libido
- Low body temperature
- PMS
- Fluid retention

- Raynaud's phenomenon
- Carpal tunnel syndrome
- Anemia
- Slow healing
- Puffy face
- Hoarse voice
- Muscle aches, tenderness, and stiffness
- Muscle weakness
- Heavier than normal menstrual periods

Hypothyroid Drugs

L-thyroxine

The main type of thyroid hormone replacement used by most conventional doctors is T4, known as L-thyroxine, generically known as levothyroxine. It is the most commonly prescribed thyroid medication. The four main nongeneric T4 prescriptions include:

Synthroid

Levothroid

Levoxyl

Unithroid

The primary difference among these medications is that each brand has different fillers, binders, or pill dosage sizes. Some patients may have allergies to certain brands, or have problems with pill dosage sizes.

As with most hormones, L-thyroxine also is available as a compounded hormone. Pharmacies known as compounding pharmacies manufacture prescriptions such as hormones on an individual basis. L-thyroxine can be compounded to whatever dosage the patient requires.

HOW DO THESE DRUGS WORK?

L-thyroxine increases the blood levels of T4 hormone levels for those with a deficiency. It is also used to treat other thyroid conditions such as goiters (enlarged thyroid gland), nodules, thyroiditis (inflammation of the thyroid), and thyroid cancer.

WHAT ARE THE BENEFITS?

These drugs increase thyroid hormone levels in the body and have a long history of use.

POTENTIAL SIDE EFFECTS

An overdose or a sensitivity to thyroid medication can cause headache, nervousness, trembling, sweating, increased appetite, diarrhea, weight loss, chest pain, irregular or rapid heartbeat, shortness of breath, irregular menstrual cycles in women, or insomnia. Rare cases of hair loss may occur.

MAJOR CAUTIONS

Taking too much thyroid over periods of time can lead to bone loss in children and adults and stunted growth in children. Caution for those with chest pain, angina, or high blood pressure, particularly for those taking T3 (liothyronine).

Store at room temperature (77 degrees Fahrenheit or 25 degrees Celsius) away from light and moisture.

KNOWN DRUG INTERACTIONS

The following drugs have potential interactions with thyroid hormone. Consult with your doctor if you are using warfarin, digoxin, estrogen replacement including birth control pills, diabetes medicines (e.g., insulin and oral diabetic medications), iodide, lithium, antithyroid medications (e.g., methimazole, propylthiouracil), testosterone and other anabolic hormones, glucocorticoids (e.g., dexamethasone, prednisone), high-dose aspirin, phenobarbital, rifamycins (e.g., rifampin), beta-blockers (e.g., propranolol), antidepressants, cytokines (e.g., interferon-alpha, interleukin-2), growth hormones, ketamine, theophylline, cough and cold medications, and supplements that contain caffeine.

The following medications can impair the absorption of thyroid hormone and should be taken four hours away from taking it: calcium supplements, iron supplements, aluminum, calcium or magnesium antacids, simethicone, cholestyramine, colestipol, sucralfate, and sodium polystyrene sulfonate.

FOOD OR SUPPLEMENT INTERACTIONS

The following foods can interfere with L-thyroxine absorption and should not be taken at the same time. These include soybean flour and soy infant formula, walnuts, and dietary fiber.

Data on the consumption of soy products impairing thyroid function are unclear. It is best to avoid consuming large quantities of soy foods and to not take thyroid medication within three hours of eating soy products.

Avoid using the herbal supplements lemon balm (*Melissa officinalis*) and bugleweed (*Lycopus virginicus*), as they can interfere with the activity of thyroid hormone and should be avoided.

NUTRIENT DEPLETION/IMBALANCE

Iron—have your doctor test you for iron-deficiency anemia before supplementing.

Liothyronine (T3)

A less commonly prescribed thyroid medication is T3, known as liothyronine. It is used when patients' T3 blood levels are low.

> Cytomel (liothyronine sodium)
>
> Compounded T3 (liothyronine) from a compounding pharmacy

HOW DO THESE MEDICATIONS WORK?

Liothyronine is used to treat hypothyroidism, specifically when blood T3 levels are low.

WHAT ARE THE BENEFITS?

Liothyronine effectively increases the levels of T3 for people who are deficient in this hormone.

POTENTIAL SIDE EFFECTS

Same as for L-thyroxine, except chest pain occurs more readily in those who are overdosed.

MAJOR CAUTIONS

Same as for L-thyroxine.

KNOWN DRUG INTERACTIONS

Same as for L-thyroxine.

FOOD OR SUPPLEMENT INTERACTIONS

Same as for L-thyroxine.

NUTRIENTS DEPLETION/IMBALANCE

Same as for L-thyroxine.

Combination L-thyroxine (T4) and Liothyronine (T3)

Another class of thyroid replacement medications are those containing both L-thyroxine and liothyronine. Some people require both of these thyroid hormones to maintain normal thyroid levels.

> Liotrix (Thyrolar)
>
> Compounded T4 (L-thyroxine) and T3 (liothyronine)

Natural Thyroid Hormones

The last class of thyroid replacement medications are known as the natural thyroid hormone replacement medications. They are made from desiccated (dried) pork thyroid glands. They contain T4 and T3, but also contain the thyroid hormones T1 and T2. Little is known about T1 and T2, but they do occur in the human body and may be one reason so many of our patients do well on these natural extracts.

Armour Thyroid

To ensure that Armour Thyroid tablets are consistently potent from tablet to tablet and lot to lot, analytical tests are performed on the thyroid powder (raw material) and on the actual tablets (finished product) to measure actual T4 and T3 activity.

NatureThroid

This is a natural preparation derived from porcine thyroid glands. Its T3 liothyronine is approximately four times as potent as T4 levothyroxine on a microgram for microgram basis, and it provides a standardized, guaranteed potency of 38 mcg levothyroxine (T4) and 9 mcg liothyronine (T3) for each 65 mg (1 grain) of the labeled content of thyroid.

Westhroid, produced by Western Research Laboratories, is the same product as NatureThroid.

POTENTIAL SIDE EFFECTS

Same as for L-thyroxine except that chest pain occurs more readily in those who are overdosed.

MAJOR CAUTIONS

Same as for L-thyroxine and liothyronine except that these three medications should be avoided by individuals allergic to pork.

KNOWN DRUG INTERACTIONS

Same as for L-thyroxine.

FOOD OR SUPPLEMENT INTERACTIONS

Same for as L-thyroxine, except that these three medications should be avoided by individuals allergic to pork.

NUTRIENT DEPLETION/IMBALANCE

Same for as L-thyroxine.

Natural Alternatives to Hypothyroid Drugs

It is important to note that many people with hypothyroidism require the life-long use of prescription thyroid medications. This is particularly true for those with Hashimoto's thyroiditis and those who have had their thyroid gland removed or destroyed with radioactive iodine. Some people who do not have Hashimoto's thyroiditis, particularly those in the early stages of hypothyroidism, may be able to correct their hypothyroidism with diet and lifestyle changes, and the use of specific nutritional supplements. We find that many patients feel better after switching from T4-only therapy to one of the natural thyroid hormone replacements, or to compounded T4/T3 or T3-only medications. The reason is that they are getting both active T4 and T3. Do not change any of your thyroid medications unless under the guidance of a knowledgeable physician.

Diet and Lifestyle Changes

Alcohol and nicotine are enemies of the thyroid gland and should be avoided.

Regular exercise is important to normalize stress hormones such as cortisol that can impair thyroid function. Fifteen to thirty minutes five times weekly is good. Consult with your doctor first before beginning a program. Avoid excessive consumption of soy foods. While there is no conclusive human evidence that soy foods or soy supplements suppress thyroid function, those prone to low thyroid function are advised to use soy products in moderation until further research is completed in this area.

Home Test for Low Thyroid Function

Since the thyroid gland controls metabolism and temperature, you can indirectly assess its function by temperature testing. This was originally developed by Broda O. Barnes, M.D., author of *Hypothyroidism: The Unsuspected Illness*. Here is how to take this assessment:

1. Shake down an oral glass thermometer before using it in the morning, or use an electronic version.

2. Immediately upon awakening, and with as little movement as possible, place the thermometer firmly in your armpit next to the skin. (It is even more accurate when placed under the tongue.)

3. Leave it there for 10 minutes.

4. Record the readings on three consecutive days. (For women with a menstrual cycle it is best to test on the first three days of your cycle.)

5. If the average temperature over the three days is less than 97.8°F, then, according to Dr. Barnes, you may have hypothyroidism.

Testing Tip

We recommend that while your thyroid hormone levels are being assessed, you get a complete thyroid panel. Many doctors only order a TSH test. While it is used as a general screening, it fails to detect many cases of hypothyroidism. A thorough thyroid panel would include TSH, Free T4, Free T3, and thyroid peroxidase antibodies. Do note that according to many holistic doctors and emerging studies, an optimal TSH level is 0.2 milli IU/L to 2.0 milli IU/L.

Iodine

Iodine is required for the production of T4 and T3. A deficiency of iodine can cause goiter (enlarged thyroid gland) and hypothyroidism. It is estimated that one and a half billion people living in 118 countries around the world are at risk for developing iodine deficiency. While most authorities consider iodine deficiency in the United States to be rare, it appears to be reemerging because people with high blood pressure avoid iodized table salt.

DOSAGE

Patients with hypothyroidism may benefit from 150 to 300 micrograms of iodine daily. Many multivitamins contain 150 mcg of iodine. Nutrition-oriented doctors often use much higher doses, but this requires testing and close monitoring of the patient.

SAFETY

High amounts of iodine, usually several milligrams, can suppress thyroid function. Also, higher amounts used for long periods of time may cause a metallic taste; soreness in the teeth and gums; burning in the mouth and throat; increased salivation; runny nose; sneezing; eye irritation and eyelid swelling; headache; cough; pulmonary edema; swelling of the parotid and submaxillary glands; inflammation of the pharynx, larynx, and tonsils; acneform skin lesions; stomach upset; diarrhea; anorexia; and depression.

Thyroid Glandular

Health food stores and professional lines carry thyroid glandular supplements. These supplements are similar to the natural thyroid hormone replacement medications made from desiccated (dried) pork thyroid glands. The difference is that they have thyroid hormones removed, although trace amounts likely remain in the products. The two sources are either bovine or porcine thyroid.

The theory behind these products is that they stimulate and nourish the thyroid gland to function more effectively. We find that they are effective for many people with mild hypothyroidism.

DOSAGE

The milligram amount per capsule or tablet of various brands varies. However, a typical dose is one tablet or capsule (usually 200 to 500 mg) taken three times daily on an empty stomach.

SAFETY

Sensitivity to thyroid glandular rarely causes headaches. Since these products are derived from animals, there is concern about contamination with diseased animal parts. There have been no reports of disease transmission to humans from the use of these products. Look for products derived from organic sources.

L-tyrosine

L-tyrosine is an amino acid that the thyroid gland combines with iodine to manufacture thyroid hormone.

DOSAGE

Take 300 to 500 mg twice daily on an empty stomach.

SAFETY

L-tyrosine is quite safe. Those on hypothyroid hormone replacement should consult with their doctor before using it, since it may increase their thyroid hormone levels. It should be avoided in persons with Graves disease (hyperthyroidism).

Thyroid Hormone Replacements: The Natural Advantage

For patients with moderate to severe hypothyroidism, we have seen consistently good results with more natural types of thyroid hormone replacements such as Armour Thyroid and NatureThroid. Both are available by prescription only. The advantage of these medications is that they contain both of the dominant thyroid hormones, thyroxine (T4) and triiodothyronine (T3). In addition, they contain the other thyroid hormones, known as T2 and T1.

TINA'S STORY

Tina, a 45-year-old, was in the beginnings of premenopause. She noticed her menstrual cycle changing and she felt the occasional hot flash. Of concern were increasing fatigue and weight gain. Testing of her thyroid levels showed a mild deficiency of thyroid hormones. She was prescribed a natural regimen to help her premenopausal symptoms as well one tablet three times daily of a thyroid glandular. Within two weeks she felt an increase in energy, and noticed that she had stopped gaining weight. After six weeks, repeat blood testing showed that her thyroid hormone levels had returned to normal.

Ashwagandha

Animal studies have shown that the herb ashwagandha improves the conversion of T4 into the more active T3. It is particularly helpful if low thyroid function is the result of chronic stress, as there is some evidence this herbal extract also balances cortisol levels.

DOSAGE

Take 250 to 500 mg twice daily.

SAFETY

Ashwagandha is well tolerated. Occasional digestive upset is reported. Preliminary evidence shows that ashwagandha may increase the effects of benzodiazepines; e.g., diazepam (Valium) and clonazepam (Klonopin). If you are on these medications, check with your doctor first before using.

References

Upton, R (Ed). 2000. Ashwagandha Root (Withania somnifera): Analytical, quality control, and therapeutic monograph. Santa Cruz, CA: *American Herbal Pharmacopoeia.* 1–25.

20

Menopause Drugs and Their Natural Alternatives

Menopause is a transitional time in a woman's life when menstruation stops. The medical definition of menopause is the absence of a woman's menstrual cycle for 12 months or longer. The typical age of menopause is around 50 years of age. Some women start menopause earlier, in their forties, and a small percentage go into menopause later than age 50.

The period of time leading up to menopause is known as perimenopause or premenopause. During this time the menstrual cycle begins to change. Periods occur closer together, are skipped, or are longer and heavier. During perimenopause, the ovaries do not ovulate as regularly. Ovarian production of hormones decreases, particularly of progesterone. Other hormones such as estrogen and testosterone begin to decrease as well.

Perimenopausal and menopausal women can experience a variety of symptoms. The most common are hot flashes. They are experienced by 75 percent of menopausal women for about two years, though another 25 percent continue to have them for five years or more. We have spoken with female patients who continued to experience hot flashes into their seventies! Other common symptoms of perimenopause/menopause include:

- Night sweats
- Insomnia
- Vaginal dryness and thinning

- Heart palpitations
- Fatigue
- Poor memory
- Low sex drive
- Mood changes
- Joint pain
- Headaches
- Hair loss/thinning

Due to declining hormones, bone loss can accelerate during menopause. In addition, women are more susceptible to other conditions developing such as hypothyroidism and cardiovascular disease. These conditions are covered in their respective chapters in this book.

Menopause Drugs

Hormone Therapy

A variety of different prescription hormone therapies are available to reduce the symptoms of menopause. This review will cover the most common prescription hormones prescribed by medical doctors. In the Natural Alternatives to Menopause Drugs section, we will cover important information on bioidentical, also known as natural, hormones, many of which are also available by prescription only. In this section of the drug review, we will note whether the commonly prescribed drugs by medical doctors are bioidentical or not. We do note that our preference is for the bioidentical hormones and other natural remedies discussed later in the chapter.

Estrogen

Estrogen that is not bioidentical:

- Premarin
- Estinyl
- Congest
- Cenestin
- Ortho-Est
- Menest
- Estratab
- Ogen

- Ortho Dienestrol
- Vagifem

Estrogen that is bioidentical:
- Estrace
- Estrasorb
- Delestrogen
- Gynodiol
- Estraderm
- Vivelle
- Vivelle Dot
- Climara
- Alora
- Esclim
- Estring
- Clinagen LA 40
- Depogen
- Estragyn 5
- Kestrone 5
- Valergen

HOW DO THESE DRUGS WORK?

They increase the body's levels of estrogen (synthetic versions mimic the activity of natural estrogen) and attach to cell receptors that relieve a variety of estrogen-deficiency symptoms associated with menopause.

WHAT ARE THE BENEFITS?

Estrogen therapy can relieve many common menopausal symptoms such as hot flashes, night sweats, vaginal dryness, vaginal thinning, and mood changes.

POTENTIAL SIDE EFFECTS

- Breakthrough bleeding and spotting
- Breast enlargement and pain, and unusual discharge or milk production
- Chest pain
- Gum swelling, tenderness, or bleeding
- Leg, arm, or groin pain
- Nausea, vomiting
- Severe headaches

- Abdominal pain
- Sudden shortness of breath
- Swelling of eyelids, face, lips, hands, or feet; swelling of feet and lower legs
- Vision or speech problems
- Yellowing of the eyes or skin
- Change in sexual desire
- Mood changes such as anxiety, depression, frustration, anger, or emotional outbursts
- Changes in appetite (increased or decreased)
- Skin rash
- Acne
- Bladder pain
- Brown spots on the face
- Fatigue
- Vaginal yeast infection
- Weight gain
- Water retention
- Loss or thinning of scalp hair

MAJOR CAUTIONS

- There is an increased risk of uterine (endometrial) cancer when not taken in combination with progesterone. Estrogen therapy also increases the risk of breast cancer.
- Do not smoke if you are taking estrogen, as it increases blood clot risk.
- Abnormal vaginal bleeding can occur.
- Do not use if you are pregnant or trying to get pregnant, or while breast-feeding.

KNOWN DRUG INTERACTIONS

The following drugs may interact with estrogen:

- Anastrozole (Arimidex)
- Some antibiotics
- Some medications used to treat HIV (human immunodeficiency virus) infection or AIDS
- Barbiturates or benzodiazepines used for inducing sleep or treating seizures (convulsions)
- Bromocriptine (Parlodel)
- Carbamazepine (Tegretol)

- Cimetidine (Tagamet)
- Clofibrate (Atromid-S)
- Cyclosporine (Gengraf, Neoral)
- Dantrolene (Dantrium)
- Exemestane (Aromasin)
- Griseofulvin (Grifulvin V)
- Other hormones such as thyroid or cortisone
- Some antidepressants such as imipramine (Tofranil)
- Isoniazid (Nydrazid, Laniazid)
- Letrozole
- Medications for diabetes
- Methotrexate (Rheumatrex, Trexall)
- Mineral oil
- Phenytoin (Dilantin)
- Raloxifene (Evista)
- Tamoxifen (Nolvadex)
- Rifabutin (Mycobutin)
- Theophylline
- Topiramate (Topamax)
- Warfarin (Coumadin)

FOOD OR SUPPLEMENT INTERACTIONS

- Grapefruit juice

Soy supplements may increase the potency of estrogen prescriptions. Check with your doctor before using soy supplements.

NUTRIENT DEPLETION/IMBALANCE

Estrogens can decrease the body's levels of vitamin B6, zinc, and magnesium. We recommend the following:

- Vitamin B6—take 50 mg daily.
- Zinc—take 15 mg daily.
- Magnesium—take 200 to 250 mg twice daily.

Progesterone

Progesterone that is not bioidentical:

Provera

Cycrin

Amen

Aygestin

Nor-QD

Micronor

Megace

Progesterone that is biodentical:

Prometrium

Crinone

HOW DO THESE DRUGS WORK?

They increase the body's levels of progesterone (synthetic versions mimic the activity of natural progesterone) and attach to cell receptors that relieve a variety of progesterone-deficiency symptoms associated with menopause.

WHAT ARE THE BENEFITS?

Progesterone therapy can relieve many common menopausal symptoms such as hot flashes, night sweats, mood changes, and insomnia. Progesterone also prevents the overgrowth of the uterine lining in women who are taking estrogens for menopausal symptoms.

POTENTIAL SIDE EFFECTS

- Abdominal pain
- Breast tenderness or discharge
- Dizziness
- Gum swelling, tenderness, or bleeding
- Muscle or bone pain
- Numbness or pain in the arm or leg
- Pain in the chest, groin, or leg
- Severe headache
- Sudden shortness of breath
- Unusual weakness or tiredness
- Vision or speech problems
- Yellowing of the skin or eyes
- Changes in sexual desire or ability
- Changes in vaginal bleeding
- Facial hair growth
- Fluid retention and swelling
- Headache
- Increased sweating or hot flashes

- Loss of appetite or increase in appetite
- Mood changes
- Nausea, vomiting
- Skin rash
- Weight gain or weight loss
- Vaginal yeast infection

MAJOR CAUTIONS

Progesterone (mainly associated with synthetic progesterone known as progestins) may cause blood clots, breakthrough bleeding, jaundice, depression, and possibly breast cancer.

Progesterone (synthetic or bioidentical) may cause dizziness or drowsiness. Do not drive, use machinery, or perform activities that require mental alertness until you know how it affects you.

Do not use if you are pregnant or trying to get pregnant, or while breast-feeding.

KNOWN DRUG INTERACTIONS

- Barbiturate medicines for inducing sleep or treating seizures (convulsions)
- Bromocriptine (Parlodel)
- Carbamazepine ((Tegretol)
- Ketoconazole (Nizoral)
- Phenytoin (Dilantin)
- Rifampin (Rifadin)
- Voriconazole (Vfend)

FOOD OR SUPPLEMENT INTERACTIONS

None known.

NUTRIENT DEPLETION/IMBALANCE

None known.

Combination Estrogen/Progesterone

Combination estrogen/progesterone that is not bioidentical:

Prempro

FemHRT

Premphase

Angeliq

Combination estrogen/progesterone that is bioidentical combined with non-bioidentical:

Ortho-Prefest

Activella

Combi Patch

HOW DO THESE DRUGS WORK?

The combination of estrogen and progesterone increases the body's levels of estrogen (synthetic versions mimic the activity of natural estrogen) and progesterone (synthetic versions mimic the activity of natural progesterone) and attaches to cell receptors that relieve a variety of estrogen/progesterone deficiency symptoms associated with menopause.

WHAT ARE THE BENEFITS?

Estrogen therapy can relieve many common menopausal symptoms such as hot flashes, night sweats, vaginal dryness, vaginal thinning, mood changes, and insomnia. Taking the combination is more effective at preventing uterine (endometrial) cancer.

POTENTIAL SIDE EFFECTS

- Breakthrough bleeding and spotting
- Breast enlargement and pain, and unusual discharge or milk production
- Chest pain
- Gum swelling, tenderness, or bleeding
- Leg, arm, or groin pain
- Nausea, vomiting
- Severe headaches
- Abdominal pain
- Sudden shortness of breath
- Swelling of eyelids, face, lips, hands, or feet; swelling of feet and lower legs
- Vision or speech problems
- Yellowing of the eyes or skin
- Change in sexual desire
- Mood changes such as anxiety, depression, frustration, anger, or emotional outbursts
- Changes in appetite (increased or decreased)
- Skin rash
- Acne
- Bladder pain
- Brown spots on the face

- Fatigue
- Vaginal yeast infection
- Weight gain
- Water retention
- Loss or thinning of scalp hair

MAJOR CAUTIONS

Progesterone (synthetic version studied) taken in combination with estrogen can increase the risk of heart disease (including heart attacks), stroke, serious blood clots in the lung (pulmonary embolism) or leg (deep venous thrombosis), breast cancer, or dementia. This combination may also increase the risk of cancer of the ovary.

KNOWN DRUG INTERACTIONS

- Anastrozole (Arimidex)
- Some antibiotics
- Some medications used to treat HIV (human immunodeficiency virus) infection or AIDS
- Barbiturates or benzodiazepines used for inducing sleep or treating seizures (convulsions)
- Bromocriptine (Parlodel)
- Carbamazepine (Tegretol)
- Cimetidine (Tagamet)
- Clofibrate (Atromid-S)
- Cyclosporine (Gengraf, Neoral)
- Dantrolene (Dantrium)
- Exemestane (Aromasin)
- Griseofulvin (Grifulvin V)
- Other hormones such as thyroid or cortisone
- Some antidepressants such as imipramine (Tofranil)
- Isoniazid (Nydrazid, Laniazid)
- Letrozole
- Medications for diabetes
- Methotrexate (Rheumatrex, Trexall)
- Mineral oil
- Phenytoin (Dilantin)
- Raloxifene (Evista)
- Tamoxifen (Nolvadex)
- Rifabutin (Mycobutin)

- Theophylline
- Topiramate (Topamax)
- Warfarin (Coumadin)
- Rifampin (Rifadin)
- Voriconazole (Vfend)

FOOD OR SUPPLEMENT INTERACTIONS

- Grapefruit juice

Soy supplements may increase the potency of estrogen prescriptions. Check with your doctor before using soy supplements.

NUTRIENT DEPLETION/IMBALANCE

Estrogens can decrease the body's levels of vitamin B6, zinc, and magnesium. We recommend the following:

- Vitamin B6—take 50 mg daily.
- Zinc—take 15 mg daily.
- Magnesium—take 200 to 250 mg twice daily.

Testosterone

Testosterone that is not bioidentical:

Methyltestosterone

Testosterone injections (injectables of testosterone enanthate and testosterone cypionate, as well as other esters such as acetate, propionate, phenylpropionate, isocaproate, caproate, decanoate, and undecanoate)

Testosterone combined with estrogen that is not bioidentical:

EstraTest

EstraTest HS

Menogen

Menogen HS

Bioidentical testosterone:

Compounded testosterone

HOW DO THESE DRUGS WORK?

They increase the body's levels of testosterone (synthetic versions mimic the activity of natural testosterone) and attach to cell receptors that relieve a variety of testosterone-deficiency symptoms associated with menopause.

WHAT ARE THE BENEFITS?

Testosterone therapy can relieve many common menopausal symptoms such as hot flashes, vaginal dryness, vaginal thinning, fatigue, low libido, and mood changes.

POTENTIAL SIDE EFFECTS

- Anxiety, depression
- Nausea, vomiting
- Skin rash and itching (hives)
- Stomach pain
- Unusual bleeding
- Unusual swelling
- Weight gain
- Yellowing of the eyes or skin
- Irregular vaginal bleeding/spotting
- Decrease in breast size
- Enlarged clitoris
- Hair loss
- Facial hair growth
- Voice changes (deepening or hoarseness)
- Acne
- Hair loss
- Headache
- Changes in sexual desire

MAJOR CAUTIONS

If you are diabetic, testosterone may affect your blood sugar levels.

KNOWN DRUG INTERACTIONS

- Fluconazole (Diflucan)
- Cyclosporine (Gengraf, Neoral)
- Prostate enlargement or prostate cancer drugs
- Warfarin (Coumadin)
- Dehydroepiandrosterone (DHEA), which can increase testosterone levels in women

FOOD OR SUPPLEMENT INTERACTIONS

None known.

NUTRIENT DEPLETION/IMBALANCE

None known.

Oral Contraceptive Pills

This form of hormone therapy is often prescribed for women in perimenopause to treat irregular bleeding and relieve common perimenopausal symptoms.

>   Estrin 1/20
>
>   Alesse

HOW DO THESE DRUGS WORK?

Oral contraceptives reduce the levels of two pituitary hormones known as luteinizing hormone (LH) and follicle-stimulating hormone (FSH). These two hormones become elevated during perimenopause and menopause, and are thought to contribute to menopausal symptoms. Also, small amounts of synthetic estrogen and/or synthetic progesterone (progestin) in oral contraceptives may directly relieve menopausal symptoms as well.

WHAT ARE THE BENEFITS?

Irregular vaginal bleeding can be stopped or controlled. Also, common perimenopausal symptoms such as hot flashes may be controlled.

Oral Contraceptives and Blood Levels

A study published in the *American Journal of Obstetrics and Gynecology* examined how oral contraceptives affect blood levels of fat-soluble antioxidants, including coenzyme Q10, alpha-tocopherol, and gamma-tocopherol (members of the vitamin E family), and the carotenoids: beta-carotene, alpha-carotene, and lycopene. Nonfasting blood samples were collected randomly at any day of the menstrual cycle from 15 premenopausal women who had used oral contraceptives for at least six months and from 40 women who did not use oral contraceptives. No dietary restrictions were imposed on any of the participants. Women who consumed coenzyme Q10 supplements and/or multivitamins as well as women who had irregular menstrual cycles were excluded from the study. Researchers found that in oral contraceptive users, blood levels of coenzyme Q10 were 37 percent lower and alpha-tocopherol levels were 23 percent lower than in women who did not use contraceptives. Blood levels of the other nutrients were comparable between the two groups.

POTENTIAL SIDE EFFECTS

Breast tenderness, nausea, higher blood pressure, and headaches are other possible side effects.

MAJOR CAUTIONS

Oral contraceptives can increase the risk of blood clots, breast cancer, and heart disease. They should be avoided by women with a history of these diseases. Breast cancer risk is more associated with long-term use. It is important to not smoke when using birth control pills, as this increases the risk of blood clots.

FOOD OR SUPPLEMENT INTERACTIONS

St. John's wort and grapefruit juice should be avoided by women taking birth control pills.

NUTRIENT DEPLETION/IMBALANCE

Nutrients depleted by oral contraceptives include: B1, B2, B3, B6, B12, folic acid, magnesium, zinc, vitamin C, CoQ10, and vitamin E. We recommend the following supplements:

- B complex—take daily.
- Magnesium—take 200 to 250 mg twice daily.
- Zinc—take 15 mg daily.
- Vitamin C—take 500 mg daily.
- CoQ10—take 100 to 200 mg daily.
- Vitamin E—take 200 IU of a mixed vitamin E daily.

Antidepressant Medications

In recent years, antidepressant medications have been used to control the symptoms of hot flashes in menopausal women.

Venlafaxine (Effexor)

Fluoxetine (Prozac)

Sertraline (Zoloft)

Paroxetine (Paxil)

Citalopram (Celexa)

HOW DO THESE DRUGS WORK?

Antidepressants allow more of the brain chemical serotonin to reach key receptors in the brain. Similar to estrogen, serotonin helps to regulate body temperature as well as mood, sleep, and appetite.

WHAT ARE THE BENEFITS?

These medications have been shown to be effective in controlling hot flashes in up to 60 percent of women and can relieve depression, anxiety, and insomnia as well.

POTENTIAL SIDE EFFECTS

There are a variety of potential side effects including headaches, anxiety, insomnia, drowsiness, loss of appetite, decreased libido or sexual dysfunction, weight gain, and fatigue. See chapter 12 on depression drugs for more information.

MAJOR CAUTIONS

Some antidepressants may rarely cause suicidal depression. They can also increase blood pressure, cause skin rashes, and cause vasculitis (inflammation of the blood vessels). See chapter 12 on depression drugs for more information.

KNOWN DRUG INTERACTIONS

See chapter 12 on depression drugs for more information.

FOOD OR SUPPLEMENT INTERACTIONS

See chapter 12 on depression drugs for more information.

NUTRIENT DEPLETION/IMBALANCE

See chapter 12 on depression drugs for more information.

Antiseizure Medication

Gabapentin (Neurontin)

This medication is approved for treating seizures or pain associated with shingles, and can reduce hot flashes.

HOW DOES THIS DRUG WORK?

Gabapentin is related to the brain chemical gamma-aminobutyric acid (GABA) but exactly how it works is unknown. GABA has a relaxing and inhibitory effect on the brain and nervous system.

WHAT ARE THE BENEFITS?

Some studies have found that gabapentin is moderately effective in reducing hot flashes.

POTENTIAL SIDE EFFECTS

Sleepiness, dizziness, unsteady gait, fatigue, and eye twitching.

MAJOR CAUTIONS

One may experience drowsiness, dizziness, or blurred vision. Do not drive, use machinery, or do anything that needs mental alertness until you know how gabapentin affects you.

KNOWN DRUG INTERACTIONS

Gabapentin should not be taken within two hours of antacids such as Maalox. It may increase the potency of sedative medications. There is a potential for adverse reactions if combined with cimetidine (Tagamet) or sevelamer (Renagel).

FOOD OR SUPPLEMENT INTERACTIONS

Avoid alcohol when using this medication.

NUTRIENT DEPLETION/IMBALANCE

The following may be depleted by gabapentin:

- Biotin—take 300 mcg daily.
- Calcium—take 500 to 1,200 mg daily.
- Folic acid—take 400 mcg daily.
- L-carnitine—take 500 mg daily.
- Vitamin A—take 5,000 IU daily.
- Vitamin B12—take 100 to 200 mcg daily.
- Vitamin B6—take 50 mg daily.
- Vitamin D—take 1,000 IU daily.
- Vitamin K—take 50 to 100 mcg daily.

Clonidine

Clonidine is used as a pill or patch to treat high blood pressure. It can also provide relief from hot flashes.

Side effects such as dizziness, drowsiness, dry mouth, and constipation are common, sometimes limiting the medication's usefulness for treating hot flashes.

HOW DOES THIS DRUG WORK?

Clonidine affects the circulatory system, which is thought to somehow help hot flashes.

WHAT ARE THE BENEFITS?

Clonidine may provide relief from hot flashes in menopausal women.

POTENTIAL SIDE EFFECTS

- Unusual fatigue
- Dizziness
- Tiredness
- Headache
- Constipation, nausea, vomiting, or diarrhea
- Insomnia
- Dry mouth

MAJOR CAUTIONS

- A very slow heart rate (fewer than 60 beats per minute)
- Unusually high or low blood pressure
- Severe headache
- Redness of the face, neck, and chest
- Dizziness
- Fainting

KNOWN DRUG INTERACTIONS

- Beta-blockers such as atenolol (Tenormin), acebutolol (Sectral), propranolol (Inderal), metoprolol (Lopressor), carvedilol (Coreg), carteolol (Cartrol), labetalol (Normodyne, Trandate), or nadolol (Corgard)
- Levodopa (Dopar, Larodopa, Sinemet)
- Prazosin (Minipress)
- Verapamil (Verelan, Calan, Isoptin, Covera-HS)
- Tricyclic antidepressants such as amitriptyline (Elavil, Endep), imipramine (Tofranil), nortriptyline (Pamelor), doxepin (Sinequan), and others

FOOD OR SUPPLEMENT INTERACTIONS

Do not take in conjunction with alcohol, as it may increase the potential side effects of dizziness and drowsiness.

NUTRIENT DEPLETION/IMBALANCE

- Coenzyme Q10—take 100 to 200 mg daily.

Natural Alternatives to Menopause Drugs

Diet and Lifestyle Changes

Increase your intake of plant foods such as legumes, vegetables, fruits, whole grains, nuts, and other seeds, as they contain hormone-balancing plant chemicals known as phytoestrogens. Ground flaxseeds also contain phytoestrogens and have been shown in studies to reduce hot flashes. In one positive study, women consumed 40 grams of ground flaxseed daily. Fermented soy foods such as tofu, miso, and tempeh can help reduce hot flashes. Reduce your intake of spicy foods, which may worsen hot flash frequency and intensity. Sedentary women are more likely to experience hot flashes. Mild to moderate aerobic exercise can reduce hot flashes. Women who smoke are more likely to experience hot flashes.

Black Cohosh

This herb is commonly used by North American and European women for the relief of hot flashes. Studies confirm that it relieves a variety of mild to moderate menopausal symptoms safely and effectively. For example, a study that

---

The Black Cohosh Connection

In 2006 the Australian Therapeutic Goods Administration (ATGA), a regulatory body in that country, announced that it had become concerned about a possible relationship between black cohosh and liver disease. It was then reported by the U.S. media to be a risk to the liver. Is there any merit to this warning by the ATGA? How did the Australian regulators reach their conclusion about black cohosh? They cited 47 reports of liver toxicity among black cohosh users that were collected worldwide. In Australia, four patients were hospitalized, and two of these required liver transplants. But the ATGA did not disclose what criteria it used to interpret the data. For example, the ATGA didn't say what brands or dosages of black cohosh products were involved in the cases or whether the products were analyzed to confirm their content. Some of the products involved in the ATGA's report contained a variety of herbs, not just black cohosh. All these factors make it difficult to judge the merit of the ATGA's warning. In a contradictory statement, the ATGA wrote, "Considering the widespread use of black cohosh, the incidence of liver reaction appears to be very low." This statement comports with a 2004 finding by the U.S. National Institutes of Health that there was no evidence that black cohosh causes liver toxicity. Now that it is a few years later, there have been no further reports of concern about black cohosh and liver toxicity. We have never seen a patient using black cohosh experience liver problems. An enzyme blood test by your doctor can always check to see if there are any liver problems.

---

included 131 evaluating doctors and 629 menopausal women found that 80 percent of women had relief from a variety of menopausal symptoms within six to eight weeks. Symptoms that were found to improve included hot flashes, heart palpitations, vertigo, headaches, nervousness, ringing in the ears, anxiety, insomnia, and depression. Also, a study in *Gynecology Endocrinology* found black cohosh comparable to low-dose transdermal estradiol in alleviating hot flashes.

DOSAGE

Take 80 mg one to two times daily of a 2.5 percent triterpene glycoside extract.

SAFETY

Black cohosh is quite safe, and recent studies indicate that it is safe for women who have a history of breast cancer. It appears to work by supplying phytoestrogens and by altering the secretion of luteinizing hormone by the pituitary gland.

Soy Isoflavones

Soy isoflavone supplements have been shown to reduce hot flashes. They contain phytoestrogens that attach to estrogen receptors on cells. One published systematic review included a meta-analysis of all randomized, controlled trials of isoflavone supplementation to determine the efficacy of isoflavone therapy in reducing the number of daily menopausal flushes. The results suggested that isoflavone supplementation may produce a slight to modest reduction in the number of daily flushes in menopausal women and that the benefit may be more apparent in women experiencing a high number of flushes per day.

DOSAGE

Take 40 to 150 mg daily.

SAFETY

There is debate over whether soy isoflavone supplements are safe for women who have a history of breast cancer. At this point they should be avoided by women with a history of this disease. Soy products may cause digestive upset or skin rash in a small percentage of users.

Vitex

Also referred to as chasteberry, this herb alters the secretion of the pituitary luteinizing and follicle stimulating hormones. It is commonly used in Europe to relieve hot flashes. It is effective during perimenopause to reduce heavy menstrual bleeding.

DOSAGE

Take 160 to 240 mg of a standardized product daily.

Perimenopausal Relief with Vitex

Vitex (chasteberry) is an excellent herb for women who are perimenopausal and still experiencing a period. It helps to keep menstrual flow from becoming too erratic and can alleviate premenstrual syndrome as well. This herb is best used on a daily basis and is not fully effective until used for two or more cycles.

SAFETY

Do not take in combination with oral contraceptives. It rarely causes skin rashes and digestive upset.

Bioidentical Hormone Replacement

Bioidentical hormones are commonly available over the counter and by prescription from compounding pharmacies. They refer to hormones that are identical in structure and function to those found in the human body. Currently, over-the-counter bioidentical hormones include progesterone cream and dehydroepiandrosterone (DHEA) capsules or tablets. A double-blind trial demonstrated that transdermal progesterone cream reduced hot flashes in 83 percent of women, compared to 19 percent given a placebo. Studies have also shown that it prevents the buildup of the endometrium (uterine lining) in women taking synthetic estrogen therapy.

Bioidentical forms of estrogen, progesterone, testosterone, DHEA, and most other prescription hormones are available by prescription from compounding pharmacies. The advantages of compounding pharmacies are numerous. The hormones are tailor-made to the patient, so more specific dosages can be used. A variety of different forms are available, including topical (transdermal), capsule, suppository, sublingual, and others to best meet the individual needs of the patient. Work with a doctor knowledgeable in bioidentical hormone replacement for individualized treatment.

CYNTHIA'S STORY

Cynthia, a 51-year-old housewife, had been suffering with extreme menopausal symptoms including hourly hot flashes, night sweats, vaginal dryness, depression, and fatigue. Herbal supplements were only of mild benefit. Hormone testing revealed severe deficiencies of estrogen, progesterone, DHEA, and testosterone. We prescribed a bioidentical hormone regimen that contained all these hormones. Improvements were noticed within two days, and within six weeks her symptoms were reported as being very mild.

References

Blumenthal, M. 2006. ATGA Black cohosh/liver warning. *HerbalGram*. 71:60–61.

Howes, LG, JB Howes, DC Knight. 2006. Isoflavone therapy for menopausal flushes: A systematic review and meta-analysis. *Maturitas*. 55:203–11.

Leonetti, HB, et al. 2005. Transdermal progesterone cream as an alternative progestin in hormone therapy. *Alternative Therapies in Health and Medicine*. November–December;11(6):36–8.

Leonetti, HB, S Longo, JN Anasti. 1999. Transdermal progesterone cream for vasomotor symptoms and postmenopausal bone loss. *Obstetrics and Gynecology*. 94:225–8.

Nappi, RE, et al. 2005. Efficacy of Cimicifuga racemosa on climacteric complaints: A randomized study versus low-dose transdermal estradiol. *Gynecology Endocrinology*. 20:30–5.

Palan, PR, et al. 2006. Effects of menstrual cycle and oral contraceptive use on serum levels of lipid-soluble antioxidants. *American Journal of Obstetrics and Gynecology*. 194(5):e35–8

Stolze, H. 1982. An alternative to treat menopausal complaints. *Gynecology*. 3:14–6.

21

Obesity Drugs and Their Natural Alternatives

What Is Obesity?

The number of overweight Americans continues to rise. Current statistics show that two-thirds of U.S. adults are overweight and one-third of the overweight are obese. Obesity means having excess weight and body fat. More specifically, obesity is diagnosed by one's body mass index (BMI), a ratio of body weight to height. The BMI is an indicator of body fatness. An adult who has a BMI of 30 or higher is considered obese. Anyone more than 100 pounds overweight or with a BMI greater than 40 is considered morbidly obese.

The table below shows the interpretation of BMI for adults at the Centers for Disease Control Web site (www.cdc.gov/nccdphp/dnpa/bmi/adult_BMI/about_adult_BMI.htm). See the CDC Web site to learn how to calculate BMI.

BMI	Weight Status
Below 18.5	Underweight
18.5–24.9	Normal
25.0–29.9	Overweight
30.0 and above	Obese

Obesity puts people at increased risk of many serious diseases such as diabetes, high blood pressure, arthritis, and certain cancers.

There are several risk factors for obesity. These include genetics, which can affect the amount of body fat stored, location of fat, and the rate of metabolism—how your cells convert food into energy. You have an increased chance of being obese if one or both of your parents are obese. This can be due to genetics or due to similar lifestyle habits. As people get older, their risk increases, too. People often become less active and their metabolism slows down. Lastly, women are more likely to be obese than men since they have less muscle mass and thus burn fewer calories.

There are many causes of obesity. Consuming an excess of calories is a very common problem in the United States. And we consume many calories from simple carbohydrates such as soft drinks, desserts, white bread, and pasta. Too many calories combined with inactivity is a recipe for weight gain. People must burn as many calories through activity as they take in, to maintain weight. Exercise also increases one's metabolic rate. In addition, many people gain weight when they quit smoking, which can slow the metabolism. Some women have difficulty losing weight after their pregnancy. Be aware that prescription medications such as corticosteroids (prednisone) or antidepressants may cause weight gain. Lastly, hormone imbalances such as low thyroid (hypothyroidism) or insulin resistance (high glucose and insulin levels) contribute to weight gain. Since 40 percent of the U.S. adult population has pre-diabetes, insulin resistance is quite common.

Obesity Drugs

Lipase Inhibitor

Orlistat (Xenical)

HOW DOES THIS DRUG WORK?

Orlistat (Xenical) inhibits the absorption of fat from the intestine, causing it to be excreted in the stool. This reduces the amount of calories absorbed from food. Orlistat blocks the action of the fat-digesting enzyme lipase and prevents the breakup and absorption of fat. Orlistat blocks absorption of approximately 30 percent of the fat in a meal.

WHAT ARE THE BENEFITS?

Reduced calorie intake from fat in foods and reduced weight.

POTENTIAL SIDE EFFECTS

- Stomach discomfort
- Increased number of bowel movements

- Loss of control of bowel movements
- Flatulence
- Oily/fatty stools
- Clear, orange-, or brown-colored bowel movements

MAJOR CAUTIONS

- Arthritis or joint pain or tenderness
- Back pain
- Rash or itching
- Shortness of breath
- Severe stomach pain
- Yellowing of the skin or whites of the eyes
- Weakness or fainting

KNOWN DRUG INTERACTIONS

- Warfarin (Coumadin)
- Cyclosporine (Sandimmune)

FOOD OR SUPPLEMENT INTERACTIONS

Do not take lipase enzymes at the same time with this drug.

NUTRIENT DEPLETION/IMBALANCE

Beta-carotene and vitamins A, D, E, and K. We recommend the following:

Take a high-potency multivitamin at least two hours away from using orlistat (Xenical).

Taking 6 grams of psyllium with each dose of orlistat (Xenical) has been shown in a study to significantly reduce digestive side effects associated with the drug.

Vitamin A—take 5,000 IU daily.

Vitamin D—take 1,000 IU daily.

Vitamin K—take 500 mcg daily.

Vitamin E—take 200 IU of mixed vitamin E form daily.

Noradrenergic Agents/Amphetamines

Diethylpropion (Tenuate, Tepanil)

Phentermine (Adipex-P, Fastin, Obestin-30, Phentermine resin oral)

Diethylpropion ER (Tenuate Dospan)

HOW DO THESE DRUGS WORK?

These drugs suppress appetite.

WHAT ARE THE BENEFITS?

Reduced appetite helps one ingest fewer calories.

POTENTIAL SIDE EFFECTS

- Blurred vision or itchy eyes
- Constipation
- Diarrhea
- Dry mouth
- Flushing of the skin
- Hair loss
- Headache
- Increase or decrease in sexual desire or performance
- Nausea/vomiting
- Nervousness
- Red or itchy skin
- Restlessness
- Strange taste in your mouth
- Upset stomach

MAJOR CAUTIONS

- Abnormal heart rate or rhythm
- Agitation
- Blurred vision
- Breast growth in men
- Chest pain or tightness in the chest
- Confusion
- Difficulty with balance
- Dizziness
- Hallucinations
- Menstrual irregularity
- Paranoia
- Seizures
- Shortness of breath or rapid breathing
- Tremors
- Trouble sleeping

KNOWN DRUG INTERACTIONS

- Amphetamine or dextroamphetamine
- Furazolidone (Furoxone)
- High blood pressure medications
- Linezolid (Zyvox)
- Diabetic medications
- Antidepressants, especially MAO inhibitors such as phenelzine (Nardil), tranylcypromine (Parnate), isocarboxazid (Marplan), and selegiline (Eldepryl)
- Procarbazine (Matulane)

FOOD OR SUPPLEMENT INTERACTIONS

- Caffeine
- Alcohol

NUTRIENT DEPLETION/IMBALANCE

None known.

Noradrenergic/Serotonergic Agent

Sibutramine (Meridia)

HOW DOES THIS DRUG WORK?

This drug is thought to suppress the appetite by increasing the amount of serotonin and norepinephrine in the brain.

WHAT ARE THE BENEFITS?

Users may achieve a 5 to 10 percent reduction from their baseline weight.

POTENTIAL SIDE EFFECTS

- Increased heart rate
- Increased blood pressure
- Menstrual problems
- Muscle or joint pain
- Pain, burning, or tingling in the hands or feet
- Unusual swelling of the arms or legs
- Unusual fatigue or weakness
- Visual problems

MAJOR CAUTIONS

- Bleeding, easy bruising, nosebleeds, bleeding of gums

- Chest pain
- Difficulty breathing
- Fever
- Heart palpitations
- Seizures
- Severe dizziness

KNOWN DRUG INTERACTIONS

- Ketoconazole (Nizoral)
- Cimetidine (Tagamet)
- Erythromycin (Erytab, Eryc, Ilosone)
- Clarithromycin (Biaxin)
- Danazol (Danocrine)
- Diltiazem (Cardizem, Tiazac, Dilacor)
- Fluconazole (Diflucan)
- Fluoxetine (Prozac)
- Itraconazole (Sporanox)
- Propoxyphene (Darvon), troleandomycin (Tao)
- Verapamil (Verelan, Covera, Calan, Isoptin)
- Serotonin reuptake inhibitors (SSRIs) such as fluoxetine (Prozac), fluvox-amine (Luvox), paroxetine (Paxil), and sertraline (Zoloft)
- MAO inhibitors such as phenelzine (Nardil), tranylcypromine (Parnate), isocarboxazid (Marplan), and selegiline (Eldepryl)
- Sumatriptan (Imitrex)
- Zolmitriptan (Zomig)
- Dihydroergotamine (DHE)
- Dextromethorphan (Robitussin-DM), meperidine (Demerol), penta-zocine (Talwin), fentanyl (Duragesic)
- Lithium (Eskalith)

FOOD OR SUPPLEMENT INTERACTIONS

- L-tryptophan
- 5-hydroxytryptophan (5-HTP)
- Alcohol

NUTRIENT DEPLETION/IMBALANCE

None known.

Natural Alternatives to Obesity Drugs

Diet and Lifestyle Changes

Following a diet that is reduced in calories on a consistent basis is essential to long-term weight loss. Generally, you need to consume a diet high in fiber, moderate in protein and complex carbohydrates, moderate in fat (mainly good fat such as monounsaturated and polyunsaturated fats), and low in simple carbohydrates. If you have problems staying consistent with your diet, make sure to join a support group. In addition, a regular exercise program is the second essential part of successful weight loss. A partner or trainer can help you stay with it. The key is to incorporate a few different forms of exercise that you like so that consistency is maintained. Regular exercise will help burn calories and increase your metabolism.

The following supplements can make weight loss easier when combined with diet and exercise.

Conjugated Linoleic Acid (CLA)

This supplement has been shown to improve body composition in people who are overweight or obese. For some people it can significantly decrease body fat mass, and it may increase lean body mass in some users. Several studies have shown that CLA can help reduce body fat mass. For example, a randomized, double-blind study published in the *Journal of Nutrition* looked at the effect of CLA on 60 overweight and obese people. Those taking CLA had a significantly greater reduction in body fat mass, as compared to people taking a placebo.

Other Factors Contributing to Weight Loss

There are other variables associated with weight loss. Hormone imbalance can make it more difficult to lose weight. An example is high insulin levels as found in those with pre-diabetes or diabetes, or in women with polycystic ovarian syndrome. In addition, hormone deficiencies such as thyroid, testosterone, progesterone, leptin, or DHEA can slow the metabolism and make it more difficult to burn calories. Another aspect is appetite control. Those who do not feel satisfied from a normal calorie intake will have more trouble reducing their calorie intake. Lastly, a neurotransmitter imbalance can have a negative effect on appetite. A holistic doctor can assess all these factors and develop a protocol that will optimize one's weight loss and weight management.

DOSAGE

Take 1,000 to 1,500 mg before each meal three times daily.

SAFETY

CLA may cause digestive upset. Those with diabetes should have their glucose levels monitored closely on this supplement. Also, CLA may increase lipoprotein, a risk factor for cardiovascular disease.

Pyruvate

This substance is formed in the body as a by-product of carbohydrate and protein metabolism. A six-week double-blind, placebo-controlled study was done to examine the effects of pyruvate supplementation (6 grams daily) on body weight, body composition, and vigor and fatigue levels in healthy overweight Caucasian men and women. The study included 26 participants who were randomly assigned to a placebo group (7 men, 7 women) and a pyruvate-supplemented group (3 men, 9 women). In addition, all participated in a three-day-per-week exercise program, consisting of a 45- to 60-minute aerobic/anaerobic routine. After six weeks of treatment, there was a statistically significant decrease in body weight, body fat, and percent body fat in the pyruvate group.

DOSAGE

Take 6 grams per day in divided doses.

SAFETY

This supplement is safe. Some users experience digestive upset such as gas, bloating, and diarrhea.

PolyGlycoPlex (PGX)

This is a blend of three natural water-soluble fibers derived from the konjac root (an underground stem common in Asia, rich in fiber that retains water), sodium alginate, and xanthan gum. It was developed by researchers at the University of Toronto. PGX decreases the body's level of ghrelin, a hormone that gives the message to the brain, "Let's eat." At the same time, it raises levels of the digestive hormone GLP-1 (glucagon-like peptide-1), secreted in the small intestine and colon. GLP-1 is known to improve blood sugar control, promote satiety, and regulate gastric emptying. The fiber also gives a sensation of fullness and it decreases glucose and insulin levels, making it a good choice for those with insulin resistance or pre-diabetes. A clinical trial conducted at the University of Toronto demonstrated that this fiber mixture was effective in controlling food intake.

DOSAGE

Take two capsules before each meal or as directed on the container.

SAFETY

Some users experience gas, bloating, or diarrhea.

Caralluma Fimbriata

This Indian vegetable has been historically used to suppress appetite and thirst. A supplement is available in extract form. Two human studies have been completed on it. The first, at St. John's National Academy of Health Sciences, in Bangalore, India, involved 50 participants who walked for 30 minutes daily and took caralluma or a placebo. Those taking caralluma showed only a slightly greater average weight loss after eight weeks (1.94 pounds) than a placebo group (1.12 pounds). However, the average loss in waist circumference was 2.75 inches in the caralluma group versus only a 1.29-inch loss in the placebo group. Loss of abdominal girth correlates with reduced body fat.

In the second study, at Western Geriatric Research Institute in Los Angeles, overweight patients took the regular dose of caralluma or a placebo for four weeks. Participants were instructed not to change their daily activity pattern (exercise), or their food intake, for four weeks before starting the trial and during the trial. Out of eighteen patients who took the caralluma and completed the trial, fifteen lost weight. Eleven patients lost an average of 6 pounds, with the highest loss at 9 pounds. The other four participants lost 1 to 2 pounds. Of the patients taking a placebo who completed the trial, three gained 1 pound each, one lost 1 pound, and the other two dropped out due to minor digestive upset.

Extract of Caralluma

A preliminary trial was conducted at Dr. Stengler's clinic on an extract of caralluma for those on a weight-loss program. He found that approximately 80 percent of patients reported a noticeable reduction in appetite.

DOSAGE

Take a 500-mg capsule 30 to 45 minutes before breakfast and dinner.

SAFETY

Digestive upset is a rare side effect.

Hydroxycitric Acid

This supplement, often referred to as HCA, is a compound found in the rind of a Southeast Asian fruit called *Garcinia cambogia.* Animal research has shown that HCA suppresses appetite and induces weight loss. Results of human studies with HCA have been mixed. A 2002 study published in the *International Journal of Obesity* looked at the effect of HCA on calorie intake and satiety in overweight men and women. Twelve women and twelve men consumed a placebo—100 milliliters (ml) of tomato juice—three times daily for two weeks, then returned to their normal diet for two weeks and, in a final two-week phase, consumed 100 ml of tomato juice with 300 mg of HCA in it three times daily. Researchers found that participants consumed 15 to 30 percent fewer calories daily during the final phase than they had during the placebo phase. Other studies have not found a similar benefit.

DOSAGE

Take 500 mg three times daily before meals.

SAFETY

Digestive upset is rare.

Pinolenic Acid

This extract from the Korean pine nut has an appetite-suppressant effect. In a randomized, double-blind, placebo-controlled trial, overweight women were given either 3 g of pinolenic acid or a placebo (olive oil) immediately before eating a breakfast consisting of a moderate portion of carbohydrates. Researchers measured blood levels of hormones associated with hunger, satiety, and eating behavior before taking the supplement and at regular intervals for four hours thereafter. At each interval, participants reported how hungry they felt. The pinolenic acid group reported significantly less hunger than the placebo group, rating their "desire to eat" 29 percent lower and their "prospective food intake" 36 percent lower.

DOSAGE

Take 3,000 mg 30 to 60 minutes before your highest-calorie meal of the day.

SAFETY

Side effects are rare.

POLLY'S STORY

Polly, a 68-year-old retiree, had had trouble losing weight all of her life. She was put on a 1,500-calorie diet with weight-management supplements such as caralluma and CLA. In addition, she increased her exercise to thirty minutes five times weekly. She stated, "I lost 30 pounds in three and a half months! My internist said I look 10 years younger, and to stick with the program. My glucose and cholesterol levels have gone down and my knee pain is gone."

References

Blankson, H, et al. 2000. Conjugated linoleic acid reduces body fat mass in overweight and obese humans. *Journal of Nutrition.* 130:2943–8.

Breitman, P, V Vuksan, M Lyon. 2004. Impact of meal replacement viscosity on appetite and adlibitum food consumption in normal weight adolescents. Presented at the 8th Annual Canadian Diabetes Association (CDA)/Canadian Society of Endocrinology and Metabolism (CSEM) Professional Conference, October.

Cavaliere, H, I Floriano, G Medeiros-Neto. 2001. Gastrointestinal side effects of orlistat may be prevented by concomitant prescription of natural fibers [psyllium mucilloid]. *International Journal of Obesity and Related Metabolic Disorders.* 25:1095–9.

Kalman, D, et al. 1999. The effects of pyruvate supplementation on body composition in overweight individuals. *Nutrition.* 15:337–40.

Kurpad, AV, R Rebecca, L Amaranth. 2005. Caralluma for weight loss: Paper presented at the 18th International Congress of Nutrition, Durban, South Africa, September 19.

Lawrence, R, S Choudhary. 2004. Western Geriatric Institute, Los Angeles. Paper presented at the 12th Annual Congress on Anti-Aging Medicines, Las Vegas, December 5.

Westerterp-Plantenga, MS, and EMR Kovacs. 2002. The effect of (-)-hydroxycitrate on energy intake and satiety in overweight humans. *International Journal of Obesity.* 26:870–2.

22

Osteoarthritis Drugs and Their Natural Alternatives

What Is Osteoarthritis?

Osteoarthritis refers to a degenerative condition in which the cartilage that cushions the joints wears down. This results in symptoms such as morning stiffness, painful joints, restricted range of motion, bone spurs, and in some cases deformity of the joints. It most commonly affects the joints of the hands, hips, knees, and spine. This is the main type of arthritis people experience. There are over 100 different types of arthritis. It is estimated that 40 million Americans have some degree of osteoarthritis. As people grow older, the likelihood of osteoarthritis increases, affecting 80 percent of those over the age of 50.

Osteoarthritis is caused by injuries early in life that lead to inflammation and breakdown of the cartilage. It can also be the result of obesity, biomechanical imbalances (such as foot arch problems), and nutritional deficiencies. Also, certain medications such as NSAIDs and steroids may contribute to cartilage deterioration.

Our experience is that diet and lifestyle changes combined with joint-specific nutritional supplements are quite effective for mild to moderate osteoarthritis. In many cases, this approach also provides some degree of improvement for those with severe osteoarthritis.

Osteoarthritis Drugs

Analgesics

There are two major classes of over-the-counter analgesics. These include acetaminophen (Tylenol) and nonsteroidal anti-inflammatory drugs (NSAIDs). The two types of NSAIDs are aspirin and nonaspirin. Examples of nonaspirin NSAIDs are ibuprofen (Advil, Nuprin, Motrin IB, and Medipren) and naproxen (Aleve). Some NSAIDs are available by prescription only, as they contain higher dosages. Most doctors prescribe acetaminophen as a first-line drug treatment for osteoarthritis.

Common NSAIDs:

Aspirin

Salsalate (Amigesic)

Diflunisal (Dolobid)

Ibuprofen (Motrin, Advil)

Ketoprofen (Orudis)

Nabumetone (Relafen)

Piroxicam (Feldene)

Naproxen (Aleve, Naprosyn)

Diclofenac (Voltaren)

Indomethacin (Indocin)

Sulindac (Clinoril)

Tolmetin (Tolectin)

Etodolac (Lodine)

Ketorolac (Toradol)

Oxaprozin (Daypro)

Celecoxib (Celebrex)

HOW DO THESE DRUGS WORK?

The exact mechanism of how acetaminophen works is unknown. It seems to raise the body's threshold or tolerance to pain. Unlike the NSAIDs it does not reduce inflammation.

NSAIDs work by blocking enzymes that are involved in the production of chemicals in the body known as prostaglandins. Certain prostaglandins promote pain and inflammation. By reducing the activity of cyclooxygenase (COX) enzymes, these medicines reduce pain and inflammation.

WHAT ARE THE BENEFITS?

Quick pain relief with medications that are easily accessible over the counter.

POTENTIAL SIDE EFFECTS

Acetaminophen can cause elevated liver enzymes or liver damage. This is typically at higher doses or when combined with alcohol, recreational drugs, or other pharmaceuticals.

For NSAIDs the most common side effects are nausea, vomiting, diarrhea, constipation, decreased appetite, rash, dizziness, headache, and drowsiness. They can also cause fluid retention and swelling of tissue.

MAJOR CAUTIONS

Acetaminophen can cause liver damage. This risk is increased with higher dosages and when combined with alcohol. Avoid its use for those with acute or chronic liver disease.

For NSAIDs there is a small risk of kidney failure, liver failure, ulcers, and prolonged bleeding after an injury or surgery. People allergic to NSAIDs may develop shortness of breath. People with asthma are at a higher risk for experiencing serious allergic reaction to NSAIDs. Those with a serious allergy to one NSAID are likely to experience a similar reaction to a different NSAID. The use of aspirin in children and teenagers with a viral infection or recent viral infection (especially chicken pox, common cold, or the flu) has been associated with the development of Reye's syndrome. This is a reaction in which one can suffer increased pressure within the brain and, often, massive accumulations of fat in the liver and other organs. Therefore, aspirin and nonaspirin salicylates (e.g., salsalate) should not be used in children and teenagers with suspected or confirmed chicken pox, common cold, or the flu.

KNOWN DRUG INTERACTIONS

Acetaminophen: The drugs cholestyramine (Questran), carbamazepine (Tegretol), isoniazid (INH, Nydrazid, Laniazid), and rifampin (Rifamate, Rifadin, Rimactane) can reduce the levels of acetaminophen and may decrease the effectiveness of acetaminophen. Higher-than-recommended doses of acetaminophen may result in severe liver damage. The potential for liver damage from acetaminophen is increased when it is combined with alcohol or drugs (recreational or pharmaceutical). Acetaminophen can increase the blood thinning effect of warfarin (Coumadin).

NSAIDs: These drugs can reduce blood flow to the kidneys and reduce the action of diuretics and decrease the elimination of lithium (Eskalith) and methotrexate (Rheumatrex). NSAIDs also decrease the ability of the blood to clot and therefore increase bleeding time. Bleeding complications are even more of a risk when NSAIDs are combined with other medications that have a blood-thinning effect. NSAIDs can also increase blood pressure. In February 2007, the American Heart Association issued new guidelines discouraging the use of regular nonsteroidal anti-inflammatory drugs (NSAIDs) in patients with known heart disease or those thought to be at high risk of getting heart disease.

FOOD OR SUPPLEMENT INTERACTIONS

Ibuprofen can cause salt and water retention. Therefore you should watch and minimize your sodium intake while using ibuprofen.

Hibiscus tea should not be consumed when you are taking acetaminophen, as it may decrease the levels of the drug.

Deglycyrrhizinated licorice (DGL) may help protect against ulceration of the digestive tract while using these medications, especially aspirin.

NUTRIENT DEPLETION/IMBALANCE

Milk thistle, vitamin C, and N-acetylcysteine may help prevent liver damage from acetaminophen. It should be noted that hospitals use oral and intravenous N-acetylcysteine to treat overdoses of acetaminophen. NSAIDs have been shown to deplete vitamin C and folic acid. Use the following supplements under the guidance of a doctor.

- Milk thistle—take 250 to 300 mg twice daily.
- Vitamin C—take 500 mg daily.
- N-acetylcysteine—take 500 mg daily.
- Folic acid—take 400 micrograms daily.

Tramadol (Ultram)

HOW DOES THIS DRUG WORK?

The exact mechanism of tramadol (Ultram) is unknown, but it seems to be similar to morphine. This drug binds to receptors in the brain (opioid receptors) that reduce pain messages.

WHAT ARE THE BENEFITS?

Reduced joint pain without the risk of stomach erosion and bleeding as found with NSAIDs.

POTENTIAL SIDE EFFECTS

- Digestive upset such as nausea, vomiting, diarrhea, and constipation
- Dizziness and drowsiness
- Headache
- Itching
- Sweating
- Dry mouth
- Rash
- Visual changes

MAJOR CAUTIONS

- Seizures.
- Sudden withdrawal may result in sweating, anxiety, pain, nausea, digestive upset, hallucinations, and insomnia.

KNOWN DRUG INTERACTIONS

- Carbamazepine (Tegretol)
- Quinidine (Quinaglute, Quinidex)
- Antidepressants such as monoamine oxidase(MAO) inhibitors or selective serotonin inhibitors (SSRIs)

FOOD OR SUPPLEMENT INTERACTIONS

- Alcohol
- 5-hydroxytryptophan (5-HTP)
- L-tryptophan

NUTRIENT DEPLETION/IMBALANCE

None known.

Codeine

HOW DOES THIS DRUG WORK?

Codeine is a narcotic that reduces pain.

WHAT ARE THE BENEFITS?

Codeine is a stronger pain reliever than acetaminophen or NSAIDs. It is commonly combined with analgesics, such as Tylenol.

POTENTIAL SIDE EFFECTS

- Nervousness
- Blurred vision
- Digestive upset such as constipation, nausea, vomiting, dry mouth
- Dizziness or drowsiness
- Headache
- Sweating

MAJOR CAUTIONS

- Confusion
- Light-headedness
- Fainting

KNOWN DRUG INTERACTIONS

- High blood pressure medications
- Seizure medications
- Antidepressant medications
- Certain antihistamine medications
- Barbiturate medications such as phenobarbitol

FOOD OR SUPPLEMENT INTERACTIONS

- Alcohol

Codeine may be taken with food to reduce digestive side effects.

Herbs with high tannin levels may reduce the absorption of codeine. These include green tea (*Camellia sinensis*), black tea, uva ursi (*Arctostaphylos uva-ursi),* black walnut *(Juglans nigra),* red raspberry *(Rubus idaeus),* oak *(Quercus spp.*), and witch hazel *(Hamamelis virginiana).*

NUTRIENT DEPLETION/IMBALANCE

None known.

COX-2 Inhibitor

Celecoxib (Celebrex)

HOW DOES THIS DRUG WORK?

This drug blocks the COX-2 enzyme that makes prostaglandins that result in pain and inflammation.

WHAT ARE THE BENEFITS?

More reduction of joint pain than with acetaminophen and NSAIDs.

POTENTIAL SIDE EFFECTS

- Headache
- Digestive upset including abdominal pain, heartburn, diarrhea, nausea, flatulence
- Insomnia

MAJOR CAUTIONS

- Fainting
- Kidney failure
- Cardiovascular risks including heart failure, worsening of blood pressure, angina pectoris (chest pain)
- Tinnitus (ringing in the ears)
- Deafness

- Ulcers of the stomach and intestine
- Blurred vision
- Anxiety
- Photosensitivity
- Weight gain, water retention
- Flu-like symptoms
- Drowsiness
- Weakness

KNOWN DRUG INTERACTIONS

Using this drug along with aspirin or other NSAIDs increases the chances of bleeding in the digestive tract.

- Fluconazole (Diflucan)
- Lithium (Eskalith)
- Warfarin (Coumadin)

FOOD OR SUPPLEMENT INTERACTIONS

- White willow (Salix alba)
- Alcohol

NUTRIENT DEPLETION/IMBALANCE

- Folic acid—take 400 mcg daily.
- Potassium—take under the guidance of a doctor.

Natural Alternatives to Osteoarthritis Drugs

Diet and Lifestyle Changes

A diet rich in fruits, vegetables, legumes, nuts, and seeds provides a diverse array of antioxidants that may benefit those with osteoarthritis. Essential fatty acids found in fish such as wild salmon and sardines, or in nuts such as walnuts can help decrease inflammation of the joints. Cartilage degeneration is due in part to free radical damage to the cartilage. Reduce your intake of foods that contribute to inflammation such as red meat, cow's milk, caffeine, simple sugars, and alcohol. Also, some individuals improve when they avoid nightshade plants, including tomatoes, eggplant, white potatoes, and all peppers (except black pepper).

Losing weight is important to take stress off your weight-bearing joints.

Beatrice, a 60-year-old retiree, was scheduled to get hip surgery due to the osteoarthritic pain she was experiencing. In a last-ditch attempt to avoid surgery, she consulted with our clinic. Beatrice began a supplementation program of glucosamine sulfate, high doses of MSM, and an herbal anti-inflammatory formula. Within six weeks most of her pain and stiffness were gone and she canceled her surgery. Now, five years later, she continues to do well.

Gentle exercises such as swimming, aqua-aerobics, and other low-impact exercise is recommended. Also, those with osteoarthritis of the feet, knees, hips, or low back may benefit from orthotic inserts.

Glucosamine

Several studies have demonstrated that glucosamine reduces symptoms of osteoarthritis, especially when it affects the knees. For example, a three-year, double-blind, placebo-controlled trial involving 212 people with osteoarthritis of the knees found that 1,500 mg of glucosamine sulfate daily significantly reduced symptoms. In addition, diagnostic images found that people supplementing glucosamine had no significant joint space loss. Those on placebo had joint deterioration.

A study published in *Osteoarthritis and Cartilage* found that treatment of knee osteoarthritis with glucosamine sulfate for at least 12 months and up to three years may prevent total joint replacement.

Research at McGill University in Montreal suggested that the sulfate portion of glucosamine sulfate may be more important than the glucosamine portion. Oral glucosamine does not show up in the bloodstream, but the sulfate does appear in both the blood and synovial fluid (which surrounds joints) within three hours. Sulfur is found in every cell and it is the third most abundant mineral in the body (after calcium and phosphorus). It is involved in cartilage formation and helps retain water in cartilage. Researchers have found that large numbers of people, particularly the elderly, may not get enough sulfur from their diets—which might explain why sulfur-containing supplements can have striking benefits. For nutritional sulfur, I recommend a variety of sulfur-containing foods in your diet. Egg yolk, broccoli, cauliflower, Brussels sprouts, asparagus, onions, and garlic are all good sources of sulfur.

Methylsulfonylmethane (MSM)

MSM appears to have a natural anti-inflammatory effect. It can reduce osteoarthritis symptoms such as pain and swelling, and improve joint function. A randomized, double-blind, placebo-controlled trial was conducted on 50 men and women between the ages of 40 and 76 with knee osteoarthritis. Participants were given 3,000 mg of MSM or placebo twice a day for 12 weeks. Compared to placebo, MSM produced significant decreases in pain and physical function impairment. MSM also produced improvement in performing activities of daily living when compared to placebo.

DOSAGE

Take 3,000 mg twice daily for 12 weeks, then reduce to 2,000 mg twice daily.

SAFETY

MSM has a mild blood-thinning effect, so consult with your doctor if you are on blood-thinning medication. High doses may cause digestive upset such as diarrhea. If this occurs, reduce the dosage.

Proteolytic Enzymes

Protein-digesting enzymes such as bromelain have anti-inflammatory effects when taken between meals. For example, one study found a mixture of protease enzymes including bromelain with an anti-inflammatory drug to be comparable to diclofenac (Voltaren).

DOSAGE

Take 500 mg of bromelain three times daily between meals; or take a proteolytic formula as directed on the label.

SAFETY

Do not combine with blood thinners. Do not take if you have gastritis or an active ulcer.

S-adenosylmethionine (SAMe)

Several clinical trials demonstrate that SAMe is superior to placebo and comparable to NSAIDs and the COX-2 inhibitor celecoxib (Celebrex) for decreasing symptoms associated with osteoarthritis. For example, a double-blind crossover study at the University of California at Irvine compared SAMe (1,200 mg) with celecoxib (Celebrex, 200 mg) for 16 weeks to reduce pain associated with osteoarthritis (OA) of the knee. Sixty-one adults diagnosed with OA of the knee were enrolled and 56 completed the study. Subjects were tested for pain, functional health, mood status, isometric joint function tests, and side effects. On the first month of Phase 1, the celecoxib group showed significantly more reduction in pain than the SAMe group. However, by the second month of Phase 1, there was no significant difference between the groups.

> ### SAMe
>
> SAMe is known as a "methyl donor." This means it is involved in chemical reactions in the body with a group containing one carbon and three hydrogen atoms (CH_3). Once SAMe donates this methyl group, it is converted to a substance known as SAH (S-adenosyl-homocysteine). This SAH group then donates its sulfur group to form tissues such as cartilage.

DOSAGE

Take 1,200 mg daily in divided doses.

SAFETY

Side effects are uncommon.

Fish Oil

Essential fatty acids such as those found in fish oil have natural anti-inflammatory benefits. They may also help with joint lubrication. While most studies have been done on those with rheumatoid arthritis, we also find fish oil to benefit those with osteoarthritis.

DOSAGE

Take 2,000 mg of combined EPA and DHA as listed on the label of a fish oil product.

SAFETY

Do not take high doses of fish oil if you are on blood-thinning medication. Digestive upset such as repeating may occur with fish oil.

References

Bruyere, O, et al. 2008. Total joint replacement after glucosamine sulphate treatment in knee osteoarthritis: Results of a mean 8-year observation of patients from two previous 3-year, randomised, placebo-controlled trials. *Osteoarthritis and Cartilage.* 16(2):254–60.

Kim, LS, et al. 2006. Efficacy of methylsulfonylmethane (MSM) in osteoarthritis pain of the knee: A pilot clinical trial. *Osteoarthritis and Cartilage.* 14:286–94.

Klein, G, W Kullich. 2000. Short-term treatment of painful osteoarthritis of the knee with oral enzymes. *Clinical Drug Investigations.* 19:15–23.

Najm, WI, et al. 2004. S-adenosyl methionine (SAMe) versus celecoxib for the treatment of osteoarthritis symptoms: A double-blind crossover trial. *BMC Musculoskeletal Disorders.* 5:6.

Reginster, JY, et al. 2001. Long-term effects of glucosamine sulphate on osteoarthritis progression: A randomised, placebo-controlled clinical trial. *Lancet.* January 27;357 (9252):251–6.

23

Osteoporosis Drugs and Their Natural Alternatives

What Is Osteoporosis?

Osteoporosis literally means "porous bone," and that's exactly what happens to the bones in your body over the years as osteoporosis slowly deteriorates the skeletal structure. Eventually, fragile bones predispose you to fracture and a plethora of other problems associated with bone loss including dowager's hump, loss of mobility, and pinched nerves from spinal collapse. In fact, bones affected by osteoporosis may become so fragile that fractures occur spontaneously or as the result of minor bumps, falls, or stresses associated with bending, lifting, or even coughing!

What Causes Osteoporosis?

Bone is a living tissue; as such, it is ever changing. Old bone is removed (resorption) and new bone is added (formation) to the skeleton on a constant basis. When we are young, bone formation is much higher than resorption. But as we age, formation slows. Peak bone mass is achieved at about age 30, after which bones can begin to weaken. If we do not have the right genetics, nutrition, weight-bearing exercise, and other factors in place, resorption becomes dominant and bone loss ensues.

Approximately 44 million Americans are threatened by osteoporosis and low bone mass—68 percent being women. One of every two women and one of every four men over 50 will experience an osteoporosis-related fracture in their lifetime.

We often think of osteoporosis as a normal consequence of aging, but in fact, it is the result of certain unchangeable factors combined with poor diet and lifestyle habits. It's never too early to build strong bones or be aware of the factors that contribute to bone loss. There are risk factors you cannot change, and risk factors you can control.

Risk factors you cannot change:

- Ethnicity. Due to genetic characteristics of bone density, Caucasian and Asian women have the highest risk, and African American and Hispanic women have a lower but significant risk.
- Family history. Heredity may play a significant predisposing role.
- Gender. Women have less bone tissue and lose bone faster than men.
- Age. Bones become thinner and weaker with age.
- Body size. Small, thin-boned women are at greater risk.

Risk factors you can exert some control over:

- Diet and nutrition. Calcium, magnesium, vitamin D, boron, silicon, and other nutrients play important roles in bone metabolism. On the other hand, junk foods, sodas, and caffeine promote bone loss.
- Cigarette smoking. Tobacco use and associated lifestyle factors, are correlated with increased bone loss.
- Alcohol intake. Excessive consumption increases the risk of bone loss and fractures.
- Inactivity. Inactivity tends to weaken bones, while weight-bearing exercise is one of the best ways to prevent bone loss.
- Use of certain medications. Glucocorticoids, long-term overdosing of thyroid medication, and some anticonvulsants can lead to loss of bone density.
- Hormone imbalance. Abnormal or low levels of hormones such as estrogen, testosterone, DHEA, growth hormone, cortisol, and thyroid can bring on osteoporosis.
- Eating disorders. Certain eating disorders increase your risk for osteoporosis due to poor nutrition and/or nutrient losses.
- Dysfunctional immune system. Cytokines are immune cells that initiate a type of inflammatory response leading to bone breakdown. Diet and lifestyle factors, along with hormonal balance and specific nutritional substances, help normalize cytokine activity. Osteoporosis is now considered a disease of chronic inflammation.

Osteoporosis Drugs

Many individuals who are at risk of osteoporosis or who have active osteoporosis are prescribed medications that can halt or reverse bone loss. The most common classes of osteoporosis medications include bisphosphonates, selective estrogen receptor modulators, calcitonin, and parathyroid hormone therapy.

Bisphosphonates

HOW DO THESE DRUGS WORK?

Bisphosphonates are the most widely used drugs in the treatment of osteoporosis. They are antiresorptive medications, which means they slow or stop the natural process that dissolves bone tissue. They do this by interfering with and limiting the function of osteoclasts (the bone-resorbing cells) and, perhaps indirectly, by stimulating osteoblasts (the bone-forming cells) to produce an inhibitor of osteoclast formation.

COMMON BISPHOSPHONATES

Alendronate (Fosamax)

Risedronate (Actonel)

Ibandronate (Boniva)

Zoledronic acid (Reclast) injection given only once per year

WHAT ARE THE BENEFITS?

Studies indicated that alendronate and risedronate lower the risk of fractures of the vertebrae by 50 percent and other fractures by 30 to 49 percent in people with osteoporosis. In other research, taking a bisphosphonate with hormone therapy results in increased bone mass when compared to taking either a bisphosphonate or estrogen alone. In men, alendronate increases bone density in the spine and hip as well as total body bone density, and it helps prevent spinal fractures and decreases in height.

POTENTIAL SIDE EFFECTS

Heartburn, abdominal pain, gastric ulcer, irritation of the esophagus, headache, pain in muscles and joints, digestive disturbances, and allergic reactions are all possible adverse effects.

MAJOR CAUTIONS

There have been rare reports of osteonecrosis (bone tissue death) of the jaw and visual disturbances. In addition, a possible link between bisphosphonate use and the development of atrial fibrillation is currently under investigation.

MEDICAL PRECAUTIONS

People with the following conditions or disorders should discuss their risks with their physician:

- Pregnancy or breast-feeding
- Severe kidney problems
- Severe heartburn or inflammation of the esophagus
- Low blood calcium

KNOWN DRUG INTERACTIONS

Bisphosphonate effectiveness is reduced when it is taken at the same time as parathyroid hormone (Forteo). Concomitant use with aminoglycoside antibiotics can cause severe hypocalcemia (low blood calcium).

FOOD OR SUPPLEMENT INTERACTIONS

Bisphosphonate absorption is impaired by food—especially foods containing calcium. Bisphosphonates should be taken when you are fasting, with water, and without dairy products, orange juice, or drinks containing caffeine. Generally, bisphosphonates must be taken at least 30 to 60 minutes before you eat or drink anything, take any other medicine, or take any supplements.

NUTRIENT DEPLETION/IMBALANCE

Calcium and phosphorus may be depleted with use of various bisphosphonates.

Selective Estrogen Receptor Modulators (SERMs)

There currently is one approved SERM: raloxifene (Evista).

HOW DO THESE DRUGS WORK?

The hormone estrogen is responsible for many actions, including regulating the turnover (formation and resorption) of bone. Decreases in estrogen levels after menopause, or removal of the ovaries, leads to osteoporosis. Selective estrogen receptor modulators (SERMs) are compounds that bind with estrogen receptors and exhibit estrogen action in some tissues and antiestrogen action in other tissues; that is, they selectively inhibit or stimulate estrogen-like action in various tissues.

WHAT ARE THE BENEFITS?

Increases in spine and hip bone mineral density by 2 to 3 percent in a three-year period. Reduced relative risk of first vertebral fracture by 55 percent, and 30 percent reduction in subsequent vertebral fractures.

POTENTIAL SIDE EFFECTS

The most common side effects with raloxifene are hot flashes, sinusitis, weight gain, muscle pain, leg cramps, and ankle swelling.

MAJOR CAUTIONS

Raloxifene increases the risk of blood clots, including deep vein thrombosis and pulmonary embolism (blood clots to the lung), with the greatest risk increase occurring during the first four months of use. Patients must avoid prolonged periods of restricted movement during travel. There is an increased risk of death by stroke in postmenopausal women with documented coronary heart disease.

MEDICAL PRECAUTIONS

Women with the following conditions or disorders should discuss their risks with their physician:

- Pregnancy or breast-feeding
- Active or past history of venous thromboembolism (blood clots)
- At risk of stroke or heart attack
- Kidney or liver problems

KNOWN DRUG INTERACTIONS

Cholestyramine (Questran) reduces the absorption of raloxifene, making it important to take these medications several hours apart. Raloxifene may slightly reduce the effects of blood thinners such as warfarin.

FOOD OR SUPPLEMENT INTERACTIONS

Alcohol should be avoided when taking raloxifene. Calcium and vitamin D supplements may support its effectiveness.

NUTRIENT DEPLETION/IMBALANCE

- Vitamin B6—take 50 mg daily.
- Magnesium—take 200 to 250 mg twice daily.

Calcitonin

Calcitonin-salmon nasal spray (Fortical, Miacalcin)

Calcitonin-salmon injection (Calcimar, Miacalcin)

HOW DO THESE DRUGS WORK?

Calcitonin is a naturally occurring hormone in both humans and animals that regulates the amount of calcium in the blood by acting on the skeleton. Calcitonins come from several animal species, but salmon calcitonin is the one most widely used. It inhibits bone removal by osteoclasts, and promotes bone formation by osteoblasts, thereby slowing bone remodeling.

WHAT ARE THE BENEFITS?

When compared with calcium alone, intranasal calcitonin reduces the rates of fracture by two-thirds in elderly women with moderate osteoporosis. Furthermore, it increases spinal bone mass in a dose-dependent manner. A unique

A Common Blood Thinner Increases Risk

The common blood thinner warfarin (Coumadin) increases the risk of osteoporosis. This medication reduces calcification of the bones. In addition, users are required to avoid vitamin K–rich foods and supplements. A deficiency of vitamin K may worsen bone loss.

benefit of calcitonin is its ability to relieve pain after a fresh osteoporosis-related bone fracture.

POTENTIAL SIDE EFFECTS

Injectable calcitonin may cause nausea with or without vomiting, local skin redness at the site of injection, flushing, and skin rash. Calcitonin nasal spray can cause runny nose, nosebleed, bone pain, and headaches. The nausea that can occur with injectable calcitonin does not occur with the nasal spray. A rare side effect of calcitonin is stomach upset.

MAJOR CAUTIONS

Although uncommon, serious side effects can include systemic allergic reaction or severe nasal irritation. Symptoms of a severe allergic reaction might include difficulty breathing; closing of the throat; swelling of the lips, tongue, or face; or hives.

MEDICAL PRECAUTIONS

Anyone with a known allergy to calcitonin should not use this medication. Safe use of calcitonin in children, in pregnancy, or by nursing mothers has not been studied.

KNOWN DRUG INTERACTIONS

Concomitant use of calcitonin and lithium may lead to a reduction in plasma lithium concentrations.

FOOD OR SUPPLEMENT INTERACTIONS

Calcium supplementation enhances the effects of nasal calcitonin on bone mass of the lumbar spine.

NUTRIENT DEPLETION/IMBALANCE

None known.

Parathyroid Hormone Therapy

There currently is one approved drug for parathyroid hormone therapy: teriparatide (Forteo)

HOW DOES THIS DRUG WORK?

Parathyroid hormone is a substance naturally produced by the parathyroid glands that is involved in the maintenance of calcium and phosphorus levels. When given once a day, synthetic parathyroid hormone stimulates the growth of new bone by increasing the number and activity of bone-forming cells called osteoblasts.

WHAT ARE THE BENEFITS?

A 65 percent relative risk reduction in new vertebral fractures has been observed and effectiveness is seen regardless of age, baseline rate of bone turnover, or baseline bone mass density. In other research, 72 percent of patients treated with Forteo achieved at least a 5 percent increase in spine density, and 44 percent of patients gained 10 percent or more.

POTENTIAL SIDE EFFECTS

Common side effects include dizziness and leg cramps. More serious side effects include chest pain (angina), nausea, vomiting, constipation, sluggishness, and muscle weakness. An allergic reaction to this drug can occur but is unlikely.

MAJOR CAUTIONS

Teriparatide (Forteo) has been shown to increase the rate of bone tumors (osteosarcoma) in studies using laboratory rats. It is unknown if there is a higher risk of bone tumors in humans. Patients and doctors must weigh potential benefits against potential risks.

MEDICAL PRECAUTIONS

People with the following conditions or disorders should discuss their risks with their physician:

- Paget's disease
- Unexplained high levels of alkaline phosphatase in the blood
- Active bone growth (e.g., in children or young adults)
- History of radiation therapy of the bones
- Hypercalcemia (high blood calcium levels)
- Bone cancer
- Kidney stones
- Pregnancy or breast-feeding

KNOWN DRUG INTERACTIONS

Before using teriparatide, tell your doctor if you are taking digoxin (digitalis, Lanoxin, Lanoxicaps). You may need dosage adjustments or special tests during treatment. Teriparatide may temporarily increase the amount of calcium in your blood, which is important to note before any blood tests.

FOOD OR SUPPLEMENT INTERACTIONS

Calcium and vitamin D supplements taken concomitantly with calcitonin may produce added benefits.

NUTRIENT DEPLETION/IMBALANCE

None known.

Natural Alternatives to Osteoporosis Drugs

Diet and Lifestyle Changes

Osteoporosis is certainly a disease highly associated with diet and lifestyle. Studies of cultures with a more primitive lifestyle demonstrate osteoporosis to be uncommon. A diet rich in inflammation-fighting foods such as vegetables, fruits, nuts, seeds, omega-3 rich fish such as wild salmon and sardines, and lean poultry is recommended. Inflammatory foods such as caffeine, alcohol, soda pop, and other simple sugars should be avoided for those with this disease. Studies also show that a high salt (sodium) diet contributes to calcium loss. Avoid packaged foods high in sodium (see chapter 9 on blood pressure). Fermented soy foods and protein powders have been shown to increase bone formation. Sea vegetables, surprisingly high in calcium, have become more readily available in health food stores. These include wakame ($\frac{1}{2}$ cup contains 1,700 mg), agar ($\frac{1}{4}$ cup contains 1,000 mg), nori ($\frac{1}{2}$ cup contains 600 mg), and kombu ($\frac{1}{4}$ cup contains 500 mg). It should be noted that sardines with bones are a good source not only of omega-3 fatty acids but of calcium, with 500 mg per half cup. Vitamin K is important for proper bone formation. This nutrient is abundant in dark green leafy vegetables such as lettuce, spinach, and broccoli. The form in these foods is vitamin K1. However, vitamin K2 is better absorbed and remains active in the body longer than vitamin K1. The best food source of vitamin K2 is natto (fermented soybeans) and, to a lesser degree, fermented cheeses (the type with holes, such as Swiss and Jarlsberg), butter, beef liver, chicken, and egg yolks.

Studies looking at high animal protein intake and osteoporosis are conflicting. While high protein intake increases calcium loss, it is known that adequate protein is required for bone formation. Those prone to higher blood glucose and insulin levels with diabetes or insulin resistance often benefit from high protein and reduced simple carbohydrate intake. The lower one's insulin levels, the lower the inflammatory response, including in the bones.

Regular weight-bearing exercise is critical for proper bone formation and the stimulation of increased bone density. Walking, jogging, and stair climbing are good. Optimally one should incorporate weight lifting twice weekly to stress various parts of the skeleton. Work with a certified trainer for a personalized program. Flexibility and balance exercises are helpful to prevent falls.

Smoking is a big contributor to osteoporosis and should be stopped.

Calcium

Government studies show that most American adults do not consume adequate calcium from their foods on a daily basis. Calcium has been shown to help prevent osteoporosis, and most studies show that by itself it slows bone loss. It is most effective when combined with other nutrients that work synergistically to build bone.

DOSAGE

Take 500 to 600 mg of well-absorbed calcium complexes such as citrate, citrate-malate, chelate, lactate, or hydroxyapatite twice daily.

SAFETY

Do not take more than 2,500 mg daily without the supervision of a physician. Men with prostate cancer should not supplement more than 500 mg unless instructed to do so by a physician. Those with hyperparathyroidism, kidney stones, or impaired kidney function should consult with a doctor before supplementing calcium.

Magnesium

This mineral is thought to be just as important as calcium for bone density. It is involved in parathyroid hormone production and the activation of vitamin D, both of which influence calcium metabolism and absorption. A study in *Magnesium Research* tested the effect of magnesium supplements on post-menopausal women with osteoporosis. Thirty-one women received two to six tablets daily of 125 mg each of magnesium for six months and two tablets for another 18 months in a two-year, open, controlled therapeutic trial. Another twenty-three postmenopausal women with osteoporosis who did not want treatment participated as the control group. Twenty-two patients (71 percent) responded by a 1 to 8 percent rise of bone density. The mean bone density of all treated patients increased significantly after one year and remained unchanged after two years. The mean bone density of the responders increased significantly both after one year and after two years. Those in the control group had a significantly decreased mean bone density.

DOSAGE

Take 250 to 350 mg twice daily.

SAFETY

Too much magnesium may cause digestive upset, including diarrhea. Lowering the dosage usually resolves these problems. Those with kidney disease should consult with a doctor before supplementing magnesium.

Vitamin D

Vitamin D has become a superstar nutrient in recent years. Its value for osteoporosis prevention and treatment has been upgraded to that of a critically important nutrient. Recent research has shown that vitamin D deficiency is commonplace in adults and children in the United States, particularly seniors.

The Two Faces of Vitamin D

There are two main forms of vitamin D: vitamin D2 (ergocalciferol), and vitamin D3 (cholecalciferol). Vitamin D2 is the type added to milk and other foods. It is derived from plant foods. Vitamin D3 is the best form used by the body. The D3 form is found in animal foods such as fish (and some fish oils such as cod liver oil), oils, and eggs. Also, when sunlight penetrates the skin, it forms vitamin D3.

Vitamin D plays an important role in the intestinal absorption of calcium and reducing the urinary excretion of calcium. It also reduces inflammation. A multitude of studies have demonstrated that vitamin D3 taken along with calcium decreases postmenopausal bone loss, helps prevent osteoporosis, and decreases the risk of fractures. A 2007 double-blind study in the *American Journal of Nutrition* followed 122 people with fracture of the hip or upper extremity. Participants were randomly assigned to receive 3,000 mg calcium carbonate plus 1,400 IU vitamin D or placebo (200 IU vitamin D). Participants were followed with X-rays, physical performance, and blood markers of bone turnover. Researchers found after one year a significant increase in lumbar spine bone density compared to those on placebo. The benefits of treatment were more pronounced in people less than 70 years old.

DOSAGE

A preventive dosage is 1,000 to 2,000 IU daily with meals. Those with osteoporosis should supplement 2,000 to 3,000 IU daily or higher as directed by a doctor. Blood tests can help monitor one's vitamin D level.

Vitamin K

Vitamin K is a key player in bone calcification. Vitamin K is required for the bone-forming protein osteocalcin to function properly. Studies have shown that vitamin K reduces bone loss as well as fracture rates. A report in the *Archives of Internal Medicine* reviewed previous randomized controlled trials that gave adult participants oral vitamin K supplements for longer than six months. The review included 20 trials and found that all studies but one showed an advantage of vitamin K in reducing bone loss.

DOSAGE

Studies have used up to 45 mg daily of vitamin K2. A typical dosage is 500 mcg to 2,000 mcg for those with osteoporosis.

SAFETY

If you are on blood-thinning medications, consult with a doctor before supplementing vitamin K.

Potassium

Recent research has shown that potassium is an important mineral for bone metabolism. The typical U.S. diet is high in refined carbohydrates, which increase acidity of the blood. To counter and reduce this acidity and restore the proper pH, the body robs the bones of calcium. With the resulting drop in bone mineral density (BMD), the risk of a fracture rises. Swiss researchers looked at the effects of potassium citrate supplements on blood pH and bone density. Published in the *Journal of the American Society of Nephrology*, the study involved 161 postmenopausal women, average age 59, who were known to have low bone mass. One group of women received tablets of potassium citrate—which is slightly alkaline—at a daily dose of 30 millimoles (1,173 mg). The other group got an equal dose of potassium chloride, which is nonalkaline. BMD measurements were performed at the start of the study, after six months, and after one year on the supplements. At the end of the study, the women taking potassium chloride showed an average bone-density loss in the lower spine of 1 percent—a significant loss. However, the group taking potassium citrate had a 1 percent increase in BMD in the lower spine, plus an increase in density of almost 2 percent in the hip. This group also excreted less calcium in the urine.

> ## Osteoporosis and pH Levels
>
> We ask patients with osteoporosis to monitor their urine pH values upon waking each morning (since blood pH monitoring is not practical, and urine acidity seems to reflect blood acidity). We have found that patients who eat healthfully, control stress, and take potassium citrate have urine that is less acidic, and that their urinary markers of bone loss improve.

DOSAGE

Take up to 1,200 mg daily of potassium citrate.

SAFETY

If you are on potassium-sparing high blood pressure medications or have kidney disease, do not supplement unless you are under the care of a doctor. Potassium supplements may cause stomach upset.

Ipriflavone

This is a copy of the soy isoflavone daidzein. There have been over 150 animal and human studies on ipriflavone. Several studies have shown that when combined with calcium, this supplement can increase bone density. It has also been shown to prevent osteoporosis when taken in combination with estrogen or vitamin D. Ipriflavone stimulates bone-building cells known as osteoblasts.

In an open study involving 100 postmenopausal women between the ages of 53 and 65, researchers gave the participants 200 mg of ipriflavone three times daily along with 1,000 mg of calcium. Ninety women completed the study. The average bone density was increased by 2 percent after six months and 5.8 percent after 12 months. During this time, symptoms of pain decreased and mobility improved. Only three women stopped treatment due to digestive upset.

DOSAGE

Take 600 mg daily.

SAFETY

Digestive upset, including diarrhea, may rarely occur. Consult with a doctor before using this supplement if you have kidney disease or use an asthma medication containing theophylline. Also, have your white blood cell count monitored by a doctor. One study found decreased levels in lymphocyte levels in some users.

Essential Fatty Acids

Essential fatty acids are often deficient in the U.S. diet. They work to reduce inflammation, a foundational cause of osteoporosis. A study reported in the *Journal of Aging* demonstrated that the combination of fish oil and evening primrose oil, along with 600 mg of calcium, improved bone density in senior women. During the first 18 months, thigh bone density increased 1.3 percent in the treatment group, but decreased 2.1 percent in the placebo group. During the same time period, low back spine density remained unchanged with the treatment group but decreased 3.2 percent overall in the placebo group. During the second period of 18 months, all patients receiving the essential fatty acid combination had a low back spine density increase of 3.1 percent. In addition, the thigh bone density increased an average of 4.7 percent in those supplementing the essential fatty acids.

DOSAGE

Take 1,500 mg of EPA and DHA combined daily, and 500 mg of GLA daily.

SAFETY

Do not take fish oil if you are on blood-thinning medications unless under the supervision of a physician.

Reducing Inflammation with Essential Fatty Acids

Essential fatty acids such as fish oil and evening primrose oil can reduce inflammation. Like many chronic degenerative conditions, chronic inflammation plays a major role in bone breakdown. Essential fatty acids are very powerful yet safe substances that reduce inflammation and should not be neglected in a holistic approach to osteoporosis.

Stephanie, a 62-year-old patient with severe osteoporosis, had declined drug therapy due to her concern about side effects. A comprehensive holistic program including weight-bearing exercise such as walking and weight lifting, bone-building supplements, and pharmaceutical prescriptions of bioidentical hormone replacement resulted in a 6 percent increase in her hip bone density after 18 months of treatment.

STEPHANIE'S STORY

Horny Goat Weed

Horny goat weed contains two plant estrogens, also found in soy, that combat osteoporosis.

Chinese researchers studied *Epimedium brevicornum maxim* (horny goat weed), an herb said to boost libido, and bone density in 85 postmenopausal women. After two years, participants who took horny goat weed extract daily had bone mineral density increases of 1.6 percent in the hip and 1.3 percent in the lower spine. The placebo group's bone density decreased 1.8 percent in the hip and 2.4 percent in the spine.

DOSAGE

Take a horny goat weed product standardized to containing 60 mg of icariin daily.

SAFETY

Side effects may include dizziness, dry mouth, nosebleed, or vomiting. Do not use if you take blood-thinning medication such as aspirin or warfarin (Coumadin).

Soy Isoflavones

Several studies have shown that soy isoflavones—from tofu, miso, natto, tempeh, soy milk, soy protein powders and/or supplements—can improve bone density, perhaps by weakly stimulating the estrogen receptors in bone-building cells. The phytoestrogens in soy, particularly daidzein and genistein, have been shown to stimulate bone-building cells known as osteoblasts.

Chinese researchers analyzed nine studies involving 432 menopausal women, looking at the effect of soy isoflavones (soy-derived compounds that have estrogen-like effects) on bone breakdown and bone formation, as measured by markers in urine and blood. Women (especially Asians) who consumed as little as 90 mg daily of soy isoflavones in supplement form showed decreases in bone breakdown and increases in new bone formation.

DOSAGE

Take 90 mg of soy isoflavones daily in capsule, tablet, or powder form.

SAFETY

Women with a history or high risk of breast cancer can safely consume fermented soy foods, but should avoid soy supplements until further research is done. Also, soy is a common food sensitivity, so symptoms such as digestive upset or skin rash can occur.

References

Cockayne, S, et al. 2006. Vitamin K and the prevention of fractures: Systematic review and meta-analysis of randomized controlled trials. *Archives of Internal Medicine.* June 26;166(12):1256–61.

Hitz, MF, JE Jensen, PC Eskildsen. 2007. Bone mineral density and bone markers in patients with a recent low-energy fracture: Effect of 1 y of treatment with calcium and vitamin D. *American Journal of Clinical Nutrition.* July;86(1):251–9.

Jehle, S, et al. 2006. *Journal of the American Society of Nephrology.* November.

Kruger, MC, et al. 1998. Calcium, gamma-linolenic acid and eicosapentaenoic acid supplementation in senile osteoporosis. *Aging* (Milano). October;10(5):385–94.

Ma, DF, et al. 2007. Soy isoflavone intake inhibits bone resorption and stimulates bone formation in menopausal women: Meta-analysis of randomized controlled trials. *European Journal of Clinical Nutrition.* 62(2):155–61.

Moscarini, M, et al. 1994. New perspectives in the treatment of postmenopausal osteoporosis: Ipriflavone. *Gynecology and Endocrinology.* September;8(3):203–7.

Stendig-Lindberg, G, R Tepper, I Leichter. 1993. Trabecular bone density in a two year controlled trial of peroral magnesium in osteoporosis. *Magnesium Research.* June;6(2):155–63.

Zhang, G, et al. 2007. Epimedium-derived phytoestrogen flavonoids exert beneficial effect on preventing bone loss in late postmenopausal women: A 24-month randomized, double-blind and placebo-controlled trial. *Journal of Bone and Mineral Research.* 22(7):1072–9.

24

Premenstrual Syndrome (PMS) Drugs and Their Natural Alternatives

What Is PMS?

It is estimated that three out of every four women experience premenstrual syndrome (PMS). This group of symptoms begins one to two weeks before a woman's menstrual flow. Symptoms can be both physical and emotional. Most women with PMS experience a few symptoms, while others suffer from several. The intensity of symptoms may vary month to month. Following is a list of symptoms women may experience:

Emotional symptoms:

- Depression
- Mood swings (irritability or anger, crying spells)
- Food cravings and changes in appetite
- Insomnia
- Social withdrawal
- Poor concentration

Physical symptoms:

- Headache
- Fatigue

- Water retention and weight gain
- Bloating, constipation, or diarrhea
- Breast tenderness
- Joint or muscle pain
- Acne

One type of PMS, known as premenstrual dysphoric disorder, or PMDD, is so severe that it interferes with a woman's ability to carry out daily activities and functions.

PMS Drugs

Diuretics

Diurex PMS

Lurline PMS

Midol PMS

Pamprin Multisymptom

Premsyn PMS

Spironolactone (Aldactone)

HOW DO THESE DRUGS WORK?

Diuretics increase the rate of urine production and excretion. This action reduces the water retention and bloating associated with PMS. The listed medications above are all over-the-counter except for spironolactone (Aldactone). The over-the-counter medications contain one or more of the following mild diuretic chemicals: ammonium chloride, caffeine, and pamabrom. Spironolactone (Aldactone) is a stronger diuretic and is a prescription drug.

WHAT ARE THE BENEFITS?

Quick reduction of bloating and water retention.

POTENTIAL SIDE EFFECTS

Over-the-counter PMS diuretic products: digestive upset, headache.

Spironolactone (Aldactone): diarrhea, cramps, drowsiness, rash, irregular menstrual periods, irregular hair growth, fever, chills, low back pain, nervousness, dry mouth, increased thirst, skin rash, itching, fatigue, weakness of legs.

MAJOR CAUTIONS

Spironolactone (Aldactone): fast or irregular heartbeat, palpitations, pain or difficulty passing urine, shortness of breath.

KNOWN DRUG INTERACTIONS

Spironolactone (Aldactone) increases potassium levels, so any medications that increase potassium should be avoided, such as potassium supplements, ACE inhibitors, indometacin (Indocin), or other potassium-sparing diuretics. Spironolactone should be used with caution when taken in conjunction with digoxin (Lanoxin).

FOOD OR SUPPLEMENT INTERACTIONS

Avoid potassium-rich foods and potassium supplements.

The following herbs should be avoided: buckthorn or alder buckthorn, buchu, cleavers, dandelion, digitalis, ginkgo biloba, gravel root, horsetail, juniper, licorice, uva ursi.

NUTRIENT DEPLETION/IMBALANCE

- Potassium—check with your doctor before using.
- Magnesium—take 200 to 250 mg twice daily.

Analgesics

There are different types of analgesics that can be used for headaches, pelvic pain, and menstrual cramps associated with premenstrual syndrome. Some nonsteroidal anti-inflammatory drugs (NSAIDs) are available by prescription only, as they contain higher dosages.

The most effective NSAIDs are:

Ibuprofen (Advil, Motrin)

Naproxen (Aleve, Anaprox)

Mefenamic acid (Ponstel)

HOW DO THESE DRUGS WORK?

NSAIDs work by blocking enzymes that are involved in the production of chemicals in the body known as prostaglandins. Certain prostaglandins promote pain and inflammation. By reducing the activity of cyclooxygenase (COX) enzymes, these medicines reduce pain and inflammation.

WHAT ARE THE BENEFITS?

Quick pain relief with medication that is easily accessible over the counter.

POTENTIAL SIDE EFFECTS

NSAIDs' most common side effects are nausea, vomiting, diarrhea, constipation, decreased appetite, rash, dizziness, headache, and drowsiness. They can also cause fluid retention and swelling of tissue.

MAJOR CAUTIONS

With NSAIDs there is a small risk of kidney failure, liver failure, ulcers, and prolonged bleeding after an injury or surgery. People allergic to NSAIDs may develop shortness of breath. People with asthma are at a higher risk for experiencing a serious allergic reaction to NSAIDs. Those with a serious allergy to one NSAID are likely to experience a similar reaction to a different NSAID.

KNOWN DRUG INTERACTIONS

NSAIDs can reduce blood flow to the kidneys and reduce the action of diuretics and decrease the elimination of lithium (Eskalith) and methotrexate (Rheumatrex). NSAIDs also decrease the ability of the blood to clot and therefore increase bleeding time. Bleeding complications are even more of a risk when NSAIDs are combined with other medications that have a blood-thinning effect. NSAIDs can also increase blood pressure.

FOOD OR SUPPLEMENT INTERACTIONS

Ibuprofen can cause salt and water retention. Therefore, those using ibuprofen should watch and minimize their sodium intake. Ibuprofen can be taken with food to prevent digestive upset. Do not take potassium supplements while using ibuprofen. Deglycyrrhizinated licorice (DGL) may help protect against ulceration of the digestive tract while using NSAIDs.

NUTRIENT DEPLETION/IMBALANCE

NSAIDs have been shown to deplete vitamin C and folic acid. We recommend the following:

- Vitamin C—take 500 mg daily.
- Folic acid—take 400 micrograms daily.

Birth Control Pills

Low-dose birth control pills modify hormone fluctuations associated with PMS and relieve symptoms.

Seasonale

Seasonique

Yaz

HOW DO THESE DRUGS WORK?

Birth control pills contain small amounts of synthetic estrogen and/or synthetic progesterone (progestin) that modify hormone fluctuations associated with PMS.

POTENTIAL SIDE EFFECTS

Breast tenderness, nausea, higher blood pressure, and headaches are possible side effects.

MAJOR CAUTIONS

Birth control pills can increase the risk of blood clots, breast cancer, and heart disease. They should be avoided by women with a history of these diseases. Breast cancer risk is more associated with long-term use. It is important to not smoke when using birth control pills, as this increases the risk of blood clots.

FOOD OR SUPPLEMENT INTERACTIONS

St. John's wort and grapefruit juice should be avoided by women taking birth control pills.

NUTRIENT DEPLETION/IMBALANCE

Nutrients depleted by oral contraceptives include: B1, B2, B3, B6, B12, folic acid, magnesium, zinc, vitamin C, CoQ10, and vitamin E. We recommend the following supplements:

Oral Contraceptives and Fat-Soluble Antioxidants

A study published in the *American Journal of Obstetrics and Gynecology* examined how oral contraceptives affect the blood levels of fat-soluble antioxidants, including coenzyme Q10; alpha-tocopherol and gamma-tocopherol (members of the vitamin E family); and the carotenoids beta-carotene, alpha-carotene, and lycopene. Nonfasting blood samples were collected randomly on any day of the menstrual cycle from 15 premenopausal women who had been using oral contraceptives for at least six months and from 40 women who were not using oral contraceptives. No dietary restrictions were imposed on any of the participants. Women who consumed coenzyme Q10 supplements and/or multivitamins as well as women who had irregular menstrual cycles were excluded from the study. Researchers found that for oral contraceptive users, blood levels of coenzyme Q10 were 37 percent lower and alpha-tocopherol levels were 23 percent lower than those in women who did not use contraceptives. Blood levels of the other nutrients were comparable between the two groups.

- B complex—take daily.
- Magnesium—take 200 to 250 mg twice daily.
- Zinc—take 15 mg daily.
- CoQ10—take 100 to 200 mg daily.
- Vitamin E—take 200 IU of mixed vitamin E daily.

Ovarian Suppressor

Danazol (Danocrine)

HOW DOES THIS DRUG WORK?

This synthetic hormone suppresses the ovarian production of hormones, altering the hormonal cycle associated with PMS.

WHAT ARE THE BENEFITS?

Prevents PMS symptoms from occurring.

POTENTIAL SIDE EFFECTS

- Dizziness
- Headache
- Fatigue
- Appetite changes
- Stomach upset
- Bloating
- Anxiety
- Oily skin
- Weight gain
- Flushing
- Changes in sleep patterns
- Change in sex drive
- Muscle cramps
- Chills
- Fluid retention in the hands or feet
- Nasal congestion
- Depression
- Hot flashes
- Deepening of the voice
- Abnormal growth of fine body hair or facial hair
- No or irregular menstrual periods while taking this medication

MAJOR CAUTIONS

Danazol (Danocrine) cannot be used over long periods of time because of the potential for serious side effects. These include vision changes, yellowing of the eyes or skin, one-sided weakness, slurred speech, stroke, blood clots, peliosis hepatitis (blood-filled cavities in the liver), liver tumors, and benign intracranial hypertension.

Women should be tested for pregnancy before using this medication, as it causes birth defects.

KNOWN DRUG INTERACTIONS

Warfarin (Coumadin) and carbamazepine (Tegretol).

FOOD OR SUPPLEMENT INTERACTIONS

None known.

NUTRIENT DEPLETION/IMBALANCE

None known.

Gonadotropin–Releasing Hormone (GnRH) Analogs

Goserelin—injection or implant (Zoladex)

Leuprolide—injection (Eligard, Lupron)

HOW DO THESE DRUGS WORK?

These medications affect the pituitary gland in such a way as to stop ovulation.

WHAT ARE THE BENEFITS?

They prevent PMS symptoms from occurring.

POTENTIAL SIDE EFFECTS

- Aches and pains
- Headaches
- Hot flashes
- Constipation
- Depression
- Irritation at the injection site

MAJOR CAUTIONS

- Bone pain
- Numbness
- Tingling or weakness in the legs or arms
- Bone thinning (with long-term use)

KNOWN DRUG INTERACTIONS

- Cimetidine (Tagamet)
- Hormones
- Methyldopa
- Metoclopramide (Reglan)
- Prasterone
- Reserpine (Harmonyl)

FOOD OR SUPPLEMENT INTERACTIONS

Vitex, black cohosh.

NUTRIENT DEPLETION/IMBALANCE

None known.

Antidepressants

This class of medications is becoming increasingly popular for the treatment of mood disturbances associated with PMS. These prescription drugs alter brain chemicals that affect mood. The following are antidepressants most commonly prescribed for women with PMS.

Selective Serotonin Reuptake Inhibitors (SSRIs)

Fluoxetine (Prozac)

Sertraline (Zoloft)

HOW DO THESE DRUGS WORK?

These drugs block the reuptake of serotonin so that it remains active in the brain longer before being broken down and reabsorbed. The neurotransmitter serotonin gives the sensation of well-being.

WHAT ARE THE BENEFITS?

Improvement in depression and mood changes associated with premenstrual syndrome. SSRIs have fewer side effects than other prescription antidepressants such as tricyclic antidepressants and monoamine oxidase (MAO) inhibitors.

POTENTIAL SIDE EFFECTS

- Nausea
- Diarrhea
- Agitation
- Insomnia

- Decreased sexual desire
- Delayed orgasm or inability to have an orgasm

MAJOR CAUTIONS

Tremors can be a side effect of SSRIs. Serotonergic syndrome, in which serotonin levels are too high, is a serious but rare condition associated with the use of SSRIs. Symptoms can include high fevers, seizures, and heart rhythm disturbances.

There is an association between bone loss and the use of SSRIs in older men and women.

Suicidal thoughts or increased risk of suicide may occur from these medications.

KNOWN DRUG INTERACTIONS

- Astemizole (Hismanal)
- Cisapride (Propulsid)
- Pimozide (Orap)
- Terfenadine (Seldane)
- Thioridazine (Mellaril)
- MAO inhibitors such as phenelzine (Nardil), tranylcypromine (Parnate), isocarboxazid (Marplan), selegiline (Eldepryl)

FOOD OR SUPPLEMENT INTERACTIONS

The following should be avoided while on these medications:

- Alcohol
- 5-HTP
- L-tryptophan
- St. John's wort

NUTRIENT DEPLETION/IMBALANCE

In one study, women taking 500 mcg of folic acid daily in addition to fluoxetine (Prozac) experienced significant improvement in their symptoms and fewer side effects compared to women taking the drug only.

Fluoxetine (Prozac) has been shown to significantly lower melatonin levels. It has not been determined whether simultaneous supplementation is appropriate.

Ginkgo biloba extract has been shown to reduce sexual side effects in those taking SSRIs in both elderly men and women. Participants in the study used 200 to 240 mg of ginkgo biloba extract.

Tricyclic Antidepressants (TCAs)

Clomipramine (Anafranil)

HOW DO THESE DRUGS WORK?

TCAs work mainly by increasing the level of norepinephrine in the brain. They may also increase serotonin levels. Altering these neurotransmitter levels can improve the emotional outlook of a woman with premenstrual syndrome.

WHAT ARE THE BENEFITS?

They are used to treat moderate to severe depression.

POTENTIAL SIDE EFFECTS

- Blurred vision
- Constipation
- Dizziness
- Drowsiness
- Dry mouth
- Impaired sexual function
- Weight gain

MAJOR CAUTIONS

- Low blood pressure
- Glaucoma

KNOWN DRUG INTERACTIONS

These medications should not be combined with monoamine oxidase (MAO) inhibiting drugs as described in chapter 6. Also do not combine with epinephrine, and use caution when also taking cimetidine (Tagamet).

FOOD OR SUPPLEMENT INTERACTIONS

Do not combine with alcohol.

NUTRIENT DEPLETION/IMBALANCE

The following nutrients may be depleted and should be supplemented while on this medication:

- Coenzyme Q10—take 100 to 200 mg daily
- Niacinamide
- Vitamin B1
- Vitamin B12
- Vitamin B2

- Vitamin B3
- Vitamin B5
- Vitamin B6
- Take a B complex daily to prevent a deficiency of these B vitamins

Atypical Antidepressants

Drugs in this class of antidepressants work like SSRIs and TCAs but with a different mechanism of action.

Nefazodone (Serzone)

Nefazodone (Serzone) works by inhibiting the reuptake of serotonin and norepinephrine and therefore increases the brain's levels of these neurotransmitters. This can reduce the emotional symptoms some women experience with PMS.

WHAT ARE THE BENEFITS?

These medications can relieve depression and offer treatment for people who do not respond to other pharmaceutical antidepressants.

POTENTIAL SIDE EFFECTS

- Nausea
- Dizziness
- Insomnia
- Agitation
- Tiredness
- Dry mouth
- Constipation
- Light-headedness
- Blurred vision
- Confusion

MAJOR CAUTIONS

Suicidal thinking and behavior.

KNOWN DRUG INTERACTIONS

- MAO inhibitor antidepressants such as isocarboxazid (Marplan), phenelzine (Nardil), tranylcypromine (Parnate), and procarbazine (Matulane)
- Selegiline (Eldepryl)
- Fenfluramine (Pondimin) and dexfenfluramine (Redux)
- Terfenadine (Seldane)

- Triazolam (Halcion)
- Alprazolam (Xanax)
- Digoxin (Lanoxin)

FOOD OR SUPPLEMENT INTERACTIONS

Avoid the following:

- 5-hydroxytryptophan (5-HTP)
- L-tryptophan
- Sour date nut (*Ziziphus jujube*)
- St. John's wort

NUTRIENT DEPLETION/IMBALANCE

None known.

Anti-anxiety Drugs

These medications may be prescribed for more severe anxiety-related symptoms of PMS.

Benzodiazepines

Alprazolam Extended-Release (Xanax XR)

Alprazolam Oral Solution (Alprazolam Intensol)

Alprazolam tablets (Niravam, Xanax)

HOW DO THESE DRUGS WORK?

Benzodiazepines enhance the effect of the neurotransmitter known as gamma-aminobutyric acid (GABA). They bind to GABA receptors, which slows down the activity of nerve cells. This causes an inhibitory and relaxant effect that can reduce anxiety associated with PMS.

WHAT ARE THE BENEFITS?

They provide rapid relief for those with PMS-related anxiety.

POTENTIAL SIDE EFFECTS

- Agitation
- Increased anxiety
- Confusion
- Memory impairment
- Lack of coordination
- Speech difficulties
- Light-headedness
- Constipation

MAJOR CAUTIONS

Benzodiazepines can be addictive, particularly in those with a history of drug or alcohol dependency. Also, people can experience withdrawal symptoms when stopping their use suddenly, such as blurred vision, decreased concentration, decreased mental clarity, diarrhea, increased awareness of noise or bright light, loss of appetite and weight, and seizures. Work with a doctor to gradually wean yourself off these medications to avoid these withdrawal effects. Lastly, combining these drugs with alcohol is potentially lethal.

KNOWN DRUG INTERACTIONS

- Ketoconazole (Nizoral)
- Itraconazole (Sporanox)
- Some HIV or AIDS medications

FOOD OR SUPPLEMENT INTERACTIONS

Do not combine with alcohol, as the interaction can be deadly. Do not take grapefruit juice while on this class of medications. Do not combine with kava supplements.

NUTRIENT DEPLETION/IMBALANCE

This class of drugs can deplete calcium, folic acid, vitamin D, vitamin K, melatonin, biotin, and folic acid. We recommend the following:

- Calcium—take 500 to 1,200 mg daily.
- Folic acid—take 400 mcg daily.
- Vitamin D—take 1,000 IU daily.
- Vitamin K—take 500 mcg daily.
- Melatonin—use under the guidance of a doctor if you are on an anxiety medication.

Buspirone

Buspirone is marketed under the brand name Buspar.

HOW DOES THIS DRUG WORK?

This medication works by stimulating serotonin type 1A receptors on nerves, leading to a relaxation effect and the reduction of anxiety associated with premenstrual syndrome.

WHAT ARE THE BENEFITS?

It reduces the symptoms of anxiety. Unlike benzodiazepines, it does not cause sedation and is not considered addictive.

POTENTIAL SIDE EFFECTS

- Dizziness
- Nausea
- Headache
- Nervousness
- Light-headedness
- Excitement
- Insomnia
- Nasal congestion
- Nightmares

MAJOR CAUTIONS

- Blurred vision or other vision changes
- Difficulty breathing
- Chest pain
- Confusion
- Feelings of hostility or anger
- Muscle aches and pains
- Numbness or tingling in hands or feet
- Ringing in the ears
- Skin rash and itching (hives)
- Sore throat
- Vomiting
- Weakness

KNOWN DRUG INTERACTIONS

- Monoamine oxidase (MAO) inhibitors such as isocarboxazid (Marplan), phenelzine (Nardil), tranylcypromine (Parnate), and procarbazine (Matulane)
- Trazodone (Desyrel)
- Warfarin (Coumadin)
- Phenytoin (Dilantin)

FOOD OR SUPPLEMENT INTERACTIONS

Do not combine with grapefruit juice. Do not combine with kava supplements.

NUTRIENT DEPLETION/IMBALANCE

None known.

Dopamine Agonist

Bromocriptine (Parlodel)

HOW DOES THIS DRUG WORK?

This drug blocks the release of a hormone called prolactin that is associated with breast pain and premenstrual syndrome.

WHAT ARE THE BENEFITS?

This medication is used for breast pain (mastalgia) associated with premenstrual syndrome that is not responsive to NSAID pain medications such as ibuprofen.

POTENTIAL SIDE EFFECTS

- Drowsiness
- Digestive upset (stomach cramps, nausea, vomiting, indigestion, constipation, diarrhea)
- Headache
- Fatigue
- Light-headedness
- Insomnia
- Nasal congestion

MAJOR CAUTIONS

- Vomiting blood
- Confusion
- Fainting
- Depression
- Irregular pulse
- Shortness of breath
- Rash
- Tingling of hands or feet
- Involuntary movements
- Nightmares
- Vision changes

This medication should be used with caution for those with a history of heart attack, angina (chest pain), liver disease, kidney disease, psychiatric illness, vascular disorders, ulcers, high or low blood pressure, and for breast-feeding women.

KNOWN DRUG INTERACTIONS

- Cabergoline (Dostinex)
- Cyclosporine (Gengraf, Neoral)
- Dihydroergotamine (Migranal)
- Ergoloid mesylates (Gerimal, Hydergine)
- Ergonovine or methylergonovine
- Ergotamine
- Erythromycin (clarithromycin, dirithromycin, troleandomycin)
- Birth control pills
- Imatinib (Gleevec)
- Levodopa (Carbidopa, Sinemet)
- HIV medications such as amprenavir, delavirdine, efavirenz, indinavir, nelfinavir, ritonavir, saquinavir
- High blood pressure medications
- Antidepressant medications
- Memantine (Namenda)
- Methysergide (Sansert)
- Metoclopramide (Reglan)
- Sirolimus (Rapamune)
- Tacrolimus (Prograf)
- Tamoxifen (Nolvadex)

FOOD OR SUPPLEMENT INTERACTIONS

Do not combine with alcohol. Do not use in conjunction with kava or black cohosh supplements.

NUTRIENT DEPLETION/IMBALANCE

None known.

Natural Alternatives to PMS Drugs

Diet and Lifestyle Changes

It has been our experience that natural therapies are highly effective in even the most severe cases of PMS. Most women will notice a dramatic improvement within one to two cycles.

Many women will notice an improvement in their PMS symptoms after implementing a healthier diet that promotes hormone balance. Since PMS can be related to excess estrogen levels, it is important to consume approximately 20 to 30 grams of fiber in the diet. Fiber binds and expels excess estrogen through the digestive tract. Plant foods such as salads, legumes, nuts, and seeds provide fiber. Another good idea is to consume 1 to 2 tablespoons of ground flaxseeds in the diet daily. They promote better estrogen balance. Also, minimize your intake of dairy products and red meat that are not organic. The accumulation of hormones over time from these foods may contribute to hormone imbalance. It is critical to avoid refined carbohydrates in the diet. Studies demonstrate a strong correlation between high sugar consumption and PMS. Too much sodium, caffeine, and alcohol may also worsen symptoms. Regular exercise has been shown to reduce the symptoms of PMS as well.

Vitex (Chasteberry)

Several studies have demonstrated that vitex, also known as chasteberry, is effective for the treatment of premenstrual syndrome. A two-month randomized study published in *Human Psychopharmacology* involved 41 women with premenstrual dysphoric disorder (PMDD), a more severe form of PMS. It compared the effects of vitex to that of fluoxetine (Prozac). Both treatments were found to be beneficial, with vitex more helpful for physical complaints and fluoxetine (Prozac) more effective for psychological symptoms. Another randomized, double-blind, placebo-controlled study reported in the *British Medical Journal* also found vitex to be effective for PMS. The study included 86 women receiving vitex and 84 receiving a placebo. The average age was 36 years and the study duration was three consecutive cycles. Women receiving vitex had much greater improvement compared to placebo, and it was well tolerated. Also, a study published in the *Archives of Gynecology and Obstetrics* found vitex extract to be effective in the symptomatic relief of premenstrual syndrome. Also impressive is a multicenter trial published in the *Journal of Women's Health and Gender-Based Medicine*. The trial involved 1,634 women suffering from PMS. After a treatment period with vitex of three menstrual cycles, 93 percent of patients reported a decrease in the number of symptoms or even a cessation of PMS complaints. Eighty-five percent of physicians rated the treatment as good or very good while 81 percent of patients assessed their status after treatment as very much or much better. Ninety-four percent of patients assessed the tolerance of vitex treatment as good or very good.

Vitex in Ancient History

Vitex (chasteberry) has a very interesting history. Hippocrates wrote about the many impressive medicinal benefits of vitex in the fourth century B.C. The ancient Greeks considered vitex to be a symbol of chastity during festivals that honored the goddess Demeter. Later in history, Roman Catholic monks used the herb to reduce libido. It also has the nickname "monk's pepper." Women do not report experiencing a lowering of libido from this herb.

DOSAGE

Take 40 drops of tincture or 180 to 240 mg in capsule form of a standardized extract. It should be taken daily for at least three months.

SAFETY

One may experience mild digestive upset that may be resolved by taking the herb with a meal. Also, there are reports of mild skin rash with itching. Vitex should not be used in combination with the birth control pill.

Calcium

Low dietary calcium intake is associated with premenstrual syndrome. Calcium supplements have been shown to be effective in the treatment of PMS. Healthy, premenopausal women between the ages of 18 and 45 years were recruited nationally across the United States at 12 outpatient centers and screened for moderate-to-severe recurring premenstrual symptoms, and 497 participants were randomly assigned to receive 1,200 mg of elemental calcium per day in the form of calcium carbonate or placebo for three menstrual cycles. Blood work and daily documentation of symptoms were monitored. Researchers found that by the third treatment cycle, calcium effectively resulted in an over-all 48 percent reduction in total symptom scores from baseline compared with a 30 percent reduction with placebo. A different study in the *Journal of General Internal Medicine* found that 1,000 mg of daily calcium supplementation was also effective for the treatment of PMS. After three months of supplementation, 73 percent of the women reported fewer symptoms during the treatment phase on calcium, 15 percent preferred placebo, and 12 percent had no clear preference.

Magnesium

Magnesium supplementation has been shown to help a variety of PMS symptoms including mood changes, fluid retention, and migraine headaches. For example, a double-blind, randomized-design study reported in *Obstetrics and Gynecology* looked at the benefit of magnesium for women with PMS. The study included 32 women (24 to 39 years old) who were given 360 mg of magnesium

Magnesium and Vitamin B6 Deficiency

Magnesium and vitamin B6 play an important role in the liver's metabolism of estrogen. A deficiency of these nutrients may contribute to elevated estrogen levels and set the stage for PMS.

or placebo three times daily from the fifteenth day of the menstrual cycle to the onset of menstrual flow for two cycles. Magnesium was quite effective for the relief of mood changes associated with PMS.

DOSAGE

Most women will experience benefits by taking 500 to 750 mg of magnesium daily. It can be taken all month long, and especially should be supplemented during the two weeks before menstrual flow.

SAFETY

Too much magnesium may cause diarrhea. If this occurs, reduce your dosage.

Vitamin B6

There is evidence that vitamin B6 can relieve a variety of PMS symptoms. It works particularly well in combination with magnesium. A 1999 review of published and unpublished randomized, placebo-controlled trials of the effectiveness of vitamin B6 in the management of PMS concluded that the pooled data of nine trials representing 940 patients suggest that doses of pyridoxine up to 100 mg a day are likely to be of benefit in treating premenstrual symptoms, including premenstrual depression.

Natural Progesterone

A low progesterone level during the luteal phase (second half of the cycle) is thought to be a causative factor in premenstrual syndrome. Our experience is that natural progesterone, either in topical or oral form, is effective for many women with moderate to severe symptoms of PMS. It is best used under the supervision of a doctor.

Suzanne, a 29-year-old mother of two, experienced one week of severe PMS symptoms every month. Her mood changes were the worst problem. Suzanne's irritability was heightened during this time, and she felt rage at her husband and others close to her. A hormone test revealed that she had very low progesterone levels. She was prescribed natural progesterone cream for two weeks before her cycle and experienced a dramatic improvement in her symptoms. Her family no longer avoided her during this time of her cycle. Progesterone has nerve-relaxing properties and helps many women who experience anxiety, irritability, muscle tightness, cramps, and insomnia due to low progesterone levels.

SUZANNE'S
STORY

DOSAGE

Topical: 10 to 20 mg one to two times daily, beginning after ovulation until one day before your period begins.

Oral: 50 to 100 mg one to two times daily, beginning after ovulation until one day before your period begins.

SAFETY

Too much progesterone may cause drowsiness, breast tenderness, fluid retention, or nausea.

Vitamin E

Vitamin E is often helpful to reduce symptoms of anxiety, food cravings, breast tenderness, and depression for women with PMS. A randomized, double-blind study in the *Journal of Reproductive Medicine* reviewed the effect of 400 IU of vitamin E (d-alpha tocopherol) on 41 women with PMS for three cycles. Significant improvement was noted in several mood and physical symptoms.

References

Atmaca, M, S Kumru, and E Tezcan. 2003. Fluoxetine versus Vitex agnus castus extract in the treatment of premenstrual dysphoric disorder. *Human Psychopharmacology.* 18:191–195.

Berger, D, et al. 2000. Efficacy of Vitex agnus castus L. extract Ze 440 in patients with premenstrual syndrome (PMS). *Archives of Gynecology and Obstetrics.* 264:150–3.

Childs, PA, et al. 1995. Effect of fluoxetine on melatonin in patients with seasonal affective disorder and matched controls. *British Journal of Psychiatry.* 166:196–8.

Cohen, AJ, B Bartlik. 1998. *Ginkgo biloba* for antidepressant-induced sexual dysfunction. *Journal of Sex and Marital Therapy.* 24:139–45.

Coppen, A, J Bailey. 2000. Enhancement of the antidepressant action of fluoxetine by folic acid: A randomised, placebo controlled trial. *Journal of Affective Disorders.* November;60(2):121–30.

Facchinetti, F, et al. 1991. Oral magnesium successfully relieves premenstrual mood changes. *Obstetrics and Gynecology.* August;78(2):177–81.

Loch, EG, H Selle, N Boblitz. 2000. Treatment of premenstrual syndrome with a phytopharmaceutical formulation containing Vitex agnus castus. *Journal of Women's Health and Gender-Based Medicine.* 9:315–20.

London, RS, et al. 1987. Efficacy of alpha-tocopherol in the treatment of the premenstrual syndrome. *Journal of Reproductive Medicine.* 32:400–4.

Palan, PR, et al. 2006. Effects of menstrual cycle and oral contraceptive use on serum levels of lipid-soluble antioxidants. *American Journal of Obstetrics and Gynecology.* May; 194(5):e35–8.

Schellenberg, R. 2001. Treatment for the premenstrual syndrome with agnus castus fruit extract: Prospective, randomized, placebo-controlled study. *British Medical Journal.* 322:134–7.

Thys-Jacobs, S, et al. 1989. Calcium supplementation in premenstrual syndrome: A randomized crossover trial. *Journal of General Internal Medicine.* 4:183–9.

———. 1998. Calcium carbonate and the premenstrual syndrome: Effects on premenstrual and menstrual symptoms. Premenstrual Syndrome Study Group. *American Journal of Obstetrics and Gynecology.* 179:444–52.

Wyatt, KM, et al. 1999. Efficacy of vitamin B6 in the treatment of premenstrual syndrome: Systematic review. *British Medical Journal.* 318:1375–81.

25

Prostate Drugs and Their Natural Alternatives

What Is BPH?

Benign prostatic hyperplasia (BPH) is commonly referred to as prostate enlargement. The prostate is a walnut-sized gland that lies below the urinary bladder and surrounds the urethra (the tube that carries urine from the bladder). The main role of the prostate is to make nutrient-rich fluid for the sperm that becomes part of the semen.

BPH is very common, with more than half of men in their sixties and as many as 90 percent in their seventies and eighties having some symptoms of BPH. Symptoms are rare in men in their forties or younger. As the gland enlarges, it encroaches upon the urethra and interferes with urine flow. This causes the bladder to become irritated and to thicken as a result. This irritation of the bladder causes it to contract even when it contains small amounts of urine. Common symptoms of BPH include:

- Frequent urination, especially at night
- Urgency and leaking or dribbling
- Weak stream
- Incomplete bladder emptying

Hormonal stimulation of the prostate gland appears to be the root issue with BPH. As men get older, their testosterone levels decline while their relative estrogen level increases. Estrogen stimulates the growth of prostate cells.

Another probable hormonal factor is dihydrotestosterone (DHT), a hormone metabolite of testosterone produced in the prostate. Older men tend to accumulate higher levels of DHT in the prostate, which also may encourage the growth of cells. BPH is not the same as prostate cancer and is not considered a precursor to prostate cancer.

Prostate Drugs

There are two classes of drugs used to treat BPH. These include alpha-blockers and enzyme inhibitors. They are used individually or sometimes in combination with each other.

Alpha 1 Blockers

Four alpha blockers have been approved by the Food and Drug Administration (FDA) for treatment of BPH, including:

> Terazosin (Hytrin)
>
> Doxazosin (Cardura)
>
> Tamsulosin (Flomax)
>
> Alfuzosin (Uroxatral)

HOW DO THESE DRUGS WORK?

Alpha 1 blockers target smooth muscle receptors and cause relaxation of the muscles of the prostate and around the bladder neck. This makes it easier to urinate. They do not shrink the prostate gland.

WHAT ARE THE BENEFITS?

Relaxing the smooth muscles around the bladder neck helps relieve urinary obstruction caused by an enlarged prostate. These drugs work to relieve symptoms within 24 to 48 hours.

POTENTIAL SIDE EFFECTS

- Reduced semen released during ejaculation
- Low blood pressure
- Dizziness
- Headache
- Stomach or intestinal irritation
- Stuffy or runny nose

MAJOR CAUTIONS

Alpha blockers can lower blood pressure dangerously, especially when taken with erectile dysfunction drugs such as sildenafil (Viagra), vardenafil (Levitra), or tadalafil (Cialis). Check with your doctor first before combining these medications.

In men who take tamsulosin (Flomax) or other alpha blockers, the FDA warns of the risk of a pupil disorder known as intraoperative floppy iris syndrome. If you take any alpha blockers, be sure to tell your doctor if you're planning to have eye surgery.

KNOWN DRUG INTERACTIONS

Check with your doctor first if you are using

- Clonidine
- Cimetidine
- Warfarin

FOOD OR SUPPLEMENT INTERACTIONS

None known.

NUTRIENT DEPLETION/IMBALANCE

None known.

Enzyme (5-alpha-reductase) Inhibitors

These drugs shrink your prostate gland. Two have been approved by the FDA for BPH:

Finasteride (Proscar)

Dutasteride (Avodart)

HOW DO THESE DRUGS WORK?

This group of BPH medications works by reducing the amount of testosterone that turns into dihydrotestosterone (DHT). It does this by blocking the enzyme 5-alpha-reductase that converts testosterone into DHT. They also reduce the number of receptor sites on the prostate to which DHT can attach.

WHAT ARE THE BENEFITS?

In men with moderate to severe BPH, these medications can significantly decrease the need for surgery and the incidence of urinary retention. Men with larger prostates benefit the most. Men with a normal prostate size but with symptoms of BPH do not benefit from these medications. Both drugs can either prevent progression of growth of the prostate or shrink the prostate in some men.

POTENTIAL SIDE EFFECTS

- Erection problems
- Decreased sexual desire
- Reduced semen release during ejaculation
- Breast enlargement or tenderness

MAJOR CAUTIONS

Finasteride (Proscar) has been shown to prevent or delay the onset of prostate cancer by about 25 percent in men 55 years and older. However, it has also been shown to slightly raise the risk of developing higher-grade prostate cancer. Using finasteride as a primary treatment to prevent prostate cancer is not recommended.

Finasteride and dutasteride (Avodart) lower PSA levels in your blood. Let your doctor know if you are taking these medications.

KNOWN DRUG INTERACTIONS

None known.

FOOD OR SUPPLEMENT INTERACTIONS

Do not combine with common herbs used for BPH such as African pygeum, nettle, and saw palmetto, since they have similar mechanisms and the additive effects may be too strong.

NUTRIENT DEPLETION/IMBALANCE

None known.

Natural Alternatives to Prostate Drugs

Diet and Lifestyle Changes

Consume foods rich in omega-3 fatty acids and monounsaturated fat that help to decrease inflammation of the prostate gland. Good choices include avocados, cold-water fish (wild salmon, sardines), ground flaxseeds (1 to 2 tablespoons daily), and pumpkin seeds. Tomatoes and tomato paste, watermelon, and cantaloupe contain the prostate-friendly nutrient lycopene. Consume three servings weekly.

Men with BPH should avoid caffeinated beverages as well as alcohol—they irritate and inflame the prostate. Also reduce your intake of foods that contain harmful fats, such as fried foods that contain hydrogenated or partially hydrogenated oils, which promote inflammation. Minimize your intake of dairy and red meat, as they contain saturated fat, which also may worsen inflammation of the prostate. Stay away from packaged foods that are high in sugar, which can worsen inflammation.

Regular exercise is important in the prevention and treatment of BPH. For example, a study in the *Archives of Internal Medicine* reported that men who walked two to three hours a week had a 25 percent lower risk of developing BPH.

Saw Palmetto

The berries of this plant were first used medicinally by Native Americans for prostate and urinary problems. A multitude of published clinical studies have demonstrated that saw palmetto provides improvement for mild to moderate symptoms of BPH. This includes benefit for frequent urination, hesitancy, painful urination, nighttime urination, and generally improved urinary flow.

Researchers have found that saw palmetto helps the prostate by reducing the activity of 5-alpha-reductase enzyme, which is involved in the production of DHT. It also reduces the growth effects of estrogen on prostate cells. Saw palmetto has also been shown to reduce smooth muscle contraction, allowing the bladder and sphincter muscles to relax, thus reducing urinary urgency. It also exerts an anti-inflammatory effect on the prostate gland by inhibiting the cyclooxygenase-2 (COX-2) enzyme. This enzyme is active in the inflammatory pathway.

In one study involving 1,098 men over the age of 50, researchers compared 320 mg of saw palmetto extract with the prescription drug finasteride (Proscar). At the end of the six-month trial, both treatments were shown to be equally effective in reducing the symptoms of BPH in two-thirds of participants.

A Flawed Study of Saw Palmetto

A 2006 study published in the *New England Journal of Medicine* reported that saw palmetto was not effective for symptoms of BPH. The double-blind trial randomly assigned 225 men over the age of 49 years who had moderate-to-severe symptoms of benign prostatic hyperplasia to one year of treatment with saw palmetto extract (160 mg twice a day) or placebo. The problem with the media headlines of this study is that they ignored more than 20 other well-designed studies showing the efficacy of saw palmetto. However, the biggest problem with the media coverage of this story is that it failed to report that the men with BPH in the study had moderate to severe symptoms. Saw palmetto has shown unquestionably that it is effective for mild to moderate symptoms of BPH.

However, saw palmetto was found to have far fewer problems with sexual dysfunction such as decreased libido and impotence. A 2002 review of saw palmetto studies involved 3,139 men from 21 randomized trials lasting 4 to 48 weeks. Eighteen of these trials were double-blind. The researchers concluded that the evidence suggests that saw palmetto provides mild to moderate improvement in urinary symptoms and flow measurement. It also produced similar improvement in urinary symptoms and flow compared to finasteride and was associated with fewer adverse treatment events.

DOSAGE

Take 320 mg daily of a product standardized between 80 and 85 percent fatty acids.

SAFETY

Saw palmetto is well tolerated with occasional reports of dizziness, headache, and digestive complaints.

Beta Sitosterol

This compound occurs naturally in plant foods such as rice bran, wheat germ, corn oil, soybeans, and peanuts. The supplemental extract form significantly relieves BPH urinary symptoms. Animal research shows that beta sitosterol may inhibit 5-alpha-reductase activity. It has been shown in animals to shrink the prostate, but this has not yet been demonstrated in humans.

DOSAGE

Take 60 to 130 mg of beta sitosterol divided into 2 to 3 doses daily on an empty stomach.

SAFETY

Digestive upset such as gas, nausea, or diarrhea occurs rarely with users. Beta sitosterol may reduce the absorption and blood levels of alpha- and beta-carotene and vitamin E, so it should be taken by itself on an empty stomach. Beta sitosterol should not be taken by those individuals with a rare genetic disease known as sitosterolemia. With this disease, people have an abnormally high absorption of beta sitosterol and cholesterol from the diet. Consult with your doctor before using this supplement in conjunction with cholesterol-lowering medications.

Pygeum Africanum

This BPH-specific supplement comes from an extract of the bark of the African plum tree. Research suggests that pygeum inhibits growth factors that are responsible for prostate tissue growth. It decreases inflammatory chemicals and improves bladder contractility.

A study involving three urology centers researched the benefit of pygeum extract on 85 men with BPH. Participants took 50 mg twice daily. Researchers found that nighttime frequency of urination was reduced by 32 percent and other urinary markers were statistically significantly improved.

DOSAGE

Take 50 to 100 mg twice daily of a standardized extract containing 13 percent sterols.

SAFETY

Side effects such as digestive upset are rare.

Rye Grass Pollen Extract

Rye grass pollen extract taken orally improves symptoms such as urinary frequency, nighttime urination, urgency, decreased urine flow rate, dribbling, and painful urination in patients with mild to moderate BPH. The extract seems to relax the sphincter muscles that control the bladder.

In a study published in the *British Journal of Urology,* 60 patients with urinary outflow obstruction due to BPH were entered into a double-blind, placebo-controlled study to evaluate the effect of a six-month course of the pollen extract Cernilton. There was a statistically significant subjective improvement with Cernilton (69 percent of the patients) compared with placebo (30 percent). Researchers found a significant decrease in residual urine (amount of urine left in bladder afer voiding) in the patients treated with Cernilton and in the size of the prostate on ultrasound. It is concluded that Cernilton has a beneficial effect in BPH and may have a place in the treatment of patients with mild or moderate symptoms of outflow obstruction.

In another study, 79 patients with BPH were treated with rye grass pollen extract. Patient ages ranged from 62 to 89 years. Rye grass pollen extract was administered in a dosage of 126 mg three times daily for more than 12 weeks. Researchers measured several parameters of urinary function. Urine maximum flow rate and average flow rate increased significantly, and residual urine volume decreased significantly from 54.2 mL to less than 30 mL. Also, 28 patients treated for more than one year showed a mean decrease of prostatic volume. No adverse reactions were observed.

DOSAGE

Take 126 mg three times daily.

SAFETY

Side effects are uncommon but may include abdominal distention, heartburn, and nausea.

Zinc

This mineral is necessary for normal prostate function. In addition, it reduces the activity of the enzyme 5-alpha-reductase that converts testosterone into DHT. Holistic doctors therefore recommend it for men with BPH as part of a comprehensive nutritional therapy.

DOSAGE

Take 50 mg twice daily for two months, and then use a maintenance dosage of 50 mg daily. Since zinc can impair copper absorption, make sure to supplement 2 mg of copper daily.

SAFETY

Zinc may rarely cause nausea, vomiting, or a metallic taste in the mouth. Population studies suggest that taking more than 100 mg of supplemental zinc daily or taking supplemental zinc for 10 or more years doubles the risk of developing prostate cancer. Iron and calcium can interfere with zinc absorption and should be taken at different times of the day.

JOE'S STORY

Joe, a 59-year-old bartender, had found he was getting up to urinate two to three times nightly instead of his usual once a night. He tried decreasing his fluid intake in the evening but it made little difference. After an examination, he was diagnosed with benign prostatic enlargement. We prescribed a combination of supplements including saw palmetto, pygeum, and zinc. He also reduced his caffeine and alcohol intake. Within eight weeks he was back to getting up only once a night. This was welcome relief, since his interrupted sleep had been draining his energy level.

References

Bent, S, et al. 2006. Saw palmetto for benign prostatic hyperplasia. *New England Journal of Medicine*. February 9;354(6):557–66.

Breza, J, et al. 1998. Efficacy and acceptability of tadenan (Pygeum africanum extract) in the treatment of benign prostatic hyperplasia (BPH): A multicentre trial in central Europe. *Current Medical Research and Opinion*. 14(3):127–39.

Buck, AC, et al. 1990. Treatment of outflow tract obstruction due to benign prostatic hyperplasia with the pollen extract, cernilton. A double-blind, placebo-controlled study. *British Journal of Urology*. October;66(4):398–404.

Carraro, JC, et al. 1996. Comparison of phytotherapy (Permixon) with finasteride in the treatment of benign prostate hyperplasia: A randomized international study of 1,098 patients. *Prostate.* October;29(4):231–40.

Leitzmann, MF, et al. 2003. Zinc supplement use and risk of prostate cancer. *Journal of the National Cancer Institute.* July 2;95(13):1004–7.

Platz, EA, et al. 1998. Physical activity and benign prostatic hyperplasia. *Archives of Internal Medicine.* November 23;158(21):2349–56.

Wilt, T, A Ishani, and R Mac Donald. 2002. Serenoa repens for benign prostatic hyperplasia. *Cochrane Database of Systematic Reviews.* (3).

Yasumoto, R, et al. 1995. Clinical evaluation of long-term treatment using cernitin pollen extract in patients with benign prostatic hyperplasia. *Clinical Therapeutics.* January–February;17(1):82–7.

PART THREE

Resources

A–Z List of Nutritional Supplements

Acetylcarnitine

Where it is found: Amino acid.

Active constituents: Modified form of the amino acid L-carnitine.

What it is used for:

- Age-related cognitive decline
- Alzheimer's disease
- Depression
- Male infertility
- Peripheral neuropathy

Common side effects or interactions: There are no common side effects.

Acidophilus

Where it is found: Yogurt and other cultured foods.

Active constituents: Lactobacillus acidophilus.

What it is used for:

- Cancer prevention
- Candidiasis
- Canker sores
- Constipation

Eczema

Food allergies

Immune support

Inflammatory bowel disease

Irritable bowel disease

Lactose intolerance

Leaky gut syndrome

Traveler's diarrhea

Vaginitis

Common side effects or interactions: Occasionally gas and bloating. Take at least one hour apart from antibiotics.

Adrenal Extract

Where it is found: Extract from purified bovine or sheep adrenal gland or adrenal cortex.

Active constituents: RNA and polypeptides.

What it is used for:

Allergies

Arthritis

Autoimmune conditions

Fatigue

Low back pain

Common side effects or interactions: Occasional reports of anxiety, irritability, headache, or insomnia.

Aloe Vera

Where it is found: Aloe vera leaves.

Active constituents: Polysaccharides may be responsible for topical healing effect.

What it is used for:

Applied topically for burns

Scrapes

Canker sores and general wound healing

Taken orally for inflammatory bowel disease

Ulcers

Type 2 diabetes

Candida intestinal infections

Constipation

Ulcerative colitis

Crohn's disease

Psoriasis

Diabetes

HIV

Common side effects or interactions: Use food-grade juice when taken orally. Aloe latex may cause diarrhea or cramping.

Arginine

Where it is found: Dairy, fish, nuts, poultry, chocolate, meat.

Active constituents: L-arginine.

What it is used for:

Angina

Congestive heart failure

High blood pressure

HIV

Impotence

Infertility

Interstitial cystitis

Surgical recovery

Wound healing

Common side effects or interactions: Do not use if there is a history of heart attack. Caution for those prone to herpes outbreaks.

Artichoke (*Cynara scolymus*)

Where it is found: Leaves of artichoke plant.

Active constituents: Cynarin, 1,3 dicaffeoylquinic acid, 3-caffeoylquinic acid, scolymoside.

What it is used for:

High cholesterol and triglycerides

Indigestion

Poor fat digestion

Constipation

Poor liver function

Common side effects or interactions: Higher doses may cause loose stool. Caution for those with gallstones.

Ashwagandha (*Withania somniferum*)

Where it is found: Root.

Active constituents: Withanolides.

What it is used for:

Stress hormone balance

Immune support

Memory enhancement

Osteoarthritis

Aging

Anemia

Fatigue

Libido

Menopause

Common side effects or interactions: No major side effects.

Astragalus (*Astragalus membranaceus*)

Where it is found: Root.

Active constituents: Several constituents including amino acids, flavonoids, polysaccharides, triterpene glycosides.

What it is used for:

Asthma prevention

Common cold

Sore throat

General immune support

Cancer

Stress

Fatigue

Hepatitis

Heart function

Chronic diarrhea

Chemotherapy and radiation support

Common side effects or interactions: No common side effects.

Beta Sitosterol

Where it is found: Rice bran, peanuts, soybeans, wheat germ.

Active constituents: Beta sitosterol.

What it is used for:

High cholesterol

Prostate enlargement

Common side effects or interactions: May decrease vitamin E and beta carotene absorption.

Betaine Hydrochloride

Where it is found: Beet extract.

Active constituents: Betaine hydrochloride.

What it is used for:

Acne

Anemia

Arthritis

Asthma

Candidiasis

Fatigue

Food sensitivities

Gallstones

Irritable bowel syndrome

Inflammatory bowel disease

Skin rashes

Vitiligo

Common side effects or interactions: May aggravate heartburn, gastritis, or reflux. Avoid in those with an active ulcer.

Bilberry (*Vaccinium myrtillus*)

Where it is found: Berries.

Active constituents: Anthocyanosides.

What it is used for:

Diabetes

Metinopathy

Macular degeneration

Cataracts

Diarrhea

Eyestrain

Glaucoma

Hemorrhoids

Night vision

Varicose veins

Common side effects or interactions: No common side effects.

Biotin

Where it is found: Gut bacterial synthesis, organ meats, cheese, soybeans, eggs, mushrooms, whole wheat, peanuts.

Active constituents: Biotin.

What it is used for:

Metabolism of fats, proteins, and carbohydrates

Nail and hair growth

Type 2 diabetes

Common side effects or interactions: No common side effects.

Bitter Melon (*Momordica charantia*)

Where it is found: Fruit.

Active constituents: Steroidal saponin group known as charantin, insulin-like peptides, and alkaloids.

What it is used for:

Diabetes

Indigestion

Common side effects or interactions: Diarrhea or abdominal cramping.

Black Cohosh (*Cimicifuga racemosa*)

Where it is found: Root and rhizome.

Active constituents: Triterpene glycosides, phytoestrogens.

What it is used for:

Arthritis

Fibromyalgia

Depression

Menopausal symptoms (such as hot flashes, night sweats, fatigue vaginal dryness, tinnitus)

Menstrual cramps

Premenstrual syndome

Common side effects or interactions: Large amounts may cause digestive upset such as diarrhea or headaches.

Boswellia (*Boswellia serrata*)

Where it is found: Resin of the tree branch.

Active constituents: Boswellic acids.

What it is used for:

Asthma

Sports injuries

Ulcerative colitis

Crohn's disease

Bursitis

Rheumatoid arthritis

Osteoarthritis

Common side effects or interactions: Side effects are not common but there have been occasional reports of diarrhea or rash from its use.

Bromelain

Where is it found: Pineapple stem.

Active constituents: Proteolytic and anti-inflammatory enzymes.

What it is used for:

Osteoarthritis

Rheumatoid arthritis

Burns

Atherosclerosis

Protein digestion

Injuries

Respiratory mucus

Surgery recovery

Thrombophlebitis

Varicose veins

Sinusitis

Prostatitis

Common side effects or interactions: Bromelain has blood-thinning properties, so consult with your doctor first if you are using blood-thinning medications.

Burdock (*Arctium lappa*)

Where it is found: Root.

Active constituents: Polyacetylene, inulin, mucilage.

What it is used for:

Acne rosacea

Acne vulgaris

Skin rashes

Indigestion

Common side effects or interactions: There are no common side effects.

Butcher's Broom (*Ruscus aculeatus*)

Where it is found: Root and stems.

Active constituents: Ruscogenins.

What it is used for:

Hemorrhoids

Varicose veins

Common side effects or interactions: There are occasional reports of nausea.

Calcium

Where it is found: Kelp, cheese, collards, kale, turnip greens, almonds, yogurt, milk, broccoli, soy.

Active constituents: Calcium

What it is used for:

Bone and tooth formation

Osteoporosis

Muscle contraction

Heartbeat

Blood clotting and nerve impulse

Growth retardation

Insomnia

Muscle and leg cramps

Common side effects: Normally there are no toxic effects with large doses.

Constipation may occur in some individuals. Some researchers feel that those with a tendency to kidney stones should avoid high doses of calcium, although this has not been proven.

Calendula (*Calendula officinalis*)

Where it is found: Flowers.

Active constituents: Flavonoids.

What it is used for:

Dermatitis

Eczema

Burns

Common side effects or interactions: There are no common side effects.

Carnitine

Where it is found: Dairy products, red meat.

Active constituents: L-carnitine, an amino acid.

What it is used for:

Angina

Anorexia

Arrhythmias

Athletic performance

Cardiomyopathy

Chronic fatigue syndrome

Congestive heart failure

Diabetes

Down's syndrome

Heart attack recovery

High cholesterol

HIV

Intermittent claudication

Kidney disease

Liver disease

Male infertility

Premature infants

Common side effects or interactions: There are no common side effects.

Carotenoids

Where they are found: Many fruits and vegetables. Examples include yellow vegetables (carrots, pumpkins, squash, sweet potatoes); green vegetables (broccoli, peas, collard greens, endive, kale, lettuce, peppers, spinach, turnip greens); fruits (apricots, cantaloupe, papaya, peaches, watermelon, cherries, tomatoes).

Active constituents: There are over 600 known carotenoids. Examples include beta carotene, alpha carotene, gamma carotene, beta zeacarotene, cryptoxanthin, lycopene, zeaxanthin, lutein, canthaxanthin, crocetin, capsanthin.

What they are used for:

Antioxidants

Precursor to vitamin A

Absorb ultraviolet rays

Immune support

Normal growth and development

Vision

Common side effects or interactions: High doses may cause carotenemia (yellowing of skin, especially palms of hands and face) which disappears after reduction of carotenoid intake.

Cascara (*Rhamnus purshiana*)

Where it is found: Bark.

Active constituents: Hydroxyanthraquinone glycosides.

What it is used for:

Constipation

Common side effects or interactions: Abodminal cramping, diarrhea. It should be avoided by women who are pregnant.

Cayenne (*Capsicum frutescens*)

Where it is found: Fruit.

Active constituents: Capsaicin.

What it is used for:

Osteoarthritis

Rheumatoid arthritis

Shingles

Atherosclerosis

Congestive heart failure

Varicose veins

Topical use for shingles pain

Psoriasis

Low back pain

Common side effects or interactions: Caution for those with history of gastritis or ulcers. Topical use may cause a burning or stinging pain, or allergic reaction. Cayenne has a blood-thinning effect, so caution for those on blood-thinning medications.

Chamomile (*Matricaria recutita*)

Where it is found: Flowers.

Active constituents: Flavonoids, including chamuzelene.

What it is used for:

Indigestion

Nervousness

Colic

Gingivitis

Diarrhea

Insomnia

Anxiety

Ulcers and inflammatory bowel disease

Topically for wound healing and eczema

Common side effects or interactions: There are no common side effects. Rare cases of allergy are reported.

Choline

Where it is found: Grains, legumes, egg yolks, whole grains, soy.

Active constituents: Choline.

What it is used for:

Elevated homocysteine

Liver cirrhosis

Hepatitis

Common side effects or interactions: There are no common side effects.

Chondroitin Sulfate

Where it is found: Cow trachea.

Active constituents: Chondroitin sulfate.

What it is used for:

Osteoarthritis

Common side effects or interactions: There are no common side effects.

Chromium

Where it is found: Whole grains, meats, potatoes, liver, brewer's yeast.

Active constituents: Chromium.

What it is used for:

Pre-diabetes

Type 2 diabetes

Polycystic ovarian syndrome

High cholesterol

High triglycerides

Low HDL cholesterol

Depression

Weight management

Sweet cravings

Common side effects or interactions: Caution when combined with diabetic medications, as chromium use may decrease the amount of prescription required.

Cinnamon (*Cinnamomum zeylanicum*)

Where it is found: Inner bark.

Active constituents: Volatile oils.

What it is used for:

Common cold

Diarrhea

Indigestion

Bleeding

Heavy menstruation

Menstrual cramps

Type 2 diabetes

High cholesterol

Common side effects or interactions: Rare cases of skin rash or bronchial constriction are reported in those sensitive to cinnamon.

Coenzyme Q10 (CoQ10)

Where it is found: Meat, fish.

Active constituents: Coenzyme Q10.

What it is used for:

Alzheimer's disease

Angina

Gingivitis

Congestive heart failure

Chronic fatigue

Hypertension

Heart attack recovery

Atherosclerosis

Cardiomyopathy

Mitral valve prolapse

Immune support

Breast cancer

Male infertility

Migraine headache prevention

Type 2 diabetes

Common side effects or interactions: Caution when using with blood-thinning medications, as CoQ10 has a mild blood-thinning effect.

Conjugated Linoleic Acid (CLA)

Where it is found: Beef (especially free range), dairy products, poultry, eggs, corn oil.

Active constituents: CLA.

What it is used for:

Cancer prevention

Weight loss

Common side effects or interactions: May increase blood glucose levels.

Copper

Where it is found: Whole grains, shellfish, nuts, eggs, poultry, organ meats, peas, dark green leafy vegetables, legumes.

Active constituents: Copper.

What it is used for:

Burns

High cholesterol

Osteoporosis

Wound healing

Common side effects or interactions: Amounts higher than 3 mg should be monitored by a physician. Those with Wilson's disease should avoid copper supplementation.

Cranberry (*Vaccinium macrocarpon*)

Where it is found: Fruit.

Active constituents: Proanthocyanidins.

What it is used for:

Prevention and treatment of urinary tract infections

Common side effects or interactions: There are no common side effects.

Creatine

Where it is found: fish, animal products.

Active constituents: Arginine, glycine, and methionine.

What it is used for:

Athletic support

Congestive heart failure

Muscle mass maintenance in seniors

Common side effects or interactions: Avoid in those with kidney disease.

Dandelion (*Taraxacum officinalis*)

Where it is found: Root and leaves.

Active constituents: Sesquiterpene lactones.

What it is used for:

Constipation

Edema

High blood pressure

Indigestion

Premenstrual syndrome

Hepatitis

Common side effects or interactions: Do not use if you have gallstones unless under the direction of a doctor. Rarely diarrhea results from using dandelion root.

Devil's Claw (*Harpagophytum procumbens*)

Where it is found: Root.

Active constituents: Harpagoside, harpagide, and procumbide.

What it is used for:

Arthritis

Low back pain

Indigestion

Common side effects or interactions: Caution for those with gallstones, gastritis, or active ulcers.

DHEA (Dehydroepiandrosterone)

Where it is found: It is naturally produced by adrenal glands, synthesized in laboratory.

Active constituents: DHEA.

What it is used for:

Alzheimer's disease

Arthritis

Chronic fatigue syndrome

Depression

Diabetes

Erectile dysfunction

Heart disease prevention

Immune support

Inflammatory bowel disease

Lupus

Menopause

Osteoporosis

Prednisone withdrawal

Common side effects or interactions: Facial hair and acne breakout. Do not use in persons with active cancer or history of cancer.

Echinacea (*Echinacea purpurea* or *angustifolia*)

Where it is found: Root, rhizome, flowers.

Active constituents: Polysaccharides, alkylamides, cichoric acid.

What it is used for:

Common cold

Sore throat

Influenza

Vaginal yeast infections

Ear infections

General immune support

Cancer

Common side effects or interactions: Caution for those with autoimmune diseases.

Elderberry (*Sambucus nigra*)

Where it is found: Berries, flowers.

Active constituents: Flavonoids.

What it is used for:

Common cold

Influenza

Bronchitis

Common side effects or interactions: There are no common side effects.

Evening Primrose Oil

Where it is found: Evening primrose plant seeds.

Active constituents: Gamma linolenic acid (GLA).

What it is used for:

Arthritis

Attention deficit hyperactivity disorder

Fibrocystic breast syndrome

Diabetes

Dry skin

Eczema

Multiple sclerosis

Peripheral neuropathy

PMS

Common side effects or interactions: Occasional digestive upset.

Fennel (*Foeniculum vulgare*)

Where it is found: Seed.

Active constituents: Volatile oils.

What it is used for:

Flatulence

Colic

Respiratory tract infections

Increasing nursing mother's breast milk supply

Common side effects or interactions: There are no common side effects.

Feverfew (*Tanacetum parthenium*)

Where it is found: Leaves.

Active constituents: Sesquiterpene lactones.

What it is used for:

Migraine headache

Common side effects or interactions: Digestive upset is a rare occurrence.

Fish Oil

Where it is found: A number of fish sources including salmon, cod, anchovy, and other fish. Modern techniques allow the oil to be extracted and purified.

Active constituents: Omega-3 fatty acids DHA (docosahexanoic acid) and EPA (eicosapentaenoic acid). Both DHA and EPA have anti-inflammatory effects.

What it is used for:

DHA plays an important role in brain function and joint health

EPA regulates inflammation

Immune system

Blood clotting and circulation

Arthritis

Asthma

Bipolar disorder

Cancer

Cardiovascular disease

Chronic obstructive pulmonary disease

Depression

Diabetes

High blood pressure

High cholesterol and triglycerides

Inflammatory bowel disease

Lupus

Osteoporosis

Preeclampsia

Pregnancy

Schizophrenia

Common side effects or interactions: Digestive upset such as heartburn, reflux, or diarrhea occasionally occurs. Those on blood-thinning medications should check with their doctor before supplementing fish oil, as it has blood-thinning effects.

Flaxseed Oil (*Linum usitatissimum*)

Where it is found: Seeds.

Active constituents: Omega-3, omega-6, and omega-9 fatty acids.

What it is used for:

Constipation

Eczema

Dry skin

Arthritis

Benign prostatic hyperplasia

Common side effects or interactions: Too much flax oil may cause nausea, vomiting, and diarrhea.

Folic Acid

Where it is found: Dark green vegetables (spinach, kale, broccoli, asparagus), organ meats, kidney beans, beets, yeast, orange juice, whole grains.

Active constituents: Folic acid.

What it is used for:

It is a methyl donor that is required for many processes in the body

Prevents neural tube defects (must be taken by mother in early pregnancy)

Helps with elevated homocysteine

Depression

Memory

Red blood cell production

Skin and nail health

Common side effects or interactions: No common side effects.

GABA (*Gamma-Amino Butyric Acid*)

Where it is found: Made from glutamine and glucose.

Active constituents: GABA.

What it is used for:

Attention deficit hyperactivity disorder

Anxiety

Epilepsy

Muscle tightness

Common side effects or interactions: Do not combine with pharmaceutical antidepressant or anti-anxiety medications.

Garlic (*Allium sativa*)

Where it is found: Cloves.

Active constituents: S-allylcysteine.

What it is used for:

Atherosclerosis

High cholesterol

High triglcyerides

Warts

Ear infections (topical)

Respiratory tract infections

High blood pressure

Yeast infections

General immune support

Cancer prevention

Common side effects or interactions: Digestive upset including heartburn. Consult with your doctor first before using if taking blood-thinning medications.

Ginger (*Zingiber officinalis*)

Where it is found: Rhizome.
Active constituents: Volatile oils.
What it is used for:
  Osteoarthritis
  Morning sickness
  Motion sickness
  Irritable bowel syndrome
  Indigestion
Common side effects or interactions: Heartburn is occasionally reported.

Ginkgo (*Ginkgo biloba*)

Where it is found: Leaves.
Active constituents: Flavones, glycosides, and terpene lactones.
What it is used for:
  Age-related cognitive decline
  Alzheimer's disease
  Attention deficit hyperactivity disorder
  Atherosclerosis
  Raynaud's disease
  Intermittent claudication
  Depression
  High blood pressure
  Erectile dysfunction
  Premenstrual syndome
  Radiation toxicity
  Tinnitus
  Stroke recovery and prevention
  Macular degeneration
  Cataracts
  Retinopathy
  Vertigo

Meniere's disease

Migraine

Normal tension glaucoma

Common side effects or interactions: Consult with your doctor before using if you are taking blood-thinning medications, since ginkgo has blood-thinning properties. Occasional digestive upset is reported.

Ginseng, American (*Panax quinquefolius*)

Where it is found: Root.

Active constituents: Ginsenosides.

What it is used for:

Asthma

Type 2 diabetes

Chronic fatigue

Menopausal symptoms

Stress

Common side effects or interactions: There are no common side effects.

Ginseng, Asian (*Panax ginseng*)

Where it is found: Root.

Active constituents: Ginsenosides.

What it is used for:

Cancer prevention (particularly breast cancer)

General immune support

Erectile dysfunction

Male infertility

Type 2 diabetes

Menopausal symptoms

Chronic fatigue

Low libido

Stress

Congestive heart failure

Common side effects or interactions: Occasional reports of increased blood pressure or insomnia.

Ginseng, Eleuthero (*Eleutherococcus senticosus*)

Where it is found: Root.

Active constituents: Eleutherosides.

What it is used for:

Immune support

Cold and flu prevention

Stress

Athletic training

Chronic fatigue

Age-related cognitive decline

Low libido

Common side effects or interactions: There are no common side effects.

Glucosamine

Where it is found: Outer covering of shellfish.

Active constituents: Glucosamine sulfate or glucosamine hydrochloride.

What it is used for:

Disc herniation

Osteoarthritis

Sprains/strains

Common side effects or interactions: Occasionally causes diarrhea.

Goldenseal (*Hydrastis canadensis*)

Where it is found: Root.

Active constituents: Alkaloids berberine, hydrastine, canadine.

What it is used for:

Colds

Sore throats

Flu

Ear infections

Digestive tract infections

Fungal infections

Sinusitis

Diarrhea

Urinary tract infections

Parasite infections

Vaginitis

Common side effects or interactions: Dry mucous membranes, heartburn.

Green Tea

Where it is found: Leaves.

Active constituents: Polyphenols, particularly epigallocatechin gallate (EGCG).

What it is used for:

Cancer

Cardiovascular disease

Detoxification

Digestive health

Gingivitis

High cholesterol

Tooth decay

Weight management

Common side effects or interactions: Several cups may cause caffeine-related symptoms such as anxiety, insomnia, heart palpitations.

Green Tea (*Camellia sinensis*)

Where it is found: Leaves.

Active constituents: Flavonoids, amino acid L-theanine.

What it is used for:

Atherosclerosis

Cervical dysplasia

Cancer prevention (especially colon, prostate, and breast)

Influenza

Leukoplakia

Gingivitis

Weight loss

Common side effects or interactions: Occasional reports of insomnia and anxiety.

Guggul (*Commiphora mukul*)

Where is it found: Stem.

Active constituents: Guggulsterones.

What it is used for:

Atherosclerosis

Elevated triglycerides and cholesterol

Hypothyroidism

Cystic acne

Common side effects or interactions: Do not combine with pharmaceutical cholesterol lowering drugs.

Gymnema (*Gymnema sylvestre*)

Where it is found: Leaves.

Active constituents: Gymnemic acids.

What it is used for:

Type 1 diabetes

Type 2 diabetes

Common side effects or interactions: Caution when combining with pharmaceutical glucose-lowering medications.

Hawthorn (*Crataegus oxyacantha*)

Where it is found: Berries, flowers, leaves.

Active constituents: Flavonoids.

What it is used for:

Atherosclerosis

High blood pressure

Congestive heart failure

Heart arrhythmias

Angina

Cardiomyopathy

Common side effects or interactions: Consult with a doctor first before using if you are taking pharmaceutical blood-thinning medications or other cardiovascular medications.

Horse Chestnut (*Aesculus hippocastanum*)

Where it is found: Seeds.

Active constituents: Aescin.

What it is used for:

  Back pain

  Hemorrhoids

  Varicose veins

  Edema

Common side effects or interactions: Caution for those with kidney or liver disease.

Huperzia (*Qian ceng ta*)

Where it is found: Moss.

Active constituents: Huperzine A.

What it is used for:

  Age-related cognitive decline

  Alzheimer's disease

Common side effects or interactions: Do not combine with pharmaceuticals used for memory enhancement.

Hydroxycitric Acid (HCA)

Where it is found: Fruit of *Garcinia cambogia*.

Active constituents: HCA.

What it is used for:

  Weight loss

Common side effects or interactions: There are no common side effects.

5-Hydroxytryptophan (5-HTP)

Where it is found: Seeds of the plant *Griffonia simplicifolia*.

Active constituents: 5-HTP, an amino acid.

What it is used for:

Anxiety

Depression

Fibromyalgia

Food cravings (carbohydrates)

Insomnia

Migraine headaches

Seasonal affective disorder

Weight loss

Common side effects or interactions: Do not combine with pharmaceutical antidepressant, anti-anxiety, or other psychiatric medications.

Inositol

Where it is found: Citrus fruit, whole grains, nuts, seeds, legumes.

Active constituents: Inositol.

What it is used for:

Depression

Diabetes

Liver detoxification support

Common side effects or interactions: No common side effects.

Iodine

Where is it found: Iodized salt and water, seafood, seaweed such as kelp.

Active constituents: Iodine.

What it is used for:

Goiter

Hypothyroidism

Fibrocystic breast disease

Common side effects or interactions: High doses can suppress thyroid function.

Ipriflavone

Where it is found: Synthesized.

Active constituents: Ipriflavone.

What it is used for:

Hyperparathyroidism

Kidney failure (to maintain bone density for those in kidney failure)

Osteoporosis

Otosclerosis

Paget's disease

Common side effects or interactions: Decreased white blood cell (lymphocyte) count, diarrhea.

Iron

Where it is found: Liver and organ meats, beef, legumes, dark green leafy vegetables, kelp, blackstrap molasses.

Active constituents: Iron.

What it is used for:

Iron deficiency anemia and conditions related to iron deficiency

Common side effects or interactions: High levels of iron are associated with increased risk of certain cancers and heart disease. Calcium hinders iron absorption. A common form of iron known as iron sulfate can be constipating and irritating to the digestive tract. Gentler forms of iron chelates are available.

Kava (*Piper methysticum*)

Where it is found: Rhizome.

Active constituents: Kava lactones.

What it is used for:

Anxiety

Insomnia

Hyperactivity

Muscle spasms

Common side effects or interactions: Do not combine with pharmaceutical anti-anxiety or antidepressant medications. Have liver enzymes monitored while using. Do not combine with alcohol.

L-carnitine

Where is it found: Meat, dairy products.

Active constituents: L-carnitine.

What it is used for:

  Angina

  Congestive heart failure

  Attention deficit hyperactivity disorder

  Erectile dysfunction

  High triglycerides

  Male infertility

  Mitral valve prolapse

  Weight loss

Common side effects or interactions: No common side effects.

Lemon Balm (*Melissa officinalis*)

Where it is found: Stems, leaves, flowers.

Active constituents: Volatile oils.

What it is used for:

  Respiratory tract infections

  Fevers

  Depression

  Antiviral

  Cold sores

  Genital herpes

  Hyperthyroidism (Grave's disease)

  Insomnia

Common side effects or interactions: There are no common side effects.

Licorice (*Glycyrrhiza glabra*)

Where it is found: Root

Active constituents: Flavonoids and glycyrrhizin.

What it is used for:

  Immune system support

  Antiviral

  Coughs

  Sore throats

  Digestive tract inflammation

  Gastritis

Adrenal gland support

Liver support

Antispasmodic

Anti-inflammatory

Asthma

Chronic fatigue syndrome

Ulcers

Reflux

Hepatitis

Shingles

Cancer

Common side effects or interactions: Large amounts can lead to water retention and increase blood pressure. This effect does not occur with the DGL (deglycyrrhizinated licorice) form, used for digestive ailments.

Lipoic Acid

Where it is found: Liver, yeast, potatoes, spinach, red meat.

Active constituents: Lipoic acid.

What it is used for:

Type 1 and type 2 diabetes

Hepatitis

Diabetic neuropathy

Low glutathione levels

Common side effects or interactions: There are no common side effects. Caution when combining with diabetic medications, as the dosage may need to be lowered.

Lomatium (*Lomatium dissectum*)

Where it is found: Root.

Active constituents: Unknown.

What it is used for:

Antiviral

Antibacterial

Common cold

Influenza

Shingles

Upper respiratory tract infections

Urinary tract infections

Common side effects or interactions: Skin rash observed in small percentage of users.

L-theanine

Where it is found: Green tea.

Active constituents: Amino acid L-theanine.

What it is used for:

Anxiety

Insomnia

Common side effects or interactions: There are no common side effects.

Lutein

Where it is found: Spinach, kale, collard greens, romaine lettuce, peas, egg yolks.

Active constituents: Lutein.

What it is used for:

Cataracts

Macular degeneration

Common side effects or interactions: There are no common side effects.

Lysine

Where it is found: Chicken, cottage cheese, avocados, wheat germ.

Active constituents: The amino acid L-lysine.

What it is used for:

Cold sores

Genital herpes

Osteoporosis

Shingles

Common side effects or interactions: There are no common side effects.

Magnesium

Where it is found: Whole grains, nuts, legumes, soy, green leafy vegetables.

Active constituents: Magnesium.

What it is used for:

    Bone and teeth formation

    Osteoporosis

    Fatigue

    Type 2 diabetes

    Pre-diabetes

    Muscle and nerve impulses

    Premenstrual syndrome

    Muscle cramps

    Heart arrhythmias

    Congestive heart failure

    High blood pressure

Common side effects or interactions: Too high of a dose may cause loose stool. Those with kidney disease or on medications for cardiovascular disease such as high blood pressure should check with their doctor first before supplementing.

Manganese

Where it is found: Liver, kidney, whole grains, nuts, spinach, green leafy vegetables.

Active constituents: Manganese.

What it is used for:

    Tardive dyskinesia

    Osgood-Schlatter disease

    Osteoporosis

    Sprains and strains

    Type 2 diabetes

Common side effects or interactions: People with cirrhosis of the liver should avoid manganese supplements unless under a doctor's care. High levels of manganese may impair iron, calcium, and zinc absorption.

Melatonin

Where it is found: Pineal gland in brain, synthesized for supplement manufacturing.

Active constituents: Melatonin.

What it is used for:

    Aging

Cancer (breast and prostate)

Cluster headaches

Insomnia

Jet lag

Radiation exposure

Seasonal affective disorder

Tardive dyskinesia

Common side effects or interactions: Do not use long term with children.

Milk Thistle (*Silybum marianum*)

Where it is found: Fruit and seeds.

Active constituents: Group of flavonoids known as silymarin.

What it is used for:

Liver disease related to alcoholism and drug use

Hepatitis

Liver cirrhosis

Type 2 diabetes

Common side effects or interactions: There are no common side effects.

Molybdenum

Where it is found: Meats, whole grain breads, legumes, leafy vegetables, organ meats, brewer's yeast.

Active constituents: Molybdenum.

What it is used for:

Asthma

Sulfite detoxification

Common side effects or interactions: No common side effects.

MSM (*Methylsulfonylmethane*)

Where it is found: Green vegetables.

Active constituents: MSM.

What it is used for:

Allergies

Arthritis

Asthma

Autoimmune diseases

Fibromyalgia

Hair and nail health

Headaches

Heartburn

Muscle spasm

Sports injuries

Common side effects or interactions: Higher dosages may cause loose stool. Has mild blood-thinning effect, so consult with doctor before using if taking blood-thinning medications.

N-acetylcysteine

Where it is found: Human body and foods.

Active constituents: Altered form of the amino acid cysteine.

What it is used for:

Angina

Antioxidant support (glutathione)

Bronchitis

Chronic obstructive pulmonary disease

Cystic fibrosis

Gastritis

HIV

Pneumonia

Postnasal drip

Common side effects or interactions: Long-term use may deplete zinc and copper levels.

Nettle (*Urtica dioica*)

Where it is found: Leaves and root.

Active constituents: Unknown.

What it is used for:

Leaves are used for allergies, hay fever, osteoarthritis

The root for benign prostatic hyperplasia

Common side effects or interactions: Mild digestive upset is occasionally reported.

Oregano (*Origanum vulgare*)

Where it is found: Leaves and dried herb.

Active constituents: Volatile oils and flavonoids.

What it is used for:

Candida infection

Yeast infections

Topically for athlete's foot

General antimicrobial action

Common side effects or interactions: Heartburn or digestive upset. May cause skin irritation when used topically. Do not use during pregnancy.

Peppermint (*Mentha piperita*)

Where it is found: Leaf.

Active constituents: Volatile oils including menthol and menthone.

What it is used for:

Colic

Indigestion

Nausea

Fevers

Irritable bowel syndrome

Headaches (topically)

Gallstones

Headaches

Common side effects or interactions: Reflux.

Phosphatidylserine (PS)

Where it is found: Soy.

Active constituents: PS.

What it is used for:

Age-associated memory impairment

Alzheimer's disease

Attention deficit hyperactivity disorder

Brain injury

Dementia

Depression

Stress hormone imbalance

Common side effects or interactions: There are no common side effects.

Phosphorus

Where it is found: Meats, fish, eggs, poultry, milk products.

Active constituents: Phosphorus.

What it is used for:

Growth

Bone production

Energy production

Kidney function

Common side effects or interactions: High amounts of phosphorus in the form of phosphoric acid leads to urinary calcium loss from the bones. Phosphorus should not be supplemented by those with kidney disease.

Potassium

Where it is found: Fruits and vegetables, especially apples, bananas, carrots, oranges, potatoes, tomatoes, cantaloupes, peaches, plums, strawberries, meat, milk, fish.

Active constituents: Potassium.

What it is used for:

High blood pressure

Heart arrhythmias

Osteoporosis

Fatigue

Muscle cramps

Common side effects or interactions: Do not supplement with potassium-sparing high blood pressure medications. Check with your doctor first before supplementing if you have heart arrhythmia or kidney disease.

Progesterone Cream (Natural)

Where it is found: Synthesized from wild yam.

Active constituents: Progesterone.

What it is used for:

    Autoimmune conditions

    Endometriosis

    Fibrocystic breasts

    Infertility (female)

    Irregular menses

    Menopausal symptoms

    Osteoporosis

    Ovarian cysts

    PMS

    Uterine fibroids

Common side effects or interactions: May cause drowsiness.

Propolis

Where it is found: Bark of trees and buds of leaves.

Active constituents: Flavonoids and phenols.

What it is used for:

    Genital herpes and rheumatoid arthritis (topical)

    Common cold

    Upper respiratory tract infections

    Parasites

    Cold sores (topical)

Common side effects or interactions: There are no common side effects.

Pygeum (Pygeum africanum)

Where it is found: Bark.

Active constituents: Phytosterols such as beta sitosterol, pentacyclic terpenes, ferulic esters.

What it is used for:

    Benign prostatic hyperplasia

    Prostatitis

Common side effects or interactions: Mild digestive upset.

Red Yeast Rice

Where it is found: Red yeast.

Active constituents: Monacolins.

What it is used for:

High cholesterol

Heart disease prevention

Common side effects or interactions: Do not combine with pharmaceutical cholesterol-lowering statin drugs.

SAMe (S-adenosylmethionine)

Where it is found: Occurs naturally in the body, made from the amino acid methionine.

Active constituents: SAMe.

What it is used for:

Depression

Detoxification

Fibromyalgia

Hepatitis

Liver cirrhosis

Osteoarthritis

Common side effects or interactions: Do not use with those who have bipolar disorder.

Saw Palmetto (*Serenoa repens, Sabal serrulata*)

Where it is found: Berries.

Active constituents: Sterols and fatty acids.

What it is used for:

Acne

Baldness

Benign prostatic hyperplasia

Bladder infection prevention (men)

Polycystic ovarian syndrome

Prostatitis

Common side effects or interactions: There are no common side effects.

Selenium

Where it is found: Liver, kidney, meats, seafood, grains, vegetables.

Active constituents: Selenium.

What it is used for:

Asthma

Atherosclerosis

Cancer prevention (colon, lung, prostate)

Depression

Immune support (especially against viral infections, including HIV support)

Male infertility

Rheumatoid arthritis

Common side effects or interactions: Blood glucose levels should be monitored when supplementing selenium.

Senna (*Cassia senna*)

Where it is found: Leaves and pods.

Active constituents: Hydroxyanthracene glycosides.

What it is used for:

Constipation

Common side effects or interactions: May cause diarrhea or abdominal cramping. Avoid during pregnancy.

Silicon

Where it is found: Unrefined grains, cereals, root vegetables.

Active constituents: Silicon.

What it is used for:

Osteoporosis

Sprains and strains

Brittle hair and nails

Common side effects or interactions: There are no common side effects.

Slippery Elm (*Ulmus fulva*)

Where it is found: Inner bark.

Active constituents: Mucilage.

What it is used for:

Bronchitis

Colitis

Ulcers

Heartburn

Gastritis

Sore throats

Urinary tract infections

Common side effects or interactions: There are no common side effects.

Soy Isoflavones

Where it is found: Soy.

Active constituents: Daidzein, genistein, and glycitein.

What it is used for:

High cholesterol

Menopause

PMS

Prostate enlargement

Vaginitis

Common side effects or interactions: Do not use in those with estrogen-sensitive cancers.

St. John's Wort (*Hypericum perforatum*)

Where it is found: Flowers.

Active constituents: Hypericin and hyperforin.

What it is used for:

Anxiety

Depression

Viral infections

Topically for burns

Scrapes

Nerve pain

Bruises

Seasonal affective disorder

Menopausal depression

Common side effects or interactions: Do not combine with pharmaceutical anti-anxiety or antidepressant medications. Rare reports of increased sensitivity to light.

Tea Tree (*Melaleuca alternifolia*)

Where it is found: Leaves.

Active constituents: Terpenoids.

What it is used for:

Topically for skin fungus

Burns

Acne

Cold sores

Mouth and gum infections

Skin infections

Vaginitis

Warts

Common side effects or interactions: Skin irritation if too concentrated a product is used. Do not take internally.

Turmeric (*Curcuma longa*)

Where it is found: Rhizome.

Active constituents: Curcuminoids.

What it is used for:

Indigestion

Rheumatoid arthritis

Osteoarthritis

Ulcerative colitis

Crohn's disease

Alzheimer's disease prevention

Common side effects or interactions: Caution for those with gallstones.

Valerian (*Valeriana officinalis*)

Where it is found: Root.

Active constituents: Volatile oils.

What it is used for:

Insomnia

Anxiety

Restlessness

Spasms

Pain

Common side effects or interactions: Do not combine with pharmaceutical antidepressant, anti-anxiety, or sleep medications.

Vanadium

Where it is found: Shellfish, mushrooms, black pepper, buckwheat.

Active constituents: Vanadium.

What it is used for:

Type 2 diabetes

Common side effects or interactions: People with manic depression should avoid its use unless under the supervision of a doctor. High amounts may cause diarrhea.

Vitamin A

Where it is found: Liver, chile peppers, carrots, vitamin A fortified milk, butter, sweet potatoes, parsley, kale, spinach, mangoes, broccoli, squash.

Active constituents: Vitamin A.

What it is used for:

Acne

Antioxidant

Vision (especially night blindness)

Growth and development

Immunity

Wound healing

Heavy menstruation

Common side effects or interactions: Too-high doses of vitamin A may cause vomiting, joint pain, abdominal pain, bone abnormalities (possibly osteoporosis), cracking or dry skin, headache, irritability, and fatigue. Symptoms disappear after supplementation has been discontinued. Pregnant women or those with liver disease should avoid vitamin A supplementation dosages above 2,500 IU (500 RE).

Vitamin B1 (Thiamin)

Where it is found: Pork, beef, liver, brewer's yeast, whole grains, brown rice, legumes.

Active constituents: Vitamin B1.

What it is used for:

Energy metabolism (carbohydrate metabolism)

Neurological activity

Brain and heart function

Peripheral neuropathy

Common side effects or interactions: No common side effects.

Vitamin B2 (Riboflavin)

Where it is found: Organ meats such as liver, milk products, whole grains, green leafy vegetables, eggs, mushrooms, broccoli, asparagus, fish.

Active constituents: Vitamin B2.

What it is used for:

Energy production

Fatty acid and amino acid synthesis

Migraine headache prevention

Common side effects or interactions: No common side effects.

Vitamin B3 (Niacin)

Where it is found: Organ meats, peanuts, fish, yeast, poultry, legumes, milk, eggs, whole grains, orange juice.

Active constituents: Vitamin B3 (niacin).

What it is used for:

Energy production

Formation of steroid compounds

Red blood cell formation

Cognitive function and mood

High total and LDL cholesterol

Low HDL cholesterol

Common side effects or interactions: Dilation of the blood vessels and flushing of the skin. Occasionally elevated liver enzymes.

Vitamin B5 (Pantothenic Acid)

Where it is found: Meats, fish, chicken, eggs, cheese, whole grains, avocados, cauliflower, sweet potatoes, oranges, strawberries, yeast, legumes.

Active constituents: Vitamin B5 (pantothenic acid, pantethine).

What it is used for:

    Metabolism of carbohydrates

    Proteins and fats for energy production

    Production of adrenal hormones and red blood cells

    High triglycerides (pantethine form)

Common side effects or interactions: No common side effects.

Vitamin B6 (Pyridoxine)

Where it is found: Meats, poultry, egg yolk, soy, peanuts, bananas, potatoes, whole grains, cauliflower.

Active constituents: Vitamin B6.

What it is used for:

    Formation of body proteins

    Neurotransmitters

    Red blood cells

    Immunity

    Detoxification

Common side effects or interactions: Doses above 200 mg for extended periods of time may cause nerve symptoms such as numbness and tingling.

Vitamin B12 (Cobalamin)

Where it is found: Gut bacteria synthesis, organ meats, clams, oysters, soy, milk products, cheese.

Active constituents: Vitamin B12.

What it is used for:

    Synthesis of DNA and red blood cells

    Nerve development

    Depression

    Dementia

    Fatigue

    Neuropathy

Shingles

Stress

Common side effects or interactions: There are no common side effects.

Vitamin C (Ascorbic Acid)

Where it is found: Citrus fruits, tomatoes, green peppers, dark green leafy vegetables, broccoli, cantaloupe, strawberries, Brussels sprouts, potatoes, asparagus.

Active constituents: Vitamin C.

What it is used for:

Antioxidant

Immunity

Collagen formation

Bone development

Cancer prevention and treatment

Gum health

Hormone and amino acid synthesis

Adrenal gland hormones

Wound healing

Stress

Athletic training

Glaucoma

Cataracts

Common side effects or interactions: Too high a dose can cause loose stool. In rare cases it may increase the formation of kidney stones.

Vitamin D

Where it is found: Cod liver oil, cold-water fish (salmon, herring, sardines, mackerel), milk (fortified with vitamin D), egg yolk, small amounts in dark green leafy vegetables and mushrooms. Sunlight is converted into vitamin D.

Active constituents: Vitamin D2 is derived from plant sources and vitamin D3 is derived from animal sources. D3 is the preferred supplemental form.

What it is used for:

Absorbs calcium and phosphorus from intestines

Increases calcium deposition into bones

Mobilizes calcium and phosphorus from bones

Optimizes immune system function and may prevent certain cancers and prevent autoimmunity

Supports normal balance in seniors

Common side effects or interactions: Vitamin D is not as toxic as once thought. Check with your doctor before using daily doses above 2,000 IU. High doses for long periods of time may contribute to nausea, anorexia, weakness, headache, digestive disturbance, kidney damage, calcification of soft tissues, and hypercalcemia.

Vitamin E

Where it is found: Vegetable oils, seeds, nuts, brown rice, whole grains.

Active constituents: Tocopherols and tocotrienols.

What it is used for:

Antioxidant

Immunity

Wound healing

Red blood cell formation

Estrogen metabolism

Nerve health

Detoxification

Alzheimer's disease

Common side effects or interactions: Check with your physician before taking along with blood-thinning medications such as warfarin (Coumadin). Mixed vitamin E products are generally a better choice than single tocopherol vitamin E formulas. Avoid synthetic vitamin E known as d-l alpha tocopherol.

Vitamin K

Where it is found: Dark green leafy vegetables, parsley, broccoli, cabbage, spinach, soy, egg yolks, liver, natto, legumes; and it is synthesized by intestinal bacteria.

Active constituents: There are three forms—phylloquinone (K1—derived from plants), menaquinone (K2—derived from gut bacteria), and menadione (K3—derived synthetically).

What it is used for:

Blood clotting

Bone formation

Osteoporosis

Antioxidant

Atherosclerosis

Common side effects or interactions: Check with your physician before taking along with blood-thinning medications such as warfarin (Coumadin).

Vitex (*Vitex agnus-castus*)

Where it is found: Dried fruit.

Active constituents: Flavonoids, iridoid glycosides, and terpenoids.

What it is used for:

Acne

Amenorrhea

Fibrocystic breast disease

Infertility

Irregular menses

Dysmenorrhea

Improved lactation

Hot flashes

Ovarian cysts

Premenstrual syndrome

Uterine fibroids

Female infertility

Common side effects or interactions: Do not take in combination with birth control pills.

Willow (Salix alba)

Where it is found: Bark.

Active constituents: Salicin.

What it is used for:

Osteoarthritis

Rheumatoid arthritis

Pain

Common side effects or interactions: Do not use with children who have a fever. Consult with your doctor if you are on blood-thinning medications before using willow.

Witch Hazel (*Hammamelis virginiana*)

Where it is found: Bark.

Active constituents: Tannins and volatile oils.

What it is used for:

Topically for cold sores

Eczema

Hemorrhoids

Varicose veins

Common side effects or interactions: There are no common side effects.

Zinc

Where it is found: Oysters, herring, shellfish, red meat, whole grains, legumes, nuts.

Active constituents: Zinc.

What it is used for:

Acne

Anorexia

Attention deficit hyperactivity disorder

Benign prostatic hyperplasia

Burns

Common cold

Type 1 and type 2 diabetes

Hepatitis

Macular degeneration

Male infertility

Osteoporosis

Wilson's disease

Wound healing

Common side effects or interactions: Zinc can reduce the absorption of calcium, magnesium, iron, and copper. High, prolonged doses above 150 mg may impair immunity or increase risk of prostate cancer.

At-a-Glance List of Pharmaceuticals

This section lists pharmaceuticals in alphabetical order by their generic names. A chart of commercial names and their generic equivalents appears on page 470.

Acetaminophen

Commercial name: Tylenol

Prescribed for: Fever, pain and swelling, arthritis

Common side effects: Side effects are not common but may include digestive upset.

Drug, food, or supplement interactions: Cholestyramine (Questran), carbamazepine (Tegretol), isoniazid (INH, Nydrazid, Laniazid), rifampin (Rifamate, Rifadin, Rimactane), warfarin (Coumadin), alcohol, hibiscus tea

Acyclovir

Commercial name: Zovirax

Prescribed for: Viral infections that cause cold sores or genital herpes, shingles, chicken pox, mononucleosis

Common side effects:

Digestive upset (nausea, vomiting)

Headache

Drug, food, or supplement interactions: Amphotericin B Fungizone); amino-glycoside antibiotics such as amikacin (Amikin), gentamicin (Garamycin), kanamycin (Kantrex), neomycin (Nes-RX, Neo-Fradin), paramomycin (Humatin), streptomycin, and tobramycin (Tobi, Nebcin); aspirin and other nonsteroidal anti-inflammatory medications such as ibuprofen (Advil, Motrin) and naproxen (Aleve, Naprosyn); cyclosporine (Neoral, Sandim-mune); medications to treat HIV or AIDS such as zidovudine (Retrovir, AZT); pentamidine (NebuPent); cimetidine (Tagamet); probenecid (Bene-mid); sulfonamides such as sulfamethoxazole and trimethoprim (Bactrim); tacrolimus (Prograf); vancomycin; digoxin (Lanoxin); St. John's wort

Alendronate

Commercial name: Fosamax

Prescribed for: Osteoporosis

Common side effects:

Digestive upset (abdominal pain, gas, nausea)

Constipation

Drug, food, or supplement interactions: Parathyroid hormone (Forteo), amino-glycoside antibiotics, calcium, food

Alfuzosin

Commercial name: Uroxatral

Prescribed for: Urinary symptoms related to benign prostatic hyperplasia

Common side effects:

Dizziness

Low blood pressure

Drug, food, or supplement interactions: Clonidine, cimetidine, warfarin

Alginate

Commercial name: Gaviscon

Prescribed for: Gastroesophageal reflux disease (GERD)

Common side effects:

Loss of appetite

Constipation or diarrhea

Weakness

Headache

Drug, food, or supplement interactions: Cellulose sodium phosphate (Calcibind), isoniazid (Rifamate), ketoconazole (Nizoral), mecamylamine (Inversine), methenamine (Mandelamine), sodium polystyrene sulfonate resin (Kayexalate), tetracycline antibiotics (Achromycin, Minocin), Cherokee rosehip, rosehip, strontium

Alprazolam

Commercial names: Niravam, Xanax

Prescribed for: Anxiety

Common side effects:

Agitation

Increased anxiety

Confusion

Memory impairment

Lack of coordination

Speech difficulties

Light-headedness

Constipation

Drug, food, or supplement interactions: Ketoconazole (Nizoral), itraconazole (Sporanox), some HIV or AIDS medications, alcohol, grapefruit juice, kava

Aluminum and Magnesium Hydroxide

Commercial names: Maalox, Mylanta

Prescribed for: Heartburn

Common side effects:

Diarrhea

Drug, food, or supplement interactions: None known

Amiloride

Commercial name: Midamor

Prescribed for: High blood pressure, edema

Common side effects:

Dry mouth

Headaches

Dizziness

Fatigue

Depression

Irritability

Reduced sex drive

Excessive urination

Electrolyte imbalance

Drug, food, or supplement interactions: ACE-inhibitor medications; large amounts of potassium-rich foods such as bananas, oranges, and green leafy vegetables; or using salt substitutes that contain potassium

Amitriptyline

Commercial names: Elavil, Endep, Vanatrip

Prescribed for: Depression

Common side effects:

Constipation

Dizziness

Drowsiness

Dry mouth

Changes in sexual function

Weight gain

Drug, food, or supplement interactions: Do not combine with monoamine oxidase (MAO) drugs or alcohol

Amlodipine

Commercial name: Norvasc

Prescribed for: High blood pressure, angina pectoris (chest pain)

Common side effects:

Edema (swelling of the lower legs)

Headaches

Drug, food, or supplement interactions: Pleurisy root, grapefruit juice

Amlodipine and Benazepril

Commercial name: Lotrel

Prescribed for: High blood pressure

Common side effects:

Edema

Headaches

Dry cough

Drug, food, or supplement interactions: See sections on amlodipine and benazepril

Amphetamine and Dextroamphetamine

Commercial name: Adderall

Prescribed for: Attention deficit hyperactivity disorder, narcolepsy

Common side effects:

Digestive upset (diarrhea, nausea, loss of appetite)

Difficulty sleeping

Dry mouth

Weight loss

Stomachache

Headache

Overstimulation/anxiety

Nervousness

Dizziness

Tics

Listlessness/lethargy

Angina

Mood changes

Drug, food, or supplement interactions: Alcohol, vitamin C, L-tyrosine

Atenolol

Commercial name: Tenormin

Prescribed for: Hypertension, congestive heart failure, heart arrhythmias, social phobias, performance anxiety

Common side effects:

Digestive upset (abdominal cramps, diarrhea, constipation, nausea)

Fatigue

Insomnia

Depression

Memory loss

Fever

Erectile dysfunction

Light-headedness

Slow heart rate

Low blood pressure

Numbness

Tingling

Cold extremities

Sore throat

Shortness of breath or wheezing

Drug, food, or supplement interactions: Caution with digoxin (Lanoxin) and calcium channel blockers, alcohol, potassium supplements, pleurisy root

Atorvastatin

Commercial name: Lipitor

Prescribed for: To reduce cholesterol and triglyceride levels, atherosclerosis, artery inflammation after a heart attack

Common side effects:

Headache

Nausea

Vomiting

Constipation

Diarrhea

Rash

Weakness

Muscle and joint pain

Increased liver enzymes

Drug, food, or supplement interactions: Cholestyramine (Questran), colestipol (Colestid), grapefruit juice, alcohol, large doses of vitamin A

Beclomethasone Nasal Inhalation

Commercial name: Beconase AQ

Prescribed for: Allergies

Common side effects:

Burning, dryness, or irritation inside the nose

Headache

Nosebleed

Unpleasant taste

Throat irritation

Drug, food, or supplement interactions: None known

Benazepril

Commercial name: Lotensin

Prescribed for: High blood pressure, heart failure

Common side effects:

　Dry cough

Drug, food, or supplement interactions: High-potassium foods, potassium supplements

Benzoyl Peroxide

Commercial names: Benoxyl, Benzac AC, Benzagel, Brevoxyl, Persa-Gel

Prescribed for: Acne vulgaris

Common side effects:

　Stinging, dryness, and peeling (tend to occur initially)

　Irritation

　Redness

　Scaly eruptions

　Darkening or lightening of the skin or rash

　Sun sensitivity

Drug, food, or supplement interactions: Caution combining with other topical acne treatments such as tretinoin (Avita, Renova, Retin-A)

Betaxolol

Commercial names: Betoptic, Betoptic S

Prescribed for: Glaucoma

Common side effects:

　Burning, stinging, or itching of the eyes or eyelids

　Vision changes

　Light sensitivity

Drug, food, or supplement interactions: None known

Bimatoprost

Commercial name: Lumigan

Prescribed for: Glaucoma

Common side effects:

Burning, stinging, or itching of the eyes or eyelids; changes in eye, eyelash, or eyelid color

Dry eyes

Increased flow of tears

Light sensitivity

Drug, food, or supplement interactions: None known

Brimonidine

Commercial name: Alphagan

Prescribed for: Glaucoma

Common side effects:

Red eyes

Irritated eyes

Dry eyes

Headache

Blurred vision

Pain in the eye

Drowsiness

Drug, food, or supplement interactions: None known

Brompheniramine

Commercial names: BroveX, BroveX CT, Lodrane 12-Hour ER Tablet

Prescribed for: Allergies

Common side effects:

Dizziness

Headache

Loss of appetite

Stomach upset

Vision changes

Irritability

Dry mouth

Dry eyes

Dry nose

Drug, food, or supplement interactions: Barbiturate medicines; doxercalciferol (Hectorol); anxiety medications, antidepressants, and other psychiatric medications; Parkinson's disease medications; alcohol

Budesonide Nasal Inhaler

Commercial name: Rhinocort Aqua

Prescribed for: Allergies

Common side effects:

Burning, dryness, or irritation inside the nose

Headache

Nosebleed

Unpleasant taste

Throat irritation

Drug, food, or supplement interactions: None known

Bupropion

Commercial name: Wellbutrin

Prescribed for: Depression, seasonal affective disorder, quitting smoking

Common side effects:

Headache

Nausea

Agitation

Dry mouth

Insomnia

Constipation

Tremor

Drug, food, or supplement interactions: Caution for those on seizure medications or coming off benzodiazepines; 5-hydroxytryptophan (5-HTP); L-tryptophan; Sour date nut (*Ziziphus jujube*); St. John's wort

Buspirone

Commercial name: Buspar

Prescribed for: Anxiety

Common side effects:

Dizziness

Headache

Nausea

Nervousness

Light-headedness

Insomnia

Drug, food, or supplement interactions: Monoamine oxidase (MAO) inhibitors. trazodone (Desyrel), warfarin (Coumadin), phenytoin (Dilantin), grapefruit juice, kava

Calcitonin Nasal Spray

Commercial names: Fortical, Miacalcin

Prescribed for: Osteoporosis

Common side effects:

Bone pain

Headache

Runny nose

Nosebleed

Drug, food, or supplement interactions: None known

Calcitonin (Injectable)

Commercial names: Calcimar, Miacalcin

Prescribed for: Osteoporosis, Paget's disease

Common side effects:

Nausea

Vomiting

Flushing of the skin, rash, and irritation at the site of injection

Drug, food, or supplement interactions: None known

Calcium Carbonate

Commercial names: Tums, Titralac, Calcium Rich Rolaids

Prescribed for: Heartburn

Common side effects:

Constipation

Drug, food, or supplement interactions: Antibiotics (e.g., tetracyclines, quinolones), demeclocycline, methacycline, verapamil (a calcium channel blocker), quinidine, sodium polystyrene sulfonate, iron-containing products, thyroid medications

Candesartan

Commercial name: Atacand

Prescribed for: High blood pressure, heart failure

Common side effects:

Dizziness

Drug, food, or supplement interactions: None known

Captopril

Commercial name: Capoten

Prescribed for: High blood pressure, heart failure, kidney disease associated with diabetes, post–heart attack recovery

Common side effects:

Dry cough

Drug, food, or supplement interactions: High-potassium foods, potassium supplements

Carbinoxamine

Commercial name: Histex CT

Prescribed for: Allergies

Common side effects:

Dizziness

Headache

Loss of appetite

Stomach upset

Vision changes

Irritability

Dry mouth

Dry eyes

Dry nose

Drug, food, or supplement interactions: Anxiety medications, antidepressants and other psychiatric medications, Parkinson's disease medications, alcohol

Carteolol

Commercial name: Ocupress

Prescribed for: Glaucoma

Common side effects:

Burning

Stinging or itching of the eyes or eyelids

Vision changes

Light sensitivity

Drug, food, or supplement interactions: None known

Celecoxib

Commercial name: Celebrex

Prescribed for: Pain and swelling, arthritis

Common side effects:

Digestive upset (heartburn, diarrhea, nausea, gastrointestinal pain, flatulence)

Headache

Insomnia

Drug, food, or supplement interactions: Willow bark

Cetirizine

Commercial name: Zyrtec

Prescribed for: Allergies

Common side effects:

Dizziness

Headache

Loss of appetite

Stomach upset

Vision changes

Irritability

Dry mouth

Dry eyes

Dry nose

Drug, food, or supplement interactions: Anxiety medications, antidepressants and other psychiatric medications, Parkinson's disease medications, alcohol

Chlorpheniramine

Commercial names: Aller-Chlor, Allergy, Chlo-Amine, Chlor-Trimeton, Chlor-Trimeton Allergy, Efidac 24

Prescribed for: Allergies

Common side effects:

Dizziness

Headache

Loss of appetite

Stomach upset

Vision changes

Irritability

Dry mouth

Dry eyes

Dry nose

Drug, food, or supplement interactions: Doxercalciferol (Hectorol), anxiety medications, antidepressants and other psychiatric medications, Parkinson's disease medications, alcohol

Chlorpropamide

Commercial name: Diabinese

Prescribed for: Type 2 diabetes

Common side effects:

Dizziness

Diarrhea

Gas

Headache

Drug, food, or supplement interactions: Alcohol; cholestyramine; fluconazole (Diflucan); nonsteroidal anti-inflammatory drugs such as ibuprofen; sulfa drugs; warfarin (Coumadin); miconazole; beta-blockers such as propranolol; thiazide diuretics; corticosteroids; thyroid medicines; estrogens; niacin; phenytoin (dilantin); calcium channel blocking drugs (e.g., diltiazem); niacin; magnesium; glucose-lowering supplements such as chromium, vanadium, cinnamon extract, fenugreek, *Gymnema sylvestre*, bitter melon extract, ginseng, and others may enhance the effect of a diabetic medication. Check with your doctor before combining together.

Cimetidine

Commercial names: Tagamet, Tagamet HB

Prescribed for: Gastroesophageal reflux disease (GERD), ulcers

Common side effects:

Diarrhea

Fatigue

Headache

Insomnia

Muscle pain

Nausea

Vomiting

Drug, food, or supplement interactions: Warfarin (Coumadin), phenytoin, theophylline, lidocaine, amiodarone, metronidazole, loratadine, calcium channel blockers (e.g., diltiazem, felodipine, nifedipine), bupropion, carbamazepine and fluvastatin, ketoconazole, caffeine, magnesium

Citalopram

Commercial name: Celexa

Prescribed for: Depression, panic disorder, anxiety, post-traumatic stress disorder, premenstrual dysphoric syndrome (PMDD), obsessive compulsive disorder (OCD)

Common side effects:

Nausea

Diarrhea

Agitation

Insomnia

Decreased sexual desire

Delayed orgasm or inability to have an orgasm

Drug, food, or supplement interactions: Astemizole (Hismanal), cisapride (Propulsid), pimozide (Orap), terfenadine (Seldane), thioridazine (Mellaril), monoamine oxidase (MAO) inhibitors, 5-hydroxytryptophan (5-HTP), L-tryptophan, St. John's wort

Clemastine

Commercial names: Dayhist-1, Tavist, Tavist Allergy

Prescribed for: Allergies

Common side effects:

Dizziness

Headache

Loss of appetite

Stomach upset

Vision changes

Irritability

Dry mouth

Dry eyes

Dry nose

Drug, food, or supplement interactions: Anxiety medications, antidepressants and other psychiatric medications, Parkinson's disease medications, alcohol

Clonazepam

Commercial name: Klonopin

Prescribed for: Anxiety, seizures

Common side effects:

Agitation

Increased anxiety

Confusion

Memory impairment

Lack of coordination

Speech difficulties

Light-headedness

Constipation

Drug, food, or supplement interactions: Ketoconazole (Nizoral), itraconazole (Sporanox), some HIV or AIDS medications, alcohol, grapefruit juice, kava

Clopidogrel

Commercial name: Plavix

Prescribed for: Prevention of blood clots associated with heart attack and stroke.

Common side effects:

Rash or itching

Diarrhea

Stomach pain

Drug, food, or supplement interactions: Ibuprofen (Motrin, Advil, Nuprin), naproxen (Naprosyn, Aleve), diclofenac (Voltaren), etodolac (Lodine), nabumetone (Relafen), fenoprofen (Nalfon), flurbiprofen (Ansaid), indomethacin (Indocin), ketoprofen (Orudis; Oruvail), oxaprozin, piroxicam (Feldene), sulindac (Clinoril), tolmetin (Tolectin), mefenamic acid (Ponstel). It should also not be combined with warfarin (Coumadin) or alcohol. Caution with high doses of vitamin E or fish oil.

Codeine

Commercial name: Codeine

Prescribed for: Pain

Common side effects:

Nausea

Vomiting

Diarrhea

Constipation

Decreased appetite

Rash

Dizziness

Headache

Drowsiness

Flushing of face

Drug, food, or supplement interactions: High blood pressure medications, seizure medications, antidepressant medications, certain antihistamine medications, barbiturate medications such as phenobarbitol, alcohol.

Codeine may be taken with food to reduce digestive side effects.

Herbs with high tannin levels may reduce the absorption of codeine. These include green tea (*Camellia sinensis*), black tea, uva ursi (*Arctostaphylos uva-ursi),* black walnut *(Juglans nigra),* red raspberry *(Rubus idaeus),* oak *(Quercus spp.*), and witch hazel *(Hamamelis virginiana).*

Cromolyn

Commercial name: Nasalcrom

Prescribed for: Allergies

Common side effects:

Bad taste in the mouth

Cough

Dry throat

Headache

Nosebleeds or runny nose

Sneezing

Stinging, burning, or irritation inside the nose

Drug, food, or supplement interactions: None known

Desloratadine

Commercial name: Clarinex

Prescribed for: Allergies

Common side effects:

Dizziness

Headache

Loss of appetite

Stomach upset

Vision changes

Irritability

Dry mouth

Dry eyes

Dry nose

Drug, food, or supplement interactions: Anxiety medications, antidepressants and other psychiatric medications, Parkinson's disease medications, alcohol

Dessicated Thyroid

Commercial names: Armour thyroid, Naturethroid, Westhroid

Prescribed for: Hypothyroidism (low thyroid)

Common side effects:

Headache

Nervousness

Diarrhea

Chest pain

Drug, food, or supplement interactions: The following medications can impair the absorption of thyroid hormone and should be taken four hours away from it: calcium supplements, iron supplements, aluminum, calcium or magnesium antacids, simethicone, cholestyramine, colestipol, sucralfate, sodium polystyrene sulfonate.

The following foods should not be taken at the same time: soybean flour and soy infant formula, walnuts, dietary fiber.

Dexchlorpheniramine ER

Commercial name: Dexchlorpheniramine ER

Prescribed for: Allergies

Common side effects:

Dizziness

Headache

Loss of appetite

Stomach upset

Vision changes

Irritability

Dry mouth

Dry eyes

Dry nose

Drug, food, or supplement interactions: Anxiety medications, antidepressants and other psychiatric medications, Parkinson's disease medications, alcohol

Dextroamphetamine

Commercial name: Dexedrine

Prescribed for: Attention deficit hyperactivity disorder, narcolepsy

Common side effects:

Digestive upset (nausea, stomach upset, loss of appetite, diarrhea, constipation)

Dry mouth

Headache

Nervousness

Dizziness

Sleep problems

Irritability or restlessness

Drug, food, or supplement interactions: Monoamine oxidase (MAO) inhibitors used for depression, clonidine (Catapres), blood thinners, anticonvulsant medications

Diazepam

Commercial name: Valium

Prescribed for: Anxiety, seizures

Common side effects:

Agitation

Increased anxiety

Confusion

Memory impairment

Lack of coordination

Speech difficulties

Light-headedness

Constipation

Drug, food, or supplement interactions: Ketoconazole (Nizoral), itraconazole (Sporanox), some HIV or AIDS medications, alcohol, grapefruit juice, kava

Diclofenac

Commercial name: Voltaren

Prescribed for: Pain and swelling, arthritis

Common side effects:

Nausea

Vomiting

Diarrhea

Constipation

Decreased appetite

Rash

Dizziness

Headache

Drowsiness

Drug, food, or supplement interactions: Blood thinners such as warfarin (Coumadin), lithium, diuretics, nonsteroidal anti-inflammatory drugs, alcohol, willow bark

Diltiazem

Commercial names: Cardizem, Dilacor XR, Tiazac

Prescribed for: High blood pressure, angina pectoris (chest pain)

Common side effects:

Constipation

Nausea

Headache

Rash

Breathing problems

Coughing

Edema (swelling of the legs with fluid)

Low blood pressure

Drowsiness

Dizziness

Drug, food, or supplement interactions: Digoxin, carbamazepine (Tegretol), cimetidine (Tagamet), grapefruit juice, pleurisy root

Diphenhydramine

Commercial names: AllerMax, Banophen, Benadryl, Diphenhist, Genahist

Prescribed for: Allergies

Common side effects:

Dizziness

Headache

Loss of appetite

Stomach upset

Vision changes

Irritability

Dry mouth

Dry eyes

Dry nose

Drug, food, or supplement interactions: Anxiety medications, antidepressants and other psychiatric medications, Parkinson's disease medications, alcohol

Doxazosin

Commercial name: Cardura

Prescribed for: Urinary symptoms related to benign prostatic hyperplasia

Common side effects:

Dizziness

Low blood pressure

Drug, food, or supplement interactions: None known

Duloxetine

Commercial name: Cymbalta

Prescribed for: Depression, anxiety

Common side effects:

Nausea

Dry mouth

Constipation

Diarrhea

Fatigue

Difficulty sleeping

Dizziness

Drug, food, or supplement interactions: Monoamine oxidase (MAO) inhibitors, haloperidol (Haldol), digoxin, warfarin (Coumadin), 5-hydroxytryptophan (5-HTP), L-tryptophan, sour date nut (*Ziziphus jujube*), St. John's wort

Dutasteride

Commercial name: Avodart

Prescribed for: Benign prostatic hyperplasia, reduced libido

Common side effects: Side effects are not common but some men experience decreased sexual function and desire.

Drug, food, or supplement interactions: African pygeum, nettle, saw palmetto

Enalapril

Commercial name: Vasotec

Prescribed for: High blood pressure, heart failure

Common side effects:

Dry cough

Headache

Light-headedness

Weakness

Nausea

Dizziness

Drug, food, or supplement interactions: Potassium-sparing diuretics; lithium (Eskalith); rifampin (Rifadin, Rimactane); losartan (Cozaar); fluconazole (Diflucan); foods high in potassium such as bananas, green leafy vegetables, and oranges; potassium supplements

Escitalopram

Commercial name: Lexapro

Prescribed for: Depression, anxiety

Common side effects:

Nausea

Diarrhea

Agitation

Insomnia

Decreased sexual desire

Delayed orgasm or inability to have an orgasm

Drug, food, or supplement interactions: Astemizole (Hismanal), cisapride (Propulsid), pimozide (Orap), terfenadine (Seldane), thioridazine (Mellaril), monoamine oxidase (MAO) inhibitors, 5-hydroxytryptophan (5-HTP), L-tryptophan, St. John's wort

Esomeprazole

Commercial name: Nexium

Prescribed for: Gastroesophageal reflux disease (GERD), esophageal damage (ulcers, erosions, strictures, or Barrett's esophagus), stomach ulcers, combination with antibiotics for treating *Helicobacter pylori*

Common side effects:

Headache

Diarrhea

Constipation

Abdominal pain

Nausea

Rash

Drug, food, or supplement interactions: Reduces the absorption of ketoconazole (Nizoral), and St. John's wort may decrease the blood levels of this drug. Can increase the absorption and concentration of digoxin (Lanoxin).

Estrogen (Bioidentical)

Commercial names: Estriol, Estradiol, Biest, Triest, Estrace, Estrasorb, Delestrogen, Gynodiol, Estraderm, Vivelle, Climara, Alora, Esclim, Estring, Clinagen LA 40, Depogen, Estragyn 5, Kestrone 5, Valergen

Prescribed for: Menopausal symptoms, osteoporosis

Common side effects:

Breakthrough vaginal bleeding and spotting

Weight gain (without using natural progesterone)

Drug, food, or supplement interactions: Thyroid, grapefruit juice

Estrogen (Synthetic)

Commercial names: Premarin, Cenestin, Estratab, Ogen, Menest, Ortho Dienestrol

Prescribed for: Menopausal symptoms, osteoporosis

Common side effects:

Nausea

Headache

Breakthrough vaginal bleeding and spotting

Anxiety

Abdominal pain

Back pain

Weight gain

Drug, food, or supplement interactions: Thyroid, grapefruit juice

Etodolac

Commercial name: Lodine

Prescribed for: Pain and swelling, arthritis

Common side effects:

Nausea

vomiting

Diarrhea

Constipation

Decreased appetite

Rash

Dizziness

Headache

Drowsiness

Drug, food, or supplement interactions: Lithium (Eskalith), methotrexate (Rheumatrex)

Ezetimibe

Commercial name: Zetia

Prescribed for: Lower cholesterol

Common side effects:

Headache

Dizziness

Diarrhea

Drug, food, or supplement interactions: Gemfibrozil (Lopid), fenofibrate (Tricor), clofibrate (Atromid-S), cyclosporin

Famotidine

Commercial names: Pepcid, Pepcid AC

Prescribed for: Gastroesophageal reflux disease (GERD), ulcers

Common side effects:

Diarrhea

Fatigue

Headache

Insomnia

Muscle pain

Nausea

Vomiting

Drug, food, or supplement interactions: Warfarin (Coumadin), phenytoin, theophylline, lidocaine, amiodarone, metronidazole, loratadine, calcium channel blockers (e.g., diltiazem, felodipine, nifedipine), bupropion, carbamazepine and fluvastatin, ketoconazole, caffeine, magnesium

Fexofenadine

Commercial name: Allegra

Prescribed for: Allergies

Common side effects:

Dizziness

Headache

Loss of appetite

Stomach upset

Vision changes

Irritability

Dry mouth

Dry eyes

Dry nose

Drug, food, or supplement interactions: Doxercalciferol (Hectorol); anxiety medications; antidepressants and other psychiatric medications; Parkinson's disease medications; alcohol; antacids; erythromycin; grapefruit, apple, or orange juice; ketoconazole (Nizoral); rifampin (Rifadin, Rimactane); St. John's wort

Finasteride

Commercial name: Proscar

Prescribed for: Benign prostatic hyperplasia

Common side effects:

Reduced libido

Drug, food, or supplement interactions: African pygeum, nettle root, saw palmetto

Flunisolide Nasal Inhalation

Commercial name: Nasarel

Prescribed for: Allergies

Common side effects:

Burning

Dryness or irritation inside the nose

Headache

Nosebleed

Unpleasant taste

Throat irritation

Drug, food, or supplement interactions: None known

Fluoxetine

Commercial name: Prozac

Prescribed for: Depression, panic disorder, bulimia, obsessive-compulsive disorder (OCD), premenstrual dysphoric disorder (PMDD)

Common side effects:

Nausea

Diarrhea

Agitation

Insomnia

Decreased sexual desire

Delayed orgasm or inability to have an orgasm

Drug, food or supplement interactions: Astemizole (Hismanal), cisapride (Propulsid), pimozide (Orap), terfenadine (Seldane), thioridazine (Mellaril), monoamine oxidase (MAO) inhibitors, 5-hydroxytryptophan (5-HTP), L-tryptophan, St. John's wort

Fluticasone Nasal Inhalation

Commercial name: Flonase

Prescribed for: Allergies

Common side effects:

Burning, dryness, or irritation inside the nose

Headache

Nosebleed

Unpleasant taste

Throat irritation

Drug, food, or supplement interactions: None known

Fluvastatin

Commercial name: Lescol

Prescribed for: To reduce cholesterol and triglyceride levels, atherosclerosis, to reduce artery inflammation after a heart attack

Common side effects:

Headache

Nausea

Vomiting

Constipation

Diarrhea

Rash

Weakness

Muscle and joint pain

Increased liver enzymes

Drug, food, or supplement interactions: Cholestyramine (Questran), colestipol (Colestid), grapefruit or grapefruit juice, high doses of vitamin A supplements

Furosemide

Commercial name: Lasix

Prescribed for: High blood pressure, edema, heart failure, cirrhosis, chronic kidney failure

Common side effects:

Dry mouth

Headaches

Dizziness

Fatigue

Depression

Irritability

Excessive urination

Drug, food, or supplement interactions: Aminoglycoside antibiotics, thiazide diuretics, digoxin (Lanoxin), steroids, buckthorn or alder buckthorn, buchu, cleavers, dandelion, digitalis, ginkgo biloba, gravel root, horsetail, juniper, licorice, uva ursi, potassium, sodium, magnesium

Glimepiride

Commercial name: Amaryl

Prescribed for: Type 2 diabetes

Common side effects:

Hypoglycemia (low blood sugar)

Dizziness

Diarrhea

Gas

Skin rashes

Drug, food, or supplement interactions: Alcohol, cholestyramine, fluconazole (Diflucan), nonsteroidal anti-inflammatory drugs such as ibuprofen, sulfa drugs, warfarin (Coumadin), miconazole (Monistat, Lotrimin), beta-blockers such as propranolol, thiazide diuretics, corticosteroids, thyroid medicines, estrogens, phenytoin (Dilantin), calcium channel blocking drugs (e.g., diltiazem), niacin, magnesium.

Glucose-lowering supplements such as chromium, vanadium, cinnamon extract, fenugreek, *Gymnema sylvestre*, bitter melon extract, ginseng, and others may enhance the effect of a diabetic medication.

Glipizide

Commercial name: Glucotrol

Prescribed for: Type 2 diabetes

Common side effects:

Digestive upset (flatulence and diarrhea)

Headache

Dizziness

Drug, food, or supplement interactions: Cholestyramine, fluconazole (Diflucan), nonsteroidal anti-inflammatory drugs such as ibuprofen, sulfa drugs, warfarin (Coumadin), miconazole (Monistat, Lotrimin), beta-blockers such as propranolol, thiazide diuretics, corticosteroids, thyroid medicines, estrogens, phenytoin (Dilantin), calcium channel blocking drugs (e.g., diltiazem), alcohol, niacin, magnesium

Glucose-lowering supplements such as chromium, vanadium, cinnamon extract, fenugreek, *Gymnema sylvestre*, bitter melon extract, ginseng, and others may enhance the effect of a diabetic medication.

Glipizide and Metformin

Commercial name: Metaglip

Prescribed for: Type 2 diabetes

Common side effects: See individual sections on glipizide and metformin.

Drug, food, or supplement interactions: See individual sections on glipizide and metformin.

Glyburide

Commercial names: Diabeta, Glynase, Micronase

Prescribed for: Type 2 diabetes

Common side effects:

Digestive upset (nausea, heartburn, and bloating)

Skin rashes

Drug, food, or supplement interactions: Cholestyramine, fluconazole (Diflucan), nonsteroidal anti-inflammatory drugs such as ibuprofen, sulfa drugs, warfarin (Coumadin), miconazole (Monistat, Lotrimin), beta-blockers such as propranolol, thiazide diuretics, corticosteroids, thyroid medicines, estrogens, phenytoin (Dilantin), calcium channel blocking drugs (e.g., diltiazem), alcohol, niacin, magnesium.

Glucose-lowering supplements such as chromium, vanadium, cinnamon extract, fenugreek, *Gymnema sylvestre*, bitter melon extract, ginseng, and others may enhance the effect of a diabetic medication.

Glyburide and Metformin

Commercial name: Glucovance

Prescribed for: Type 2 diabetes

Common side effects: See individual sections on glyburide and metformin.

Drug, food, or supplement interactions: See individual sections on glyburide and metformin.

Hydrochlorothiazide

Commercial names: Esidrix, HydroDiuril

Prescribed for: High blood pressure, edema, heart failure, cirrhosis, chronic kidney failure

Common side effects:

Dry mouth

Headaches

Dizziness

Fatigue

Depression

Irritability

Excessive urination

Potassium deficiency

Elevated glucose levels

Drug, food, or supplement interactions: Beta-blockers, other thiazide diuretics, carbamazepine (Tegretol), chlorpropamide (Diabinese), buckthorn or alder buckthorn, buchu cleavers, dandelion, digitalis, ginkgo biloba, gravel root, horsetail, juniper, licorice, uva ursi

Ibandronate

Commercial name: Boniva

Prescribed for: Osteoporosis

Common side effects:

Pain in the back, legs, arms, or abdomen

Diarrhea

Drug, food, or supplement interactions: Parathyroid hormone (Forteo), aminoglycoside antibiotics, food (should be taken 60 minutes away from any food, especially foods containing calcium), caffeine, calcium supplements (take at different time of day)

Ibuprofen

Commercial name: Motrin

Prescribed for: Pain and swelling, arthritis

Common side effects:

Nausea

Vomiting

Diarrhea

Constipation

Decreased appetite

Rash

Dizziness

Headache

Drowsiness

Drug, food, or supplement interactions: Diuretics, lithium (Eskalith), methotrexate (Rheumatrex), blood-thinning medications, minimize sodium intake, hibiscus tea

Indomethacin

Commercial name: Indocin

Prescribed for: Pain and swelling, arthritis

Common side effects:

Nausea

Vomiting

Diarrhea

Constipation

Decreased appetite

Rash

Dizziness

Headache

Drowsiness

Drug, food, or supplement interactions: Diuretics, lithium (Eskalith), methotrexate (Rheumatrex), blood-thinning medications, minimize sodium intake, hibiscus tea

Insulin

Commercial names: Humalog (lispro, lispro protamine injection), Humulin, Iletin, NovoLog (aspart, aspart protamine injection), Novolin, Exebera, Levemir (detemir injection), Velosulin, Apidra (glulisine injection), Regular Iletin, Regular Insulin, Lantus (glargine injection)

Prescribed for: Type 1 diabetes, uncontrolled Type 2 diabetes

Common side effects:

Hypoglycemia (low blood sugar)

Skin reactions (redness, swelling, itching, or rash at the site of injection)

Drug, food, or supplement interactions: Monoamine oxidase (MAO) inhibitors such as phenelzine (Nardil), beta-blockers such as propranolol (Inderal), salicylates such as aspirin (Bayer) or salsalate (Disalcid), anabolic steroids such as methyltestosterone (Android), tetracycline antibiotics such as doxycycline (Vibramycin), guanethidine (Ismelin), oral hypoglycemic drugs such as glyburide (Diabeta), sulfa antibiotics (e.g., sulfadiazine), ACE inhibitors such as captopril (Capoten).

Drugs that may reduce the effectiveness of insulin include: Diltiazem (Cardizem), niacin, corticosteroids (e.g., prednisone), estrogens, oral contraceptives, thyroid hormones such as levothyroxine (Synthroid), isoniazid, epinephrine, thiazide diuretics such as hydrochlorothiazide and furosemide (Lasix), alcohol, niacin, chromium (may reduce the amount of insulin required), tobacco (smoking).

Glucose-lowering supplements such as chromium, vanadium, cinnamon extract, fenugreek, *Gymnema sylvestre*, bitter melon extract, ginseng, and others may enhance the effect of a diabetic medication. Check with your doctor before combining together.

Ipratropium Nasal

Commercial name: Atrovent nasal

Prescribed for: Allergies

Common side effects:

Cough

Dry mouth

Metallic taste in the mouth

Dry nose

Irritation, burning, or itching in the nose

Stuffy nose

Dizziness

Headache

Infection in the respiratory tract

Nausea

Nosebleeds

Drug, food, or supplement interactions: None known

Irbesartan

Commercial name: Avapro

Prescribed for: High blood pressure, heart failure

Common side effects:

Digestive upset (abdominal pain, diarrhea, heartburn)

Drug, food, or supplement interactions: Avoid drugs containing (or sparing) potassium and lithium.

Avoid salt substitutes and supplements containing potassium.

Large amounts of foods high in potassium such as bananas, green leafy vegetables, and oranges.

Ketoprofen

Commercial name: Orudis

Prescribed for: Pain and swelling, arthritis

Common side effects:

Nausea

Vomiting

Diarrhea

Constipation

Decreased appetite

Rash

Dizziness

Headache

Drowsiness

Drug, food, or supplement interactions: Diuretics, lithium (Eskalith), methotrexate (Rheumatrex), blood-thinning medications, minimize sodium intake, hibiscus tea

Ketorolac

Commercial name: Toradol

Prescribed for: Pain and swelling, arthritis

Common side effects:

Nausea

Vomiting

Diarrhea

Constipation

Decreased appetite

Rash

Dizziness

Headache

Drowsiness

Drug, food, or supplement interactions: Diuretics, lithium (Eskalith), methotrexate (Rheumatrex), blood-thinning medications, minimize sodium intake, hibiscus tea

Lansoprazole

Commercial name: Prevacid

Prescribed for: Gastroesophageal reflux disease (GERD), esophageal damage (ulcers, erosions, strictures, or Barrett's esophagus), stomach ulcers, combination with antibiotics for treating *Helicobacter pylori*

Common side effects:

Headache

Diarrhea

Constipation

Abdominal pain

Nausea

Rash

Drug, food, or supplement interactions: Lansoprazole (Prevacid) may interfere with the absorption of ketoconazole (Nizoral) and increase the absorption and concentration of digoxin (Lanoxin), St. John's wort

Latanoprost

Commercial name: Xalatan

Prescribed for: Glaucoma

Common side effects:

Burning, stinging, or itching of the eyes or eyelids

Changes in eye, eyelash, or eyelid color

Dry eyes

Increased flow of tears

Light sensitivity

Drug, food, or supplement interactions: None known

Levobunolol

Commercial names: AKBeta, Betagan

Prescribed for: Glaucoma

Common side effects:

Burning, stinging, or itching of the eyes or eyelids

Vision changes

Light sensitivity

Drug, food, or supplement interactions: None known

Levothyroxine

Commercial names: Synthroid, Levothroid, Levoxyl, Unithroid

Prescribed for: Hypothyroidism (low thyroid)

Common side effects:

Headache

Nervousness

Diarrhea

Chest pain

Drug, food, or supplement interactions: Warfarin (Coumadin), digoxin (Lanoxin), estrogen replacement including birth control pills, diabetes medicines (e.g., insulin and oral diabetic medications), iodide, lithium (Eskalith), anti-thyroid medications (e.g., methimazole, propylthiouracil), testosterone, glucocorticoids (e.g., dexamethasone, prednisone), high-dose aspirin, phenobarbital, rifamycins (e.g., Rifampin), beta blockers (e.g., propranolol), antidepressants, cytokines (e.g., interferon-alpha, interleukin-2), growth hormones, ketamine, theophylline, cough and cold medications, caffeine.

The following should be taken four hours away from thyroid medications: calcium supplements, iron supplements, aluminum, calcium or magnesium antacids, simethicone, cholestyramine, colestipol, sucralfate, sodium polystyrene sulfonate.

The following foods should not be eaten within three hours of thyroid medications: soybean flour and soy infant formula, walnuts, dietary fiber.

Liothyronine Sodium

Commercial name: Cytomel

Prescribed for: Hypothyroidism (low thyroid)

Common side effects:

Headache

Nervousness

Diarrhea

Chest pain

Drug, food, or supplement interactions: Warfarin (Coumadin), digoxin (Lanoxin), estrogen replacement including birth control pills, diabetes medicines (e.g., insulin and oral diabetic medications), iodide, lithium (Eskalith), anti-thyroid medications (e.g., methimazole, propylthiouracil), testosterone, glucocorticoids (e.g., dexamethasone, prednisone), high-dose aspirin, phenobarbital, rifamycins (e.g., rifampin), beta blockers (e.g., propranolol), antidepressants, cytokines (e.g., interferon-alpha, interleukin-2), growth hormones, ketamine, theophylline, cough and cold medications, caffeine.

The following should be taken four hours away from thyroid medications: calcium supplements, iron supplements, aluminum, calcium or magnesium antacids, simethicone, cholestyramine, colestipol, sucralfate, sodium polystyrene sulfonate.

The following foods should not be eaten within three hours of thyroid medications: soybean flour and soy infant formula, walnuts, dietary fiber.

Lisinopril

Commercial names: Prinivil, Zestril

Prescribed for: High blood pressure, heart failure, post–heart attack recovery

Common side effects:

Nausea

Insomnia

Anxiety

Fatigue

Sexual dysfunction

Nasal congestion

Dizziness

Drug, food, or supplement interactions: Potassium-sparing diuretics, lithium (Eskalith), rifampin (Rifadin, Rimactane), losartan (Cozaar), fluconazole (Diflucan).

Avoid salt substitutes and supplements containing potassium, as well as large amounts of foods high in potassium such as bananas, green leafy vegetables, and oranges

Loratadine

Commercial names: Alavert, Claritin, Triaminic

Prescribed for: Allergies

Common side effects:

Dizziness

Headache

Loss of appetite

Stomach upset

Vision changes

Irritability

Dry mouth

Dry eyes

Dry nose

Drug, food, or supplement interactions: Doxercalciferol (Hectorol), anxiety medications, antidepressants and other psychiatric medications, Parkinson's disease medications, alcohol

Lorazepam

Commercial name: Ativan

Prescribed for: Anxiety

Common side effects:

    Agitation

    Increased anxiety

    Confusion

    Memory impairment

    Lack of coordination

    Speech difficulties

    Light-headedness

    Constipation

Drug, food, or supplement interactions: Ketoconazole (Nizoral), itraconazole (Sporanox), some HIV or AIDS medications, alcohol, kava

Losartan

Commercial name: Cozaar

Prescribed for: High blood pressure, left ventricular hypertrophy, kidney disease associated with diabetes

Common side effects:

    Chronic cough

    Diarrhea

    Dizziness

    Nasal congestion

    Muscle cramps

Drug, food, or supplement interactions: Potassium-sparing diuretics, lithium (Eskalith).

    Avoid salt substitutes and supplements containing potassium, as well as large amounts of foods high in potassium such as bananas, green leafy vegetables, and oranges, due to risk of hyperkalemia (elevated blood potassium).

Losartan and Hydrochlorothiazide

Commercial name: Hyzaar

Prescribed for: High blood pressure, left ventricular hypertrophy

Common side effects:

    Chronic cough

    Diarrhea

    Dizziness

Nasal congestion

Muscle cramps

Dry mouth

Headaches

Fatigue

Depression

Irritability

Excessive urination

Potassium deficiency

Elevated glucose levels

Drug, food, or supplement interactions: See individual sections on losartan and hydrochlorothiazide.

Lovastatin

Commercial name: Mevacor

Prescribed for: To reduce cholesterol and triglyceride levels, atherosclerosis, reduce artery inflammation after a heart attack

Common side effects:

Headache

Nausea

Vomiting

Constipation

Diarrhea

Rash

Weakness

Muscle and joint pain

Increased liver enzymes

Drug, food, or supplement interactions: Cholestyramine (Questran), colestipol (Colestid), grapefruit or grapefruit juice, high doses of vitamin A

Magnesium Hydroxide

Commercial name: Phillips' Milk of Magnesia

Prescribed for: Heartburn

Common side effects:

Diarrhea

Drug, food, or supplement interactions: None known

Metformin

Commercial name: Glucophage

Prescribed for: Pre-diabetes, type 2 diabetes, polycystic ovary syndrome

Common side effects:

Digestive upset (vomiting, gas, bloating, nausea, diarrhea, low appetite)

Drug, food, or supplement interactions: Alcohol, cephalexin (Keflex, Keftab), cimetidine (Tagamet), digoxin (Lanoxin), dofetilide (Tikosyn), entecavir, morphine (Kadian, Avinza), nifedipine (Adalat, Procardia), procainamide (Pronestyl, Procan-SR, Procanbid), propantheline (Pro-Banthine), quinidine (Quinaglute, Quinidex, Quinora), quinine (Quinerva, Quinite, QM-260), ranitidine (Zantac), trimethoprim (Trimpex, Proloprim, Primsol), trospium (Sanctura), vancomycin (Vancocin), diuretics, alcohol, dehydroepiandros-terone (DHEA), guar gum.

Ginkgo biloba (may be combined under doctor's supervision).

Glucose-lowering supplements such as chromium, vanadium, cinnamon extract, fenugreek, *Gymnema sylvestre*, bitter melon extract, ginseng, and others may enhance the effect of a diabetic medication. Check with your doctor before combining together.

Methylphenidate

Commercial names: Ritalin, Concerta, Metadate

Prescribed for: Attention deficit hyperactivity disorder

Common side effects:

Loss of appetite

Difficulty sleeping

Dry mouth

Weight loss

Stomachache

Headache

Overstimulation/anxiety

Dizziness

Tics

Listlessness/lethargy

Angina

Mood changes

Drug, food, or supplement interactions: Monoamine oxidase (MAO) inhibitors; anticonvulsants (e.g., phenobarbital, phenytoin, primidone); tricyclic drugs (e.g., imipramine, clomipramine, desipramine); clonidine (Catapres), SSRIs (selective serotonin reuptake inhibitors) such as fluoxetine, citalopram, and paroxetine; NRIs (norepinephrine reuptake inhibitors) such as Strattera; bupropion (Wellbutrin); amphetamine and tricyclic antidepressants; alcohol; magnesium hydroxide supplements; vitamin C; lithium (Eskalith)

Metoclopramide

Commercial name: Reglan

Prescribed for: Gastroesophageal reflux disease (GERD)

Common side effects:

Nausea

Diarrhea

Dry mouth

Headache

Dizziness

Drowsiness

Restlessness

Insomnia

Drug, food, or supplement interactions: Cimetidine (Tagamet), insulin, cabergoline, cyclosporine, digoxin (Lanoxin), levodopa, monoamine oxidase (MAO) inhibitors, alcohol, N-acetylcysteine, vitex (chasteberry)

Metipranolol Opthalmic

Commercial name: OptiPranolol

Prescribed for: Glaucoma

Common side effects:

Burning, stinging, or itching of the eyes or eyelids

Vision changes

Light sensitivity

Drug, food, or supplement interactions: None known

Mometasone Nasal Spray

Commercial name: Nasonex

Prescribed for: Allergies

Common side effects:

Burning, dryness, or irritation inside the nose

Headache

Nosebleed

Unpleasant taste

Throat irritation

Drug, food, or supplement interactions: None known

Montelukast

Commercial name: Singulair

Prescribed for: Allergies

Common side effects:

Cough

Insomnia

Dizziness

Drowsiness

Headache

Heartburn

Hoarseness or sore throat

Indigestion or stomach upset

Muscle aches or cramps

Nausea

Runny nose

Unusual dreams

Drug, food, or supplement interactions: Carbamazepine (Tegretol), paclitaxel (Taxol), phenobarbital, phenytoin (Dilantin), repaglinide (Prandin), rifabutin (Mycobutin), rifampin (Rifadin, Rimactane), rosiglitazone (Avandia)

Nabumetone

Commercial name: Relafen

Prescribed for: Pain and swelling, arthritis

Common side effects:

Nausea

vomiting

Diarrhea

Constipation

Decreased appetite

Rash

Dizziness

Headache

Drowsiness

Drug, food, or supplement interactions: Diuretics, lithium (Eskalith), methotrexate (Rheumatrex), blood-thinning medications, minimize sodium intake,
hibiscus tea

Nadolol

Commercial name: Corgard

Prescribed for: High blood pressure, angina, rapid heart rate, arrhythmias,
migraine headaches, tremors

Common side effects:

Digestive upset (abdominal cramps, diarrhea, constipation, nausea)

Fatigue

Insomnia

Depression

Memory loss

Fever

Erectile dysfunction

Light-headedness

Slow heart rate

Low blood pressure

Numbness

Tingling

Cold extremities

Sore throat

Shortness of breath or wheezing

Drug, food, or supplement interactions: Calcium channel blockers such as
digoxin (Lanoxin) and haloperidol (Haldol), phenytoin (Dilantin), phenobarbital, rifampin, cimetidine (Tagamet), chlorpromazine, theophylline, lidocaine, potassium. Use with caution for those on diabetic medications.
Alcohol and aluminum-containing antacids may reduce absorption.

Naproxen

Commercial names: Aleve, Naprosyn

Prescribed for: Fever, pain and swelling, arthritis

Common side effects:

Nausea

Vomiting

Diarrhea

Constipation

Decreased appetite

Rash

Dizziness

Headache

Drowsiness

Tinnitus (ringing in the ears)

Drug, food, or supplement interactions: Diuretics, lithium (Eskalith), methotrexate (Rheumatrex), blood-thinning medications, minimize sodium intake, hibiscus tea

Nicardipine

Commercial name: Cardene

Prescribed for: High blood pressure, angina pectoris (chest pain)

Common side effects:

Light-headedness

Dizziness

Fatigue

Drug, food, or supplement interactions: Beta-blockers, anti-seizure medicines, digitalis heart medicines, certain immune-suppressing drugs, diuretics, grapefruit, grapefruit juice, calcium, vitamin D, St. John's wort, pleurisy root

Nicotinic Acid

Commercial names: Niaspan, Niacor, Slo-Niacin

Prescribed for: High cholesterol and triglyceride levels, low HDL cholesterol

Common side effects:

Warmth and flushing of the neck, ears, and face along with itching, tingling

Headache

Stomach upset

Drug, food, or supplement interactions: Caution with diabetic, blood pressure, and statin cholesterol drugs. Drinking hot liquids or alcohol shortly before or after niacin is taken may increase the occurrence of flushing.

Nifedipine

Commercial names: Adalat, Procardia

Prescribed for: High blood pressure, angina pectoris (chest pain)

Common side effects:

Flushing of the face

Edema

Headache

Dizziness

Drug, food, or supplement interactions: Beta-blockers, antiseizure medicines, digitalis heart medicines, certain immune-suppressing drugs, diuretics, grapefruit, grapefruit juice, calcium, vitamin D, St. John's wort, pleurisy root

Nitroglycerin ER

Commercial name: Nitroglyn

Prescribed for: Angina pectoris (chest pain)

Common side effects:

Throbbing headache

Flushing of the head and neck

Increased heart rate or heart palpitations

Nausea

Vomiting

Drug, food, or supplement interactions: Benzodiazepines such as Valium, migraine medications such as Imitrex, pseudoephedrine such as Sudafed, antidepressants or antipsychotic medications, alcohol

Nizatidine

Commercial name: Axid

Prescribed for: Gastroesophageal reflux disease (GERD), ulcers

Common side effects:

Diarrhea

Fatigue

Headache

Insomnia

Muscle pain

Nausea

Vomiting

Drug, food, or supplement interactions: Warfarin (Coumadin), phenytoin, theophylline, lidocaine, amiodarone, metronidazole, loratadine, calcium channel blockers (e.g., diltiazem, felodipine, nifedipine), bupropion, carba-mazepine and fluvastatin, ketoconazole, caffeine, magnesium

Omeprazole

Commercial name: Prilosec

Prescribed for: Gastroesophageal reflux disease (GERD), esophageal damage (ulcers, erosions, strictures, or Barrett's esophagus), stomach ulcers, combination with antibiotics for treating *Helicobacter pylori*

Common side effects:

Headache

Diarrhea

Constipation

Abdominal pain

Nausea

Rash

Drug, food, or supplement interactions: may decrease absorption of ketoconazole (Nizoral), St. John's wort, and increase the absorption and concentration of digoxin (Lanoxin)

Orlistat

Commercial name: Xenical

Prescribed for: Weight loss

Common side effects:

Stomach discomfort

Increased number of bowel movements

Loss of control of bowel movements

Flatulence

Oily/fatty stools

Clear, orange, or brown-colored bowel movements

Drug, food, or supplement interactions: Warfarin (Coumadin), cyclosporine (Sandimmune), lipase enzymes

Oxaprozin

Commercial name: Daypro

Prescribed for: Fever, pain and swelling, arthritis

Common side effects:

Fever

Nausea

Vomiting

Diarrhea

Constipation

Decreased appetite

Rash

Dizziness

Headache

Drowsiness

Drug, food, or supplement interactions: Lithium (Eskalith), methotrexate (Rheumatrex), blood-thinning medications

Oxazepam

Commercial name: Serax

Prescribed for: Anxiety

Common side effects:

Agitation

Increased anxiety

Confusion

Memory impairment

Lack of coordination

Speech difficulties

Light-headedness

Constipation

Drug, food, or supplement interactions: Ketoconazole (Nizoral), itraconazole (Sporanox), some HIV or AIDS medications, alcohol, grapefruit juice, kava

Oxymetazoline

Commercial name: Afrin

Prescribed for: Nasal decongestant

Common side effects:

Burning, stinging, dryness, or irritation of the nose

Drug, food, or supplement interactions: Atropine, bromocriptine (Parlodel), linezolid (Zyvox), maprotiline (Ludiomil), antidepressants, migraine medications, high blood pressure medications, oxytocin, vasopressin, diuretic medications

Pantoprazole

Commercial name: Protonix

Prescribed for: Gastroesophageal reflux disease (GERD), esophageal damage (ulcers, erosions, strictures, or Barrett's esophagus), stomach ulcers, combination with antibiotics for treating *Helicobacter pylori*

Common side effects:

Headache

Diarrhea

Constipation

Abdominal pain

Nausea

Rash

Drug, food, or supplement interactions: Reduces the absorption of ketoconazole (Nizoral), and St. John's wort may decrease the blood levels of this drug. Can increase the absorption and concentration of digoxin (Lanoxin).

Paroxetine

Commercial names: Paxil, Paxil CR, Pexeva

Prescribed for: Depression, panic attacks, obsessive-compulsive disorder (OCD), social anxiety disorder (social phobia), post-traumatic stress disorder (PTSD), anxiety

Common side effects:

Nausea

Diarrhea

Agitation

Insomnia

Decreased sexual desire

Delayed orgasm or inability to have an orgasm

Drug, food, or supplement interactions: Astemizole (Hismanal), cisapride (Propulsid), pimozide (Orap), terfenadine (Seldane), thioridazine (Mellaril), monoamine oxidase (MAO) inhibitors, 5-hydroxytryptophan (5-HTP), L-tryptophan, St. John's wort

Pemoline

Commercial name: Cylert

Prescribed for: Attention deficit hyperactivity disorder

Common side effects:

Loss of appetite

Difficulty sleeping

Dry mouth

Weight loss

Stomachache

Headache

Overstimulation/anxiety

Dizziness

Tics

Listlessness/lethargy

Angina

Mood changes

Drug, food, or supplement interactions: Monoamine oxidase (MAO) inhibitors; anticonvulsants (e.g., phenobarbital, phenytoin, primidone); tricyclic drugs (e.g., imipramine, clomipramine, desipramine); clonidine (Catapres); SSRIs (selective serotonin reuptake inhibitors) such as fluoxetine, citalopram, and paroxetine; NRIs (norepinephrine reuptake inhibitors) such as Strattera; bupropion (Wellbutrin); amphetamine and tricyclic antidepressants; alcohol; magnesium hydroxide supplements; vitamin C; lithium (Eskalith)

Phentermine

Commercial names: Adipex-P, Fastin, Obestin-30, Phentermine resin oral

Prescribed for: Appetite suppression for weight loss

Common side effects:

High blood pressure

Heart palpitations

Restlessness

Tremor

Dizziness

Digestive upset (constipation, nausea, diarrhea)

Drug, food, or supplement interactions: Amphetamine or dextroamphetamine; furazolidone (Furoxone); high blood pressure medications; linezolid (Zyvox); diabetic medications; antidepressants, especially monoamine oxidase (MAO) inhibitors such as phenelzine (Nardil), tranylcypromine (Parnate), isocarboxazid (Marplan), selegiline (Eldepryl); procarbazine (Matulane); caffeine; alcohol

Pilocarpine Ophthalmic

Commercial names: Isopto Carpine, Pilocar, Pilopine HS

Prescribed for: Glaucoma

Common side effects:

Headache

Blurred vision

Eye irritation, burning, or itching

Drug, food, or supplement interactions: Antihistamines, atropine, acetazolamide, epinephrine, timolol

Pioglitazone Hydrochloride

Commercial name: Actos

Prescribed for: Type 2 diabetes

Common side effects:

Headache

Low blood sugar (hypoglycemia)

Fatigue

Sinusitis

Muscle ache

Drug, food, or supplement interactions: Rifampin (Rifadin, Rimactane), gemfibrozil (Lopid).

Glucose-lowering supplements such as chromium, vanadium, cinnamon extract, fenugreek, *Gymnema sylvestre*, bitter melon extract, ginseng, and others may enhance the effect of a diabetic medication. Check with your doctor before combining together.

Pioglitazone Hydrochloride and Glimepiride

Commercial name: Duetact

Prescribed for: Type 2 diabetes

Common side effects: See individual sections on pioglitazone hydrochloride and glimepiride.

Drug, food, or supplement interactions: See individual sections on pioglitazone hydrochloride and glimepiride.

Piroxicam

Commercial name: Feldene

Prescribed for: Pain and swelling, arthritis

Common side effects:

Nausea

Vomiting

Diarrhea

Constipation

Decreased appetite

Rash

Dizziness

Headache

Drowsiness

Drug, food, or supplement interactions: Diuretics, lithium (Eskalith), methotrexate (Rheumatrex), blood-thinning medications, minimize sodium intake, hibiscus tea

Pravastatin

Commercial name: Pravachol

Prescribed for: To reduce cholesterol and triglyceride levels, atherosclerosis, to reduce artery inflammation after a heart attack

Common side effects:

Headache

Nausea

Vomiting

Constipation

Diarrhea

Rash

Weakness

Muscle and joint pain

Increased liver enzymes

Drug, food, or supplement interactions: Cholestyramine (Questran), colestipol (Colestid), grapefruit or grapefruit juice, high doses of vitamin A

Progesterone (Bioidentical)

Commercial names: Prometrium, Crinone

Prescribed for: menopausal symptoms, premenstrual syndrome, breakthrough vaginal bleeding and spotting, irregular menstrual cycle, primary amenorrhea, combined with estrogen for preventing endometrial cancer, insomnia, anxiety, facial hair, hair loss

Common side effects:

Breast tenderness

Drug, food, or supplement interactions: Barbiturate medicines for inducing sleep or treating seizures (convulsions), bromocriptine (Parlodel), carbamazepine (Tegretol), ketoconazole (Nizoral), phenytoin (Dilantin), rifampin (Rifadin), voriconazole (Vfend)

Progesterone (Synthetic)

Commercial names: Provera, Cycrin, Amen, Aygestin, Nor-QD, Micronor, Megace

Prescribed for: Menopausal symptoms, premenstrual syndrome, breakthrough vaginal bleeding and spotting, irregular menstrual cycle, primary amenorrhea, combined with estrogen for preventing endometrial cancer

Common side effects:

Breast tenderness

Headache

Water retention

Weight gain

Mood changes

Drug, food, or supplement interactions: Barbiturate medicines for inducing sleep or treating seizures (convulsions), bromocriptine (Parlodel), carbamazepine (Tegretol), ketoconazole (Nizoral), phenytoin (Dilantin), rifampin (Rifadin), voriconazole (Vfend)

Propranolol

Commercial name: Inderal

Prescribed for: High blood pressure, angina, rapid heart rate, arrhythmias, migraine headaches, tremors

Common side effects:

Digestive upset (abdominal cramps, diarrhea, constipation, nausea)

Fatigue

Insomnia

Depression

Memory loss

Fever

Erectile dysfunction

Light-headedness

Slow heart rate

Low blood pressure

Numbness

Tingling

Cold extremities

Sore throat

Shortness of breath or wheezing

Drug, food, or supplement interactions: Calcium channel blockers such as digoxin (Lanoxin) and haloperidol (Haldol). Use with caution for those on diabetic medications. Alcohol and aluminum-containing antacids may reduce absorption.

Pseudoephedrine

Commercial names: Pseudoephedrine, Sudafed

Prescribed for: Nasal and sinus congestion

Common side effects:

Dizziness

Insomnia

Headache

Loss of appetite

Nausea

Stomach upset

Restlessness or nervousness

Drug, food, or supplement interactions: Ammonium chloride; amphetamine or other stimulant drugs; bicarbonate, citrate, or acetate products such as sodium bicarbonate, sodium acetate, sodium citrate, sodium lactate, and potassium citrate; bromocriptine (Parlodel); cocaine; furazolidone (Furoxone); linezolid (Zyvox); some cough and cold medicines; diabetic medications; antidepressants including monoamine oxidase (MAO) inhibitors such as phenelzine (Nardil), tranylcypromine (Parnate), isocarboxazid (Marplan), and selegiline (Carbex, Eldepryl); migraine medications; procarbazine (Matulane); cardiovascular medications for high blood pressure, chest pain, heart arrhythmias; theophylline (Theo-Dur, Respbid, Slo-Bid, Theo-24, Theolair, Uniphyl, Slo-Phyllin); thyroid hormones; caffeine (coffee, tea, chocolate, guarana); St. John's wort.

High-tannin-containing herbs may interfere with absorption. Examples include green tea, black tea, uva ursi *(Arctostaphylos uva-ursi)*, black walnut *(Juglans nigra)*, red raspberry *(Rubus idaeus)*, oak *(Quercus spp.)*, and witch hazel *(Hamamelis virginiana)*.

Pseudoephedrine Combined with Triprolidine

Commercial name: Actifed Daytime Allergy

Prescribed for: Nasal and sinus congestion

Common side effects:

Dizziness

Insomnia

Headache

Loss of appetite

Nausea

Stomach upset

Restlessness or nervousness

Drug, food, or supplement interactions: Ammonium chloride; amphetamine or other stimulant drugs; bicarbonate, citrate, or acetate products such as sodium bicarbonate, sodium acetate, sodium citrate, sodium lactate, and potassium citrate; bromocriptine (Parlodel); cocaine; furazolidone (Furoxone); linezolid (Zyvox); some cough and cold medicines; diabetic medications; antidepressants including monoamine oxidase (MAO) inhibitors such as phenelzine (Nardil), tranylcypromine (Parnate), isocarboxazid (Marplan), and selegiline (Carbex, Eldepryl); migraine medications; procarbazine (Matulane); cardiovascular medications for high blood pressure, chest pain, heart arrhythmias; theophylline (Theo-Dur, Respbid, Slo-Bid, Theo-24, Theolair, Uniphyl, Slo-Phyllin); thyroid hormones; caffeine (coffee, tea, chocolate, guarana); St. John's wort.

High-tannin-containing herbs may interfere with absorption. Examples include green tea, black tea, uva ursi *(Arctostaphylos uva-ursi),* black walnut *(Juglans nigra)*, red raspberry *(Rubus idaeus)*, oak *(Quercus spp.)*, and witch hazel *(Hamamelis virginiana)*.

Rabeprazole

Commercial name: Aciphex

Prescribed for: Gastroesophageal reflux disease (GERD), esophageal damage (ulcers, erosions, strictures, or Barrett's esophagus), stomach ulcers, combination with antibiotics for treating *Helicobacter pylori*

Common side effects:

Headache

Diarrhea

Constipation

Abdominal pain

Nausea

Rash

Drug, food, or supplement interactions: Reduces the absorption of ketoconazole (Nizoral), and St. John's wort may decrease the blood levels of this drug. Can increase the absorption and concentration of digoxin (Lanoxin).

Raloxifene

Commercial name: Evista

Prescribed for: Osteoporosis

Common side effects:

Hot flashes

Weight gain

Leg cramps

Sinusitis

Edema of the ankles

Drug, food, or supplement interactions: Cholestyramine (Questran), blood-thinning medications such as warfarin (Coumadin), alcohol

Ranitidine

Commercial name: Zantac

Prescribed for: Gastroesophageal reflux disease (GERD), ulcers

Common side effects:

Diarrhea

Fatigue

Headache

Insomnia

Muscle pain

Nausea

Vomiting

Drug, food, or supplement interactions: Warfarin (Coumadin), phenytoin, theophylline, lidocaine, amiodarone, metronidazole, loratadine, calcium channel blockers (e.g., diltiazem, felodipine, nifedipine), bupropion, carbamazepine and fluvastatin, ketoconazole, caffeine, magnesium

Retinoids (Tretinoin, Adapalene, Isotretinoin)

Commercial names: Retin-A, Avita, Renova, Differin, Isotrex Gel, Accutane

Prescribed for: Acne vulgaris

Common side effects:

Mild stinging, sensation of warmth, dryness, scaling, and redness at site of topical application.

Internal use of isotretinoin can cause dry nose, nosebleeds, cracks in the corners of the mouth, dry mouth, inflammation of the whites of the eyes, thinning hair, bone loss, and joint aches. Birth defects are a risk for pregnant women.

Drug, food, or supplement interactions: Avoid supplementing vitamin A in combination with isotretinoin.

Risedronate

Commercial name: Actonel

Prescribed for: Osteoporosis, Paget's disease

Common side effects:

Joint pain

Headache

Diarrhea

Abdominal pain

Nausea

Drug, food, or supplement interactions: Parathyroid hormone (Forteo), aminoglycoside antibiotics, food (should be taken 60 minutes away from any food, especially foods containing calcium), caffeine, calcium supplements (take at different time of day)

Rizatriptan

Commercial name: Maxalt

Prescribed for: Migraine headaches

Common side effects:

Flushing of face

Weakness

Dizziness

Sweating

Abdominal pain

Chest pain

Drug, food, or supplement interactions: Selective serotonin reuptake inhibitors (SSRIs) such as fluoxetine (Prozac), paroxetine (Paxil), sertraline (Zoloft), citalopram (Celexa), and fluvoxamine (Luvox); monoamine oxidase (MAO) inhibitors such as phenelzine (Nardil) and tranylcypromine (Parnate); propranolol (Inderal); cimetidine (Tagamet); 5-hydroxytryptophan (5-HTP); L-tryptophan; ginkgo biloba; alcohol

Rosiglitazone Maleate

Commercial name: Avandia

Prescribed for: Type 2 diabetes

Common side effects:

High blood sugar (hyperglycemia)

Headache

Low blood sugar (hypoglycemia)

Fatigue

Sinusitis

Back pain

Drug, food, or supplement interactions: Rifampin (Rifadin, Rimactane), gemfibrozil (Lopid)

Glucose-lowering supplements such as chromium, vanadium, cinnamon extract, fenugreek, *Gymnema sylvestre*, bitter melon extract, ginseng, and others may enhance the effect of a diabetic medication. Check with your doctor before combining together.

Rosiglitazone Maleate and Glimepiride

Commercial name: Avandaryl

Prescribed for: Type 2 diabetes

Common side effects: See individual sections on rosiglitazone maleate and glimepiride.

Drug, food, or supplement interactions: See individual sections on rosiglitazone maleate and glimepiride.

Rosiglitazone Maleate and Metformin Hydrochloride

Commercial name: Avandamet

Prescribed for: Type 2 diabetes

Common side effects: See individual sections on rosiglitazone maleate and metformin hydrochloride.

Drug, food, or supplement interactions: See individual sections on rosiglitazone maleate and metformin hydrochloride.

Rosuvastatin

Commercial name: Crestor

Prescribed for: To reduce cholesterol and triglyceride levels, atherosclerosis, to reduce artery inflammation after a heart attack

Common side effects:

Nausea

Vomiting

Diarrhea

Rash

Muscle and joint pain

Headache

Drug, food, or supplement interactions: Cholestyramine (Questran), colestipol (Colestid), grapefruit or grapefruit juice, high doses of vitamin A

Salicylates

Commercial names: Aspirin, acetylsalicylic acid, Acuprin, Alka-Seltzer, Ascriptin A/D, Bayer, Bufferin, Easprin, Ecotrin, Empirin, Zorprin

Prescribed for: Conditions that involve pain and inflammation such as arthritis. Also used as a blood thinner for the prevention of blood clots associated with heart attack and stroke.

Common side effects:

Disorders of the digestive tract (stomach ulceration, abdominal burning, pain, cramping, nausea, and gastritis)

Tinnitus (ringing in the ears)

Drug, food, or supplement interactions: Blood-thinning medications such as warfarin (Coumadin), ginkgo biloba, high doses of vitamin E

Salicylic Acid Topical

Commercial names: Oxy Clean Maximum Strength, Oxy Clean Medicated, Salex, Sebasorb, Stri-Dex

Prescribed for: Acne vulgaris

Common side effects: Burning, stinging, itching, dryness, redness, peeling, or irritation of the skin

Drug, food, or supplement interactions: Caution with other topical treatments.

Sertraline

Commercial name: Zoloft

Prescribed for: Depression, social anxiety disorder, panic disorder, obsessive-compulsive disorder (OCD), post-traumatic stress disorder (PTSD), and pre-menstrual dysphoric disorder (PMDD)

Common side effects:

Nausea

Diarrhea

Agitation

Insomnia

Decreased sexual desire

Delayed orgasm or inability to have an orgasm

Drug, food, or supplement interactions: Astemizole (Hismanal), cisapride (Propulsid), pimozide (Orap), terfenadine (Seldane), thioridazine (Mellaril), monoamine oxidase (MAO) inhibitors, 5-hydroxytryptophan (5-HTP), L-tryptophan, St. John's wort

Sibutramine

Commercial name: Meridia

Prescribed for: Appetite suppression for weight loss

Common side effects:

Insomnia

Headache

Dry mouth

Constipation

Drug, food, or supplement interactions: Ketoconazole (Nizoral); cimetidine (Tagamet); erythromycin (Erytab, Eryc, Ilosone); clarithromycin (Biaxin); danazol (Danocrine); diltiazem (Cardizem, Tiazac, Dilacor); fluconazole (Diflucan); fluoxetine (Prozac); itraconazole (Sporanox); propoxyphene (Darvon); troleandomycin (Tao); verapamil (Verelan, Covera, Calan, Isoptin); serotonin reuptake inhibitors (SSRIs) such as fluoxetine (Prozac), fluvoxamine (Luvox), paroxetine (Paxil), sertraline (Zoloft); monoamine oxidase (MAO) inhibitors such as phenelzine (Nardil), tranylcypromine (Parnate), isocarboxazid (Marplan), selegiline (Eldepryl); sumatriptan (Imitrex); zolmitriptan (Zomig); dihydroergotamine (DHE); dextromethorphan (Robitussin-DM), meperidine (Demerol), pentazocine (Talwin), and fentanyl (Duragesic); lithium (Eskalith); L-tryptophan; 5-hydroxytryptophan (5 HTP); alcohol

Sildenafil Tablets

Commercial name: Viagra

Prescribed for: Erectile dysfunction

Common side effects:

Flushing of the face

Headaches

Digestive upset (nausea and diarrhea)

Pain

Nasal congestion

Drug, food, or supplement interactions: Isosorbide dinitrate (Isordil), isosorbide mononitrate (Imdur, Ismo, Monoket), nitroglycerin (Nitro-Dur, Transderm-Nitro), cimetidine (Tagamet), erythromycin, ketoconazole (Nizoral), itraconazole (Sporanox), mibefradil (Posicor), grapefruit juice

Simvastatin

Commercial name: Zocor

Prescribed for: To reduce cholesterol and triglyceride levels, atherosclerosis, to reduce artery inflammation after a heart attack

Common side effects:

Headache

Nausea

Vomiting

Constipation

Diarrhea

Rash

Weakness

Muscle and joint pain

Increased liver enzymes

Drug, food, or supplement interactions: Cholestyramine (Questran), colestipol (Colestid), grapefruit or grapefruit juice, high doses of vitamin A

Sulindac

Commercial name: Clinoril

Prescribed for: pain and swelling, arthritis

Common side effects:

Nausea

Vomiting

Diarrhea

Constipation

Decreased appetite

Rash

Dizziness

Headache

Drowsiness

Drug, food, or supplement interactions: Warfarin (Coumadin) and other blood-thinning medications, lithium, cyclosporine (Sandimmune), potassium, white willow

Sumatriptan

Commercial name: Imitrex

Prescribed for: Migraine headaches

Common side effects:

Flushing of the face

Weakness

Dizziness

Sweating

Abdominal pain

Chest pain

Drug, food, or supplement interactions: Selective serotonin reuptake inhibitors (SSRIs) such as fluoxetine (Prozac), paroxetine (Paxil), sertraline (Zoloft), citalopram (Celexa), and fluvoxamine (Luvox); monoamine oxidase (MAO) inhibitors such as phenelzine (Nardil) and tranylcypromine (Parnate); propranolol (Inderal); cimetidine (Tagamet); 5-hydroxytryptophan (5-HTP); L-tryptophan; ginkgo biloba; alcohol

Tadalafil

Commercial name: Cialis

Prescribed for: Erectile dysfunction

Common side effects:

Digestive upset (diarrhea, stomach upset, nausea)

Flushing of the face

Headaches

Flu-like symptoms

Drug, food, or supplement interactions: Isosorbide dinitrate (Isordil), isosorbide mononitrate (Imdur, Ismo, Monoket), nitroglycerin (Nitro-Dur, Transderm-Nitro), cimetidine (Tagamet), erythromycin, ketoconazole (Nizoral), itraconazole (Sporanox), mibefradil (Posicor), grapefruit juice

Tamsulosin

Commercial name: Flomax

Prescribed for: Urinary symptoms related to benign prostatic hyperplasia

Common side effects:

Dizziness

Low blood pressure

Drug, food, or supplement interactions: Clonidine (Catapres), cimetidine (Tagamet), warfarin (Coumadin)

Telmisartan

Commercial name: Micardis

Prescribed for: High blood pressure

Common side effects:

Dizziness

Back pain

Fatigue

Headache

Drug, food, or supplement interactions: Potassium-sparing diuretics, lithium (Eskalith)

Avoid salt substitutes and supplements containing potassium, as well as large amounts of foods high in potassium such as bananas, green leafy vegetables, and oranges.

Terazosin

Commercial name: Hytrin

Prescribed for: Urinary symptoms related to benign prostatic hyperplasia

Common side effects:

Dizziness

Low blood pressure

Drug, food, or supplement interactions: None known

Teriparatide

Commercial name: Forteo

Prescribed for: Osteoporosis, Paget's disease

Common side effects:

Dizziness

Leg cramps

Drug, food, or supplement interactions: Digoxin (digitalis, Lanoxin)

Testosterone (Biodentical)

Commercial names: AndroGel, Androderm, Testoderm, Testoderm TTS, Testim

Prescribed for: Low testosterone and conditions related to low testosterone such as erectile dysfunction, osteoporosis, congestive heart failure

Common side effects:

Hypogonadism (low testosterone)

Erectile dysfunction

Digestive upset (nausea and vomiting)

Headache

Hair loss

Acne

Mood changes (depression, irritability)

Frequent erections

Drug, food, or supplement interactions: Fluconazole (Diflucan), cyclosporine (Gengraf, Neoral), medicines for prostate enlargement or prostate cancer, warfarin (Coumadin)

Testosterone (Synthetic)

Commercial name: Methyltestosterone

Prescribed for: Low libido (male and female), menopausal symptoms

Common side effects:

Facial hair growth

Acne

Mood changes (anxiety, depression, irritability)

Drug, food, or supplement interactions: Fluconazole (Diflucan), cyclosporine (Gengraf, Neoral), medicines for prostate enlargement or prostate cancer, warfarin (Coumadin)

Ticlopidine

Commercial name: Ticlid

Prescribed for: Prevention of blood clots associated with heart attack and stroke

Common side effects:

Rash or itching

Diarrhea

Stomach pain

Drug, food, or supplement interactions: Ibuprofen (Motrin; Advil; Nuprin), naproxen (Naprosyn, Aleve), diclofenac (Voltaren), etodolac (Lodine), nabumetone (Relafen), fenoprofen (Nalfon), flurbiprofen (Ansaid), indomethacin (Indocin), ketoprofen (Orudis, Oruvail), oxaprozin, piroxicam (Feldene), sulindac (Clinoril), tolmetin (Tolectin), mefenamic acid (Ponstel), warfarin (Coumadin)

Timolol

Commercial names: Betimol, Timoptic, Timoptic-XE

Prescribed for: Glaucoma

Common side effects:

Burning

Stinging

Itching of the eyes or eyelids

Vision changes

Light sensitivity

Drug, food, or supplement interactions: Caution with high blood pressure medicines, haloperidol (Haldol), digoxin (Lanoxin)

Tolazamide

Commercial name: Tolinase

Prescribed for: Type 2 diabetes

Common side effects:

Digestive upset (reduced appetite, cramps, bloating, heartburn, diarrhea, constipation, nausea)

Weight gain

Drug, food, or supplement interactions: Cholestyramine, fluconazole (Diflucan), nonsteroidal anti-inflammatory drugs such as ibuprofen, sulfa drugs, warfarin (Coumadin), miconazole (Monistat, Lotrimin), beta-blockers (e.g., propranolol), thiazide diuretics, corticosteroids, thyroid medicines, estrogens, phenytoin (Dilantin), calcium channel blocking drugs (e.g., diltiazem), alcohol, niacin, magnesium.

Glucose-lowering supplements such as chromium, vanadium, cinnamon extract, fenugreek, *Gymnema sylvestre*, bitter melon extract, ginseng, and others may enhance the effect of a diabetic medication.

Tolmetin

Commercial name: Tolectin

Prescribed for: Pain and swelling, arthritis

Common side effects:

Fever

Nausea

Vomiting

Diarrhea

Constipation

Decreased appetite

Rash

Dizziness

Headache

Drowsiness

Drug, food, or supplement interactions: Lithium (Eskalith), methotrexate (Rheumatrex), blood-thinning medications such as warfarin (Coumadin), hibiscus tea

Tramadol

Commercial name: Ulttram

Prescribed for: Pain

Common side effects:

Nausea

Vomiting

Diarrhea

Constipation

Decreased appetite

Rash

Dizziness

Headache

Drowsiness

Drug, food, or supplement interactions: Carbamazepine (Tegretol), quinidine (Quinaglute, Quinidex), antidepressants such as monoamine oxidase (MAO) inhibitors or selective serotonin inhibitors (SSRIs), alcohol, 5-hydroxytryptophan, L-tryptophan

Travoprost

Commercial name: Travatan

Prescribed for: Glaucoma

Common side effects:

Burning, stinging, or itching of the eyes or eyelids

Changes in eye, eyelash, or eyelid color

Dry eyes

Increased flow of tears; light sensitivity

Drug, food, or supplement interactions: None known

Triamcinolone Nasal Spray

Commercial names: Nasacort AQ, Nasacort HFA

Prescribed for: Allergies

Common side effects:

Burning, dryness, or irritation inside the nose

Headache

Nosebleed

Unpleasant taste

Throat irritation

Drug, food, or supplement interactions: None known

Valacyclovir

Commercial name: Valtrex

Prescribed for: Cold sores, genital herpes, shingles

Common side effects:

Digestive upset (nausea, vomiting)

Headache

Drug, food, or supplement interactions: Amphotericin B (Fungizone); amino-glycoside antibiotics such as amikacin (Amikin), gentamicin (Garamycin), kanamycin (Kantrex), neomycin (Nes-RX, Neo-Fradin), paramomycin (Humatin), streptomycin, and tobramycin (Tobi, Nebcin); aspirin and other nonsteroidal anti-inflammatory medications such as ibuprofen (Advil,

Motrin) and naproxen (Aleve, Naprosyn); cyclosporine (Neoral, Sandimmune); medications to treat HIV or AIDS such as zidovudine (Retrovir, AZT); pentamidine (NebuPent); cimetidine (Tagamet); probenecid (Benemid); sulfonamides such as sulfamethoxazole and trimethoprim (Bactrim); tacrolimus (Prograf); vancomycin; digoxin (Lanoxin); alcohol; St. John's wort

Valsartan

Commercial name: Diovan

Prescribed for: High blood pressure, heart failure, post–heart attack recovery

Common side effects:

Digestive upset (diarrhea, abdominal pain, diarrhea, nausea)

Headache

Dizziness

Fatigue

Drug, food, or supplement interactions: Potassium-sparing diuretics such as amiloride (Midamor), buckthorn or alder buckthorn, buchu, cleavers, dandelion, digitalis, ginkgo biloba, gravel root, horsetail, juniper, licorice, uva ursi

Vardenafil

Commercial name: Levitra

Prescribed for: Erectile dysfunction

Common side effects:

Digestive upset (diarrhea, stomach upset, nausea)

Flushing of the face

Headaches

Flu-like symptoms

Drug, food, or supplement interactions: Isosorbide dinitrate (Isordil), isosorbide mononitrate (Imdur, Ismo, Monoket), nitroglycerin (Nitro-Dur, Transderm-Nitro), cimetidine (Tagamet), erythromycin, ketoconazole (Nizoral), itraconazole (Sporanox), mibefradil (Posicor), grapefruit juice

Venlafaxine

Commercial name: Effexor

Prescribed for: Depression, anxiety

Common side effects:

Nausea

Anxiety

Insomnia

Headaches

Drowsiness

Reduced appetite

Drug, food, or supplement interactions: Monoamine oxidase (MAO) inhibitors, haloperidol, digoxin, warfarin, 5-hydroxytryptophan (5-HTP), L-tryptophan, sour date nut *(Ziziphus jujube)*, St. John's wort

Verapamil

Commercial names: Calan, Isoptin, Verelan

Prescribed for: High blood pressure, angina pectoris (chest pain), arrhythmia, atrial fibrillation

Common side effects:

Headache

Constipation

Dizziness

Weakness

Fainting

Drug, food, or supplement interactions: Caution with beta-blockers, anti-seizure medicines, digitalis, certain immune-suppressing drugs, diuretics, grapefruit and grapefruit juice, calcium, vitamin D, and St. John's wort

Warfarin

Commercial names: Coumadin, Jantoven

Prescribed for: Prevention and treatment of blood clots

Common side effects:

Bleeding gums

Bruising

Nosebleeds

Heavy menstrual bleeding

Cuts that bleed too long

Drug, food, or supplement interactions: Acetaminophen; allopurinol; amiodarone; antibiotics; anti-inflammatory drugs; NSAIDs such as ibuprofen; aprepitant; aspirin; azathioprine; barbiturate medicines for inducing sleep or treating seizures; bosentan; cimetidine (Tagamet); cyclosporine; disulfiram; hormones, including testosterone, estrogen, and contraceptive or birth control pills; certain medicines for heart arrhythmia (common examples include propafenone [Rythmol] and propranolol [Inderal]); quinidine; quinine; seizure or epilepsy medicine such as carbamazepine, phenytoin, and valproic acid; thyroid medicine; tolterodine.

The following supplements enhance or interfere with blood thinning medications: American ginseng; panax (Asian) ginseng; cranberry; dan shen; devil's claw; dong quai; fenugreek; ginkgo; goji berry; grapefruit seed extract; garlic; ginger; horse chestnut; papain; red clover; reishi; pycnogenol; coenzyme Q10; green tea; iron; magnesium; St. John's wort; vitamin C; zinc; vitamin E; vitamin K; large quantities of foods rich in vitamin K such as broccoli, spinach, or kale; alcohol

Zoledronic Acid

Commercial name: Reclast

Prescribed for: Osteoporosis

Common side effects:

Muscle and joint pain

Headache

Fever

Drug, food, or supplement interactions: Parathyroid hormone (Forteo), amino-glycoside antibiotics

Zolmitriptan

Commercial name: Zomig

Prescribed for: Migraine headaches

Common side effects:

Flushing of face

Weakness

Dizziness

Sweating

Abdominal pain

Chest pain

Drug, food, or supplement interactions: Selective serotonin reuptake inhibitors (SSRIs) such as fluoxetine (Prozac), paroxetine (Paxil), sertraline (Zoloft), citalopram (Celexa), and fluvoxamine (Luvox); monoamine oxidase (MAO) inhibitors such as phenelzine (Nardil) and tranylcypromine (Parnate); propranolol (Inderal); cimetidine (Tagamet); 5-hydroxytryptophan (5-HTP); L-tryptophan; ginkgo biloba; alcohol

Commercial and Generic Names of Common Pharmaceuticals

Commercial Name	Generic Name
Accutane	retinoids (tretinoin, adapalene, isotretinion)
acetylsalicylic acid	salicylates
Aciphex	rabeprazole
Actifed Daytime Allergy	pseudoephedrine combined with triprolidine
Actonel	risedronate
Actos	pioglitazone hydrochloride
Acuprin	salicylates
Adalat	nifedipine
Adderall	amphetamine and dextroamphetamine
Adipex-P	phentermine
Afrin	oxymetazoline
AKBeta	levobunolol
Alavert	loratadine
Aleve	naproxen
Alka-Seltzer	salicylates
Allegra	fexofenadine
Aller-Chlor	chlorpheniramine

Commercial Name	Generic Name
Allergy	chlorpheniramine
AllerMax	diphenhydramine oral
Alora	estrogen (bioidentical)
Alphagan	brimonidine
Amaryl	glimepiride
Amen	progesterone synthetic
AndroGel Androderm	testosterone (bioidentical) topical gel or transdermal
Apidra	insulin
Armour thyroid	dessicated thyroid
Ascriptin A/D	salicylates
aspart, aspart injection, aspart protamine injection (NovoLog)	insulin
aspirin	salicylates
Atacand	candesartan
Ativan	Lorazepam
Atrovent nasal	ipratropium nasal

Commercial Name	Generic Name
Avandamet	rosiglitazone maleate and metformin hydrochloride
Avandaryl	rosiglitazone maleate and glimepiride
Avandia	rosiglitazone maleate
Avapro	irbesartan
Avita	retinoids (tretinoin, adapalene, isotretinion)
Avodart	dutasteride
Axid	nizatidine
Aygestin	progesterone synthetic
Banophen	diphenhydramine oral
Bayer	salicylates
Bayer	salicylates
Beconase AQ	beclomethasone nasal inhalation
Benadryl	diphenhydramine oral
Benoxyl	benzoyl peroxide
Benzac AC	benzoyl peroxide
Benzagel	benzoyl peroxide
Betagan	levobunolol
Betimol	timolol
Betoptic	betaxolol
Betoptic S	betaxolol
Biest	estrogen (bioidentical)
Boniva	ibandronate
Brevoxyl	benzoyl peroxide
BroveX	brompheniramine
BroveX CT	brompheniramine
Bufferin	salicylates
BuSpar	buspirone
Calan	verapamil
Calcimar	calcitonin (injectable)
Calcium Rich Rolaids	calcium carbonate
Capoten	captopril
Cardene	nicardipine
Cardizem	diltiazem

Commercial Name	Generic Name
Cardura	doxazosin
Celebrex	celecoxib
Celexa	citalopram
Cenestin	estrogen (synthetic)
Chlo-Amine	chlorpheniramine
Chlor-Trimeton	chlorpheniramine
Chlor-Trimeton Allergy	chlorpheniramine
Cialis	tadalafil
Clarinex	desloratadine
Claritin	loratadine
Climara	estrogen (bioidentical)
Clinagen LA 40	estrogen (bioidentical)
Clinoril	sulindac
Codeine	codeine
Concerta	methylphenidate
Corgard	nadolol
Coumadin	warfarin
Cozaar	lLosartan
Crestor	rosuvastatin
Crinone	progesterone (bioidentical)
Cycrin	progesterone synthetic
Cylert	pemoline
Cymbalta	duloxetine
Cytomel	liothyronine sodium
Dayhist-1	clemastine
Daypro	oxaprozin
Delestrogen	estrogen (bioidentical)
Depogen	estrogen (bioidentical)
detemir injection (Levemir)	insulin
Dexchlorphenir-amine ER	dexchlorpheniramine ER
Dexedrine	dextroamphetamine
Diabeta	glyburide
Diabinese	chlorpropamide
Differin	retinoids (tretinoin, adapalene, isotretinion)

Commercial Name	Generic Name	Commercial Name	Generic Name
Dilacor XR	diltiazem	Glucovance	glyburide and metformin
Diovan	valsartan	glulisine injection (Apidra)	insulin
Diphenhist	diphenhydramine oral	Glynase	glyburide
Duetact	pioglitazone hydrochloride and glimepiride	Gynodiol	estrogen (bioidentical)
Easprin	salicylates	Histex CT	carbinoxamine
Ecotrin	salicylates	Humalog	insulin
Effexor	venlafaxine	Humulin	insulin
Efidac 24	chlorpheniramine	HydroDiuril	hydrochlorothiazide
Elavil	amitriptyline	Hytrin	terazosin
Empirin	salicylates	Hyzaar	losartan and hydrochlorothiazide
Endep	amitriptyline	Iletin	insulin
Esclim	estrogen (bioidentical)	Imitrex	sumatriptan
Esidrix	hydrochlorothiazide	Inderal	propranolol
Estrace	estrogen (bioidentical)	Indocin	indomethacin
Estraderm	estrogen (bioidentical)	Isoptin	verapamil
Estradiol	estrogen (bioidentical)	Isopto Carpine	pilocarpine ophthalmic
Estragyn 5	estrogen (bioidentical)	Isotrex Gel	retinoids (tretinoin, adapalene, isotretinion)
Estrasorb	estrogen (bioidentical)		
Estratab	estrogen (synthetic)	Jantoven	warfarin
Estring	estrogen (bioidentical)	Kestrone 5	estrogen (bioidentical)
Estriol	estrogen (bioidentical)	Klonopin	clonazepam
Evista	raloxifene	Lantus	insulin
Exubera	insulin	Lasix	furosemide
Fastin	phentermine	Lescol	fluvastatin
Feldene	piroxicam	Levemir	insulin
Flomax	tamsulosin	Levitra	vardenafil
Flonase	fluticasone nasal inhalation	Levothroid	levothyroxine
Forteo	teriparatide	Levoxyl	levothyroxine
Fortical	calcitonin nasal spray	Lexapro	escitalopram
Fosamax	alendronate	Lipitor	atorvastatin
Gaviscon	alginate	lispro, lispro protamine injection (Humalog)	insulin
Genahist	diphenhydramine oral		
glargine injection (Lantus)	insulin	Lodine	etodolac
Glucophage	metformin	Lodrane 12-Hour ER Tablet	brompheniramine
Glucotrol	glipizide		

Commercial Name	Generic Name
Lotensin	benazepril
Lotrel	amlodipine and benazepril
Lumigan	bimatoprost
Maalox	aluminum and magnesium hydroxide
Maxalt	rizatriptan
Megace	progesterone synthetic
Menest	estrogen (synthetic)
Meridia	sibutramine
Metadate	methylphenidate
Metaglip	glipizide and metformin
Methyltestosterone	testosterone (synthetic)
Mevacor	lovastatin
Miacalcin	calcitonin nasal spray
Miacalcin	calcitonin (injectable)
Micardis	telmisartan
Micronase	glyburide
Micronor	progesterone synthetic
Midamor	amiloride
Motrin	ibuprofen
Mylanta	aluminum and magnesium hydroxide
Naprosyn	naproxen
Nasacort AQ	triamcinolone nasal spray
Nasacort HFA	triamcinolone nasal spray
Nasalcrom	cromolyn nasal spray
Nasarel	flunisolide nasal inhalation
Nasonex	mometasone nasal spray
Naturethroid	dessicated thyroid
Nexium	esomeprazole
Niacor	nicotinic acid
Niaspan	nicotinic acid
Niravam	alprazolam
Nitroglyn	nitroglycerin ER
Nor-QD	progesterone synthetic
Norvasc	amlodipine
Novolin	insulin

Commercial Name	Generic Name
NovoLog	insulin
Obestin-30	phentermine
Ocupress	carteolol
Ogen	estrogen (synthetic)
OptiPranolol	metipranolol ophthalmic
Ortho Dienestrol	estrogen (synthetic)
Orudis	ketoprofen
Oxy Clean Maximum Strength	salicylic acid topical
Oxy Clean Medicated	salicylic acid topical
Paxil	paroxetine
Paxil CR	paroxetine
Pepcid	famotidine
Pepcid AC	famotidine
Persa-Gel	benzoyl peroxide
Pexeva	paroxetine
Phentermine resin oral	phentermine
Phillips' Milk of Magnesia	magnesium hydroxide
Pilocar	pilocarpine ophthalmic
Pilopine HS	pilocarpine ophthalmic
Plavix	clopidogrel
Pravachol	pravastatin
Premarin	estrogen (synthetic)
Prevacid	lansoprazole
Prilosec	omeprazole
Prinivil	lisinopril
Procardia	nifedipine
Prometrium	progesterone (bioidentical)
Proscar	finasteride
Protonix	pantoprazole
Provera	progesterone synthetic
Prozac	fluoxetine
Pseudoephedrine	pseudoephedrine
Reclast	zoledronic acid
Reglan	metoclopramide

Commercial Name	Generic Name	Commercial Name	Generic Name
Regular iletin	insulin	Tolinase	tolazamide
Regular insulin	insulin	Toradol	ketorolac
Relafen	nabumetone	Travatan	travoprost
Renova	retinoids (tretinoin, adapalene, isotretinion)	Triaminic	loratadine
		Triest	estrogen (bioidentical)
Retin-A	retinoids (tretinoin, adapalene, isotretinion)	Tums	calcium carbonate
		Tylenol	acetaminophen
Rhinocort Aqua	budesonide nasal inhaler	Ultram	tramadol
Ritalin	methylphenidate	Unithroid	levothyroxine
Salex	salicylic acid topical	Uroxatral	alfuzosin
Sebasorb	salicylic acid topical	Valergen	estrogen (bioidentical)
Serax	oxazepam	Valium	diazepam
Singulair	montelukast	Valtrex	valacyclovir
Slo-Niacin	nicotinic acid	Vanatrip	amitriptyline
Stri-Dex	salicylic acid topical	Vasotec	enalapril
Sudafed	pseudoephedrine	Velosulin	insulin
Synthroid	levothyroxine	Verelan	verapamil
Tagamet	cimetidine	Viagra	sildenafil tablets
Tagamet HB	cimetidine	Vivelle	estrogen (bioidentical)
Tavist	clemastine	Voltaren	diclofenac
Tavist Allergy	clemastine	Wellbutrin	bupropion
Tenormin	atenolol	Westhroid	dessicated thyroid
Testim	testosterone (bioidentical) topical gel or transdermal	Xalatan	latanoprost
		Xanax	alprazolam
Testoderm	testosterone (bioidentical) topical gel or transdermal	Xenical	orlistat
		Zantac	ranitidine
Testoderm TTS	testosterone (bioidentical) topical gel or transdermal	Zestril	lisinopril
		Zetia	ezetimibe
Tiazac	diltiazem	Zocor	simvastatin
Ticlid	ticlopidine	Zoloft	sertraline
Timoptic	timolol	Zomig	zolmitriptan
Timoptic-XE	timolol	Zorprin	salicylates
Titralac	calcium carbonate	Zovirax	acyclovir
Tolectin	tolmetin	Zyrtec	cetirizine

GLOSSARY

Amino acids   The individual building blocks of protein. There are approximately 20 different amino acids. Ten of the amino acids are known as "essential amino acids," which means our body cannot manufacture them so it is essential we consume them from our diet. The remaining 10 nonessential amino acids can be manufactured in the body. Amino acids can be taken as individual nutrients to influence brain chemistry.

Antihistamine   A substance that reduces or blocks histamine response.

Anti-inflammatory   A substance used to relieve inflammation.

Antioxidants   Substances that neutralize or reduce the effects of cell-damaging free radicals. Common examples include vitamins A, C, and E, pycnogenol, and selenium.

Arrhythmia   An abnormal or irregular heart rhythm.

Arteriosclerosis   A hardening of the arteries created when plaque and calcium attach to the interior of the arterial wall. This causes a loss in elasticity and flexibility of the artery, resulting in reduced circulation.

Atherosclerosis   The most common type of arteriosclerosis in which fatty deposits accumulate within the blood vessel walls of medium and large arteries.

Carbohydrate   A food compound containing carbon and water molecules that provides energy to the body.

Cardiovascular disease   A disease of the heart and blood vessels.

Carotenoids   A group of fat-soluble pigments (colors) found in plants or nutritional supplements that are known to have antioxidant properties.

Cell   The smallest independently functioning unit in the structure of an organism.

Chlorophyll   A green plant pigment responsible for capturing the light energy needed for photosynthesis. Used in natural medicine for detoxification, red blood cell support, and antioxidant properties.

Dementia   A deterioration or impairment of mental functioning.

Detoxification   The process of eliminating toxins and waste products in the body.

Digestion   The chemical and physical process of breaking down and assimilating food.

Diuretic   A substance or drug that increases the amount of urine flow.

Edema   A buildup of fluid in the tissues that results in swelling.

Fat soluble   A substance that dissolves in fats and oils. Fat-soluble vitamins require a source of fat for optimal absorption.

FDA   The Food and Drug Administration. It is an agency within the U.S. Public Health Service, which is a part of the Department of Health and Human Services. It is in charge of overseeing the safety of prescription and over-the-counter drugs, foods, and nutritional supplements.

Fiber   The indigestible portion of plant food. It helps to eliminate waste from the body.

Free radicals   Unstable negatively charged molecules that are potentially damaging to the organs and tissues of the body. They are formed by the normal process of energy production within cells, as well as by pollution, toxins, and radiation. Antioxidant enzyme systems that occur within the body, as well as antioxidants from foods or supplements, protect against free radicals. Free radicals can also have beneficial properties as part of the immune response to destroying microbes.

Gastrointestinal tract   The stomach, small intestine, and large intestine.

Histamine   A chemical released by the immune system (from mast cells) in response to an allergen, resulting in allergy symptoms (runny nose, watery eyes, sneezing, skin rash, etc).

Holistic   From the Greek term *holos*, for whole. Pertaining to the whole person in mind, body, and spirit. Often used in the term "holistic medicine."

Hormone   A substance produced by an endocrine gland that regulates the function of cells and organs.

Inflammation   The immune system's reaction to an illness, irritation, or injury that results in heat, pain, redness, and/or swelling.

Melatonin   A natural hormone produced by the body at night to promote sleep. Also available in supplement form.

Mg   See **milligram**.

Microgram (mcg)   A measure of weight equivalent to 1/1000 mg or one-millionth part of a gram.

Milligram   A measurement of weight that is 1/1000 gram.

Naturopathic medicine   A system of natural medicine that focuses on working with the healing systems of the body. Naturopathic doctors are trained as primary health care providers. As general practitioners, they work to restore health using clinical nutrition, herbal medicine, homeopathy, physical medicine, counseling, nutritional supplementation, natural hormones, hydrotherapy, and other forms of natural healing. They are also trained in the use of pharmaceutical medicines and minor surgery.

Nerves   The body's complex wiring that carries messages to and from the brain.

Neuropathy   A disease or disorder that affects the nerves. Common symptoms include numbness, tingling, and/or burning.

Neurotransmitter   A chemical that carries messages between nerve cells of the brain and nervous system.

Nonsteroidal anti-inflammatory drugs (NSAID)   A class of drugs used to reduce pain and inflammation.

Over-the-counter medication   A medication that does not require a prescription from a doctor. It can be obtained directly from a store by the consumer.

Pharmaceutical   A drug preparation available from pharmacies.

Placebo   A "sugar pill" or other inactive substance that helps researchers determine the effects of a drug or substance being tested.

Protein   A nitrogen-containing compound found in plant and animal foods. The body uses protein as a fuel source and to form or repair tissues, organs, and muscles. It comprises enzymes and hormones, and is found in every cell in the body. Amino acids are the individual building blocks of protein. There are approximately 20 different amino acids.

Side effect   The adverse reaction to a substance such as a pharmaceutical medication.

Triglyceride   A chemical compound formed from a molecule of the alcohol glycerol and three molecules of fatty acids. Triglycerides constitute many of the fats and oils in the diet.

Vasoconstriction   The constriction of blood vessels resulting in less blood flow.

Vasodilation   A relaxation of blood vessel walls resulting in increased blood flow.

HOLISTIC DOCTOR ASSOCIATIONS

American College for Advancement in Medicine
24411 Ridge Route, Suite 115
Laguna Hills, CA 92653
949-309-3520 phone
www.acam.org

American Association of Naturopathic Physicians
4435 Wisconsin Avenue, NW, Suite 403
Washington, DC 20016
866-538-2267 toll-free
www.naturopathic.org

RECOMMENDED READING

Balch, James, and Mark Stengler, *Prescription for Natural Cures: A Self-Care Guide for Treating Health Problems with Natural Remedies, Including Diet and Nutrition, Nutritional Supplements, Bodywork, and More* (Hoboken, NJ: John Wiley & Sons, 2004).

Cass, Hyla, *Supplement Your Prescription: What Your Doctor Doesn't Know about Nutrition* (Laguna Beach, CA: Basic Health Publications, 2007).

Cohen, Suzy, *The 24-Hour Pharmacist: Advice, Options, and Amazing Cures from America's Most Trusted Pharmacist* (New York: HarperCollins, 2007).

Pelton, Ross, and James LaValle, *The Nutritional Cost of Drugs: A Guide to Maintaining Good Nutrition While Using Prescription and Over-the-Counter Drugs,* Second Edition (Morton Publishing, 2004).

Stengler, Mark, *Bottom Line Natural Healing* monthly newsletter (Stamford, CT: Boardroom Inc.).

———, *The Natural Physician's Healing Therapies* (Paramus, NJ: Prentice Hall, 2001).

Strand, Ray, *Death by Prescription: The Shocking Truth behind an Overmedicated Nation* (Nashville: Thomas Nelson, 2006).

INDEX